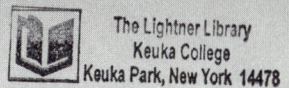
Occupational Therapy

Examination Review Guide

FOURTH EDITION

Caryn R. Johnson, MS, OTR/L, FAOTA

Academic Fieldwork Coordinator and Associate Professor
Department of Occupational Therapy
Thomas Jefferson University
Philadelphia, Pennsylvania

Tina DeAngelis, EdD, OTR/L

Program Director, Entry Level Occupational Therapy
Doctorate and Clinical Assistant Professor
Department of Occupational Therapy
Thomas Jefferson University
Philadelphia, Pennsylvania

Mary Muhlenhaupt, OTD, OTR/L, FAOTA

Assistant Professor
Department of Occupational Therapy
Thomas Jefferson University
Philadelphia, Pennsylvania

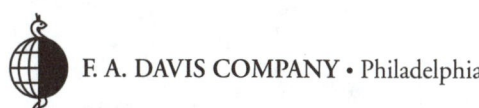

F. A. DAVIS COMPANY • Philadelphia

F.A. Davis Company
1915 Arch Street
Philadelphia, PA 19103
www.fadavis.com

Printed in the United States of America

Last digit indicates print number: 10 9 8 7 6 5 4 3 2 1

ISBN: 8=978-0-8036-3931-7

Senior Acquisitions Editor: Christa Fratantoro
Developmental Editor: Andrea Edwards
Director of Content Development: George Lang
Design and Illustration Manager: Carolyn O'Brien

Preface

The purpose of this workbook is to provide occupational therapy students a general review of occupational therapy practice and study tools to use while preparing to take the NBCOT examination. It also serves as an excellent review for occupational therapists reentering the field or changing areas of practice. This workbook's format encourages users to synthesize knowledge and become comfortable with the multiple-choice format of the National Board for Certification in Occupational Therapy (NBCOT) certification examination.

New to this edition is an online testing tool that allows users to take three practice exams that mimic both the Clinical Simulation Tests and the multiple-choice question styles used by the NBCOT. Additionally, users can customize their own multiple-choice exams to identify strengths and weaknesses in various content areas. The online testing tool and a digital version of this workbook are available at davisplus.fadavis.com (keyword: Johnson). Use the Davis*Plus* code inside the front cover of this workbook to access the online content at our Davis*Plus* website; the site will invite you to create an account (if you don't already have one).

The questions in the certification exam are designed to require the reader to call upon his/her knowledge of occupational therapy practice and to *apply* that knowledge to realistic practice situations. Questions in this book have been designed to simulate that style of question and provide a review of the material simultaneously. The reader will find that questions do not test basic knowledge alone, but require application of that knowledge to move through a reasoning process that leads to the *best* answer. While the majority of questions in the *Occupational Therapy Exam Review Guide* have been written in a style that simulates the exam, some have been written to maximize review of important content areas.

The textbooks cited as references for most answers are those most commonly required for purchase by students in occupational therapy education programs across the United States. In some cases, the authors cite less well-known references because they provide the best rationales. Students can often access these books through their own occupational therapy libraries.

Please keep in mind that this workbook is *not:*

- a comprehensive guide to practicing as an occupational therapist,
- intended to replicate the NBCOT exam or any of the questions on the NBCOT exam, or
- a tool that offers the student any guarantee of passing the NBCOT exam.

This workbook and accompanying Davis*Plus* digital resources *are designed to:*

- provide a general review of occupational therapy practice,
- help readers identify the strengths and weaknesses in their application of knowledge to practice of occupational therapy,
- acquaint the reader with the format of questions used on the examination,
- provide the reader with opportunities to practice taking computerized exams,
- help the reader organize and set priorities for study time, and
- provide the reader with a reference list from which further study may be pursued.

The Authors

Caryn Reichlin Johnson, MS, OTR/L, FAOTA, serves as Academic Fieldwork Coordinator and Associate Professor in the Occupational Therapy Program at Thomas Jefferson University in Philadelphia, Pennsylvania, where she has taught since 1983. She has held faculty positions in both OT and OTA programs. Caryn received her Bachelor's Degree in Occupational Therapy from Tufts University in 1978 and an Advanced Master's Degree in Occupational Therapy from Thomas Jefferson University in 1991. In addition, she maintains a clinical practice, specializing in aquatic rehabilitation. Past clinical experience includes working in the areas of adult physical rehabilitation and community mental health. Caryn has held leadership positions at the local, state, and national levels; coauthored the AOTA Fieldwork Educator Certificate Program curriculum; and she has published and presented extensively. Special interests include developing fieldwork opportunities in emerging practice settings, the collaborative fieldwork model, and the development of professional behaviors in OT and OTA students. In her free time, Caryn works with a wide variety of craft media.

Tina DeAngelis, EdD, OTR/L, is Program Director, Entry Level Occupational Therapy Doctorate (EOTD) and clinical assistant professor in the Occupational Therapy Program at Thomas Jefferson University in Philadelphia, Pennsylvania. She received her Associate's Degree in Occupational Therapy from Harcum College in 1987, her Bachelor's Degree in Occupational Therapy from College Misericordia in 1992, and her Advanced Master's Degree in Occupational Therapy from Thomas Jefferson University in 1997. She later completed her educational doctorate degree (EdD) in Higher Education Leadership at Widener University in 2006, with her dissertation research focusing on the entry-level doctorate degree and its impact on the future of the profession. Tina has practiced in the field of occupational therapy for over 27 years in the clinical areas of burn care, trauma, orthopedics, hands, neurological conditions, dementia, and mental health in practice settings ranging from state hospitals and general rehabilitation to home care. She is also a clinical fieldwork educator at Baker Industries, a nonprofit work rehabilitation program for individuals with emotional and physical needs, homelessness, addiction, and/or a history of incarceration in both the Malvern and Kensington, Pennsylvania, locations. Tina currently serves as the Education Special Interest Section (EDSIS) chairperson of the American Occupational Therapy Association and on the AOTA's Commission on Education (COE).

Mary Muhlenhaupt, OTD, OTR/L, FAOTA, is an Assistant Professor at Thomas Jefferson University in Philadelphia, Pennsylvania, where she teaches pediatric and program development coursework. Her work at Jefferson also includes direction of a program of professional development for administrators and providers representing multiple disciplines in the infant/toddler early intervention system in Philadelphia. Mary's occupational therapy career, sustained over more than 37 years, has included pediatric practice in hospital, school, early intervention, and private practice settings. She is an author for a variety of AOTA publications related to pediatric topics, as well as for chapters and other publications about pediatric occupational therapy practice. Recent work focuses on collaborative goal-setting practices to enhance children's engagement in the therapy process. Her service to the profession includes terms as Chairperson and as Education/Research Liaison for AOTA's School System Special Interest Section, along with a 3-year term as member of the AOTA Board of Directors. Additionally, she served in numerous leadership roles in local and state positions in the New York State Occupational Therapy Association, and served as the President of both the New York and Pennsylvania State Occupational Therapy Associations.

Acknowledgments

The input and enthusiasm of many individuals has made this book possible. We especially want to thank Christa Fratantoro, Elizabeth Stepchin, Andrea Edwards, Robert Allen, and Elizabeth Schaeffer, all at F.A. Davis, for their guidance and support. We also want to thank the students and faculty at Thomas Jefferson University for their support and contributions—in more ways than they know. Our deepest thanks to friends and family for tolerating us, present and absent, while we lost ourselves to this project for the past year.

This book would have been impossible to complete without the tremendous support provided by our graduate assistants. For that contribution, we would like to thank the following Thomas Jefferson University students and alumni:

Molly Bear
Nicole Bishara
Lacey Brinser
Rebecca Coale
Allison Duggan
Kelsey Engelstadt
Ester Goldman
Adam Remich
Lauren Rickard

Finally, we would like to recognize the efforts of those educators and practitioners from across the country who painstakingly reviewed, contributed to, critiqued, and validated every question to ensure accuracy and appropriateness.

Reviewers and Contributors

Richard Buckwalter
Occupational Therapist
Ann Klein Forensic Center
West Trenton, New Jersey

Nancy Edwards Carson, PhD, OTR/L
Assistant Professor
Occupational Therapy
Medical University of South Carolina
Charleston, South Carolina

Elaine Charest, MA, MBA, OTR/L, FACHE
Director of Therapy Operations
Administration
HealthSouth Rehabilitation Hospital of York
York, Pennsylvania

Stacey Creech, OTR/L
Occupational Therapist
Ann Klein Forensic Center
West Trenton, New Jersey

Susan Griffiths, OTR/L
Occupational Therapist
Ann Klein Forensic Center
West Trenton, New Jersey

Meredith P. Gronski, OTD, OTR/L
Instructor/ Lead Community Therapist
Occupational Therapy
Washington University School of Medicine
St. Louis, Missouri

Julia Henderson-Kalb, MS OTR/L
Instructor
Department of Occupational Science and Occupational
  Therapy
Saint Louis University
St. Louis, Missouri

E. Adel Herge, OTD, OTR/L, FAOTA
Associate Professor
Director, Combined BSMSOT Program
Thomas Jefferson University
Philadelphia, Pennsylvania

Michelle Marshina OTD, OTR/L
Therapy Manager, Brain Injury and Stroke Program
Magee Rehabilitation Hospital
Philadelphia, Pennsylvania

MaryBeth Merryman, PhD, OTR/L, FAOTA
Professor, Doctoral Program Director
Occupational Therapy & Occupational Science
Towson University
Towson, Maryland

Maryrose Mielczarek, OTR/L
Occupational Therapist
Ann Klein Forensic Center
West Trenton, New Jersey

Lauren E. Milton, OTD, OTR/L
Assistant Professor
Occupational Therapy
Maryville University
St. Louis, Missouri

Debby Nightingale, OTR/L
Adjunct Faculty
Thomas Jefferson University
Philadelphia, Pennsylvania

Robyn Otty, OTD, OTR/L, BCPR
Assistant Professor
Occupational Therapy
Maryville University
St. Louis, Missouri

Nikki Riviello OTR/L
Advanced Clinician, Brain Injury and Stroke Program
Magee Rehabilitation Hospital
Philadelphia, Pennsylvania

Janeene Sibla, OTD, OTR/L
Associate Professor, OT Program Director
Occupational Therapy
University of Mary
Bismarck, North Dakota

Christine Silverman, OTR/L
Occupational Therapist (retired)
Resources for Human Development
Philadelphia, Pennsylvania

Susan Tully, MS, OTR/L
Assistant Professor
Occupational Therapy
Midwestern University
Glendale, Arizona

Catherine Verrier Piersol, PhD, OTR/L
Associate Professor, Department of Occupational
  Therapy
Clinical Director, Jefferson Elder Care
Thomas Jefferson University
Philadelphia, Pennsylvania

Contents

Preparing for the Examination

WHAT IS THE NBCOT EXAMINATION?

The National Board for Certification in Occupational Therapy (NBCOT) examination is designed to identify those candidates who demonstrate entry-level competence for occupational therapy practice. Once you have successfully completed the examination, you are certified as an occupational therapist. Examinations are given for both certified occupational therapy assistant (COTA) and registered occupational therapist (OTR) candidates and differ according to knowledge and skill level.

Passing the National Board for Certification in Occupational Therapy (NBCOT) examination is the culmination of academic and fieldwork study. The exam requires you to apply knowledge of occupational therapy and/or synthesize bits of knowledge to select the correct answer. Questions on the certification exam are carefully constructed to test:

- Your knowledge of occupational therapy practice and the skills performed by occupational therapists.
- Your grasp of background knowledge needed to support practice.
- Your ability to apply your knowledge to practice situations.
- Your ability to understand what the question is asking.
- Your clinical reasoning skills—selecting the correct answer based on correctly prioritizing the most significant issue presented in the question.

The examination is offered at hundreds of online testing centers around the United States, as well as internationally, throughout the year. You are eligible to take online practice exams once you have registered for the NBCOT exam. More information on the NBCOT exam and practice exams is available at www.nbcot.org.

WHO CAN TAKE THE CERTIFICATION EXAMINATION?

The NBCOT oversees the certification examination and eligibility of candidates. Candidates must have graduated from an accredited occupational therapy educa-tion program and successfully completed the required fieldwork. You are required to submit an official transcript or Academic Credential Verification Form from your occupational therapy program. Because the application process is continually updated, it is best to carefully read the most current information available at www.nbcot.org for instructions.

> NOTE: Be sure to thoroughly read the NBCOT Certification Exam Handbook, available from the website.

Individuals with a history of felony or other types of criminal background history may not be eligible to take the NBCOT exam. For a fee, NBCOT will complete an "Early Determination Review" to determine eligibility.

APPLYING TO TAKE THE NBCOT EXAMINATION

You should visit www.nbcot.org for information as soon as you begin to think about taking the exam. The website provides a wealth of necessary information for completing the application to take the examination, as well as forms you will need and information to help you prepare for the exam. Some important topics include:

- Eligibility requirements
- Application process
- School codes
- Notification of eligibility to take the exam
- Fees
- Requesting reasonable accommodations
- Scheduling the exam
- Cancellation, rescheduling, consequences of lateness or no-show
- Preparing for the exam
- Retaking the exam

> NOTE: NBCOT has reported evidence that students who take the exam within 3 months after they complete academic program requirements do better than students who wait longer than 3 months to take the exam. Target your NBCOT exam test date within 3 months of your completion of coursework (including your level II fieldwork)! Develop your study plan so you are well-prepared for this test date!

According to the NBCOT website (http://proxy.nbcot.org/pdf/AOTA_2013_OTR_042013.pdf), the following points are recommended to avoid the most common problems experienced when applying to take the exam:

- Do not set up more than one account with NBCOT—doing so will cause delays.
- If you do not select a state where you wish to have your score report sent, or you fail to confirm that you are registered for the exam, licensure may be delayed.
- If the name on your "Authorization to Test (ATT)" letter does not match the names on your primary and secondary IDs needed for entry to testing on the day of exam, you will not be allowed to take the exam.
- Do not change your name and/or e-mail address during the application process. This may cause confusion. Transcripts that do not come directly from your institution's registrar's office, or are incomplete, will not be accepted

WHAT IS THE FORMAT OF THE NBCOT EXAMINATION?

■ Multiple-Choice Questions

The certification examination is composed of 170 multiple-choice questions that use the four-option format, and contains a section of clinical simulation test problems. No combination or "K" questions are used ("K" questions can include more than one answer options, such as "A and B" or "all of the above.") Questions are designed as brief practice scenarios and require the candidate to decide what the therapist *should do* based on his or her application of occupational therapy *knowledge*. Candidates have 4 hours to complete the examination.

■ Clinical Simulation Test

The Clinical Simulation Tests (CSTs) provide scenarios that have greater depth to them. A CST will typically start with a short opening paragraph containing information about an individual, his/her condition, and how it is affecting occupational performance. Several distinct sections follow, concerning evaluation, treatment planning, and intervention. In each section, you are provided with a short paragraph of information, ending with instructions to identify the actions you should take. Generally, you will need to choose from a list of six to 10 action-based options, some of which are correct choices, some of which are wrong choices, and some of which are neutral choices (doesn't help, doesn't hurt). With each option you select, you will receive "feedback" about the implications of choosing that action. Sometimes this will let you know whether you made the correct decision, but not always. You may also be able to use the feedback to guide future decisions. Once a section of answers is submitted, you cannot go back to change anything.

The second section is typically about the treatment planning process and the third section is typically about the intervention process. Any additional sections will expand on topics relevant to the scenario, and the procedure of selecting correct answers is the same.

A point is awarded for each correct option you select. A point is deducted for each incorrect option you select. No points are awarded or deducted for the neutral options, whether you select them or not.

> NOTE: Students tend to like the CST problems and do well on them, because they require the same type of thinking and reasoning they grew accustomed to during their fieldwork experiences.

The questions for the examination are developed by the NBCOT Certification Examination Validation Committee. The group consists of content experts, both occupational therapists and occupational therapy assistants, from a variety of practice settings across the United States. The format of the exam is based on the most current *NBCOT Practice Analysis*, which obtains information about current professional practice among recent OT and OTA graduates, and results in a new "Exam Blueprint" every 5 or so years.

Every time the examination is given, a new set of questions is drawn from an "item bank." The item banks for the OT and OTA examinations are separate. The questions on each examination correspond to the content outline for either OT or OTA candidates. The content outline specifies how many items should be asked for each of the identified "domains." Whereas some questions are easier and others harder, each item has the same weight in scoring, and every question on the examination has only one correct answer.

> NOTE: You should *never* leave a question unanswered. It is better to guess than to leave it blank, because then you at least have a chance (if you are lucky) of getting the right answer.

The raw scores of correct answers are statistically converted to a "scaled score," which may range from 300 to 600 points. A scaled score of 450 or more is required to pass the examination. The score does not actually reflect how many questions the candidate got right or wrong. The national pass rate for first-time test takers varies from year to year, and usually falls somewhere in the range of 82% to 88%.

DOMAINS AND CONTENT AREAS

The NBCOT *2012 Practice Analysis of the Occupational Therapist Registered* (NBCOT, 2012) examined current practice of occupational therapists and resulted in the identification of four domains of occupational therapy practice that describe what occupational therapy practitioners *do* and form the basis for the development of a new "Exam Blueprint" for the OT examination (NBCOT, 2012). Each domain is accompanied by related tasks and knowledge areas in which the entry-level occupational therapy practitioner should be competent. These knowledge areas are summarized in the "Study Guidelines" tables on pages 7 to 11. Certain concepts are emphasized throughout, such as the importance of being client-centered and occupation-based. These domains are summarized below.

■ Domain 1—Evaluation

"Acquire information regarding factors that influence occupational performance throughout the occupational therapy process" (NBCOT, 2012, p. 23).

These questions apply to skills and tasks related to collecting and analyzing data, assessment, and evaluation such as:

- Interviewing
- Observation
- Developing an occupational profile
- Screening and chart/record review
- Applying theory and evidence to the selection of screening and assessment tools
- Administering and scoring commonly used screening and assessment tools (standardized and nonstandardized)
- Documenting results

■ Domain 2—Treatment Planning

"Formulate conclusions regarding client needs and priorities to develop and monitor an intervention plan throughout the occupational therapy process" (NBCOT, 2012, p. 24).

These questions apply to the ability to design interventions based on evaluation/assessment/screening results, as well as patient/client responses to intervention, and will address skills and tasks, such as:

- Analyzing and interpreting assessment results
- Collaborating with the individual and relevant others to develop client-centered goals and interventions, taking into consideration the client's condition, context, and priorities

- Utilizing data from the assessment process to develop an intervention plan, monitor progress, and reassess the plan
- Utilizing evidence and best practice to guide clinical decision-making
- Determining program development and client advocacy needs
- Selecting/designing goal-related interventions that establish or restore function, adapt or modify tasks or the environment, or prevent negative outcomes
- Selecting appropriate service delivery methods
- Determining frequency and duration of treatment
- Selecting appropriate environments and contexts
- Appropriately identifying and referring clients to other team members/health professionals
- Documenting treatment/intervention plans and goals

■ Domain 3—Intervention

"Select interventions for managing a client-centered plan throughout the occupational therapy process" (NBCOT, 2012, p. 25).

These questions apply to tasks and skills related to using clinical reasoning to select and provide intervention to the individual and/or caregivers and will address areas such as:

- Applying, adapting, and grading intervention activities/techniques that support participation in occupations based on sensory, cognitive, perceptual, motor, and psychosocial needs, skills, and abilities
- Using remedial, compensatory, and prevention strategies to maximize occupational performance
- Providing intervention within optimal environments and times
- Adapting the environment to maximize participation
- Working and/or consulting with caregivers, teachers, and other team members
- Selecting and/or adapting/grading therapeutic equipment, tools, objects, and assistive technology
- Acquiring and teaching safe use of therapeutic equipment, tools, objects, durable medical equipment, and assistive technology
- Leading groups to enhance social, developmental, and cognitive skills
- Seating and positioning, transfers, and mobility
- Feeding and eating
- Selecting and using preparatory methods such as exercise, use of orthosis, and physical agent modalities
- Educating about wellness, health promotion, and prevention (i.e., stress management, ergonomics, falls prevention)
- Providing prevocational and vocational interventions
- Instructing in home programs
- Recommending equipment, strategies, and services
- Monitoring response to treatment

- Modifying the treatment plan as needed
- Documenting progress and response to treatment
- Assisting transition by recommending post-intervention services
- Discharge planning and documentation

■ Domain 4—Service Management and Professional Practice

"Manage and direct occupational therapy services to promote quality in practice" (NBCOT, 2012, p. 29).

Questions in this section apply to tasks and skills related to management, service delivery, and professional practice, and will address areas such as: **Coordinating a variety of services**

- Documenting services according to regulatory and funding guidelines
- Participating as a member of a team
- Understanding and complying with regulations, laws, reimbursement requirements, policies and procedures, HIPAA, AOTA Code of Ethics
- Analyzing and interpreting research and applying it to practice
- Maintaining professional practice standards in the areas of:
  - Supervision
  - Licensure
  - Recertification
  - Documentation
  - Professional development activities
  - Service competency
- Promoting occupational therapy
- Interpreting and appropriately applying management concepts such as:
  - Safety and risk management
  - Continuous quality improvement
  - Program evaluation and outcome measures
  - Scope of practice and practice standards

WHAT YOU NEED TO DO IN THE 2 WEEKS BEFORE YOUR NBCOT EXAMINATION DATE

Use this checklist to help you prepare for your exam day:

[✔] At least 2 weeks in advance, double-check the date and time on your admission notice.

[✔] One week in advance, be sure you know where you are going, how to get there, and where you will be able to park.

[✔] The day before your test, confirm your travel plan so that you arrive at the test site 30 minutes ahead of your scheduled start time.

[✔] The day before your test, ensure your admission notice is in the bag/folder you will bring to test site.

[✔] The day before your test, ensure that your two forms of identification, including one government-issued photo ID with signature (such as driver's license or passport) and a secondary form of ID with signature (such as a credit card or student ID card) that both have the *same name* as the one listed on the exam admission notice, are in the in the bag/folder you will bring to test site.

The test area is divided into individual sections much like cubicles in a library. You will be in a room with other people, and a testing center administrator and video surveillance cameras will monitor the exam. You may use earplugs provided by the facility to minimize distractions. Food and drinks, dictionaries, cell phones, and other similar items are not permitted in the testing area. Special permission is even required for bottled water. Lockers are provided for all items in your possession that are not permitted in the testing area.

> NOTE: You have 4 hours to take the test, and no breaks are included. If you need to take a break, you may leave the testing room to use the bathroom, stretch, get a drink, etc., but remember that the clock keeps ticking.

A tutorial is offered at the beginning of the exam process. Be sure to take advantage of this. Taking the tutorials does not count against your time, and this is a good time to take a break if you need it.

> NOTE: NBCOT reports that students who take the tutorials do better on the exam.

WHAT HAPPENS AFTER THE NBCOT EXAMINATION?

Typically, official test results are mailed within 4–6 weeks after the certification examination to candidates who have passed the exam, and within 2 weeks to candidates who have failed. However, unofficial, online results may be obtained within 1 to 2 days of the scoring date on the NBCOT scoring schedule. As previously stated, a score of 450 or higher is required to pass the certification examination.

You can request that results be sent to the licensing agency of the state(s) in which you plan to apply for licensure as an occupational practitioner A fee is assessed for each report you request—no reports are sent free of charge. Almost all states require a copy of the report. It is recommended that you complete an application for state licensure before taking the examination. Often, these applications require a notarized copy of transcripts from an accredited occupational therapy program, letters of reference, a picture identification, and so forth. Depending on the state licensure laws and requirements of your new employer, you may be able to work with a temporary permit until examination results are received. You should contact the licensing agency as soon as you know the state in which you will be practicing. You should learn as early as possible what information will be necessary for licensure and when applications should be submitted.

Despite all of your thoughtful preparation, you may experience unique or unusual circumstances that impact your performance on test day. NBCOT has established a grievance process that pertains to these situations. If you experience difficulty with the testing conditions, wish to contest the content of any question, or have any other complaints about your experience taking the exam, you must file a complaint at the test center, before you leave, and report it immediately to NBCOT (go to NBCOT.org for specific requirements).

Candidates who fail the examination and wish to retake it must retake the entire examination and pay the fee again. There is no limit on how many times an individual may take the exam, although there is a waiting period. In addition, failing the exam may affect employment status, and employers *must* be notified. Those who wish to appeal their results may submit an appeal to NBCOT following the procedure outlined on the NBCOT website.

HOW TO USE THE OCCUPATIONAL THERAPY EXAMINATION REVIEW GUIDE

This book has three sample exams, each with 200 multiple-choice questions that simulate the actual NBCOT examination by asking application-oriented questions in a four-option, multiple-choice format. Questions in the first three exams are organized to allow candidates to assess their performance in each of the four domains. The 200 questions in the fourth exam are grouped by content area (pediatrics, mental health, physical disabilities, and service management/ professional practice), allowing candidates to assess their competence with various age groups and diagnostic categories.

A complete set of answers with rationales follows each examination. To help you review as much as possible, the book provides a complete rationale for each answer, which explains why wrong answers are wrong and why the right answers are right. Hence, each question-answer unit is actually a mini-lesson on not one, but four concepts. In addition, each answer provides you with a reference from which further information may be obtained on the subject matter. A complete bibliography, including primary textbooks that many students are likely to own, is located after the final chapter.

The section on "Developing Your Personal Study Plan" will help you identify your strengths and weaknesses and organize and set priorities for study time. At the end of the section is a tool for developing a study plan.

HOW TO USE THE DAVISPLUS ONLINE TESTING WEBSITE

The online testing environment accessible at davisplus .fadavis.com (keyword: Johnson) can be used in various ways. At first, you may choose to select questions from our multiple-choice question bank for personalized study. You can customize exams by domain (evaluation, treatment planning, intervention, professional practice) or content area (pediatric, physical dysfunction, or mental health/cognitive) and take them either in review or exam mode. Review mode allows you to view feedback upon answering each question. Exam mode simulates the real testing environment but offers feedback when reviewing your exam results. This customizable option allows you to create short quizzes for targeted review or, if so desired, simulate a full exam.

The preset exams (Exams A through C) on the website are each composed of 170 multiple-choice questions and three clinical simulation tests. For realistic testing conditions, give yourself 4 hours to complete each of the exams. These exams enable you to evaluate how well you have retained information and been able to implement your study plan. The mix of questions in each test covers the range of entry-level occupational therapy practice, thus providing a general review of professional practice.

The NBCOT establishes a Blueprint for the exam, which determines how many questions to use from each domain. For example, the *2012 Practice Analysis* uses the following percentages:

- 17% evaluation
- 28% treatment planning

- 45% intervention
- 10% professional practice

Note that the default option for building your own exam by domain is set to approximate the 2012 percentages. When you customize, you may weigh the domains any way you wish, ultimately adding up to 100%.

WHERE TO BEGIN

Viewed as one task, preparing to take the examination can seem overwhelming. Breaking the process into smaller parts makes it easier to manage. The first step is to identify your areas of strength and weakness. The "Personal Study Plan Tables" can help you through this process. Once you have completed this step, the second step is to complete your study plan. The final step is to pull all of the information together to take the practice examinations. It may be helpful to review the test-taking tips occasionally.

DEVELOPING YOUR PERSONAL STUDY PLAN

The question most frequently asked by occupational therapy students preparing for the examination is, "How do I start?" The *Occupational Therapy Examination Review Guide* was specifically developed to be a primary source for exam preparation. It will help you put all your educational preparation together and organize your study time. It will also promote your comfort with multiple-choice questions. All students preparing for the examination should have their coursework at their fingertips, including books, notes, and handouts. Once you have assembled the stacks of information you have accumulated over the years, the question arises, "Where do I start?"

One way to use this book is to develop a study plan based on your performance on the simulation examinations. Start by taking simulation Examination 1 and record how many correct answers you score in each Domain. This will give you some idea of the Domains on which you need to concentrate. The next step is to define your strengths and weaknesses. To do this, turn to the Personal Study Plan Tables on pages 7 to 11. Starting with the Evaluation section, go through all the component parts of that area as well as the background knowledge areas suggested for review. Classify the areas in which you are weakest as "D" and those in which you are strongest as "A." Assign "B" or "C," with "B" being stronger than "C," to the remaining practice areas. Within each letter grouping, identify the

weakest subject with the number 4, and sequentially number through to the strongest subject—the larger the number, the higher your study priority will be. Repeat this with the tables for Treatment Planning, Intervention, and Management/Professional Practice. Once this has been completed, your personal plan for study needs to be organized and priorities set for accomplishment.

After completing simulation Examinations 2 and 3, record the numbers of your correct answers for each Domain. This will further indicate areas for which you still need review.

Now that you have set your priorities for studying, set target dates for completing your review of each area or subject. For instance, you may choose to work on Domain 1 (evaluation) during the month of January. Another individual may choose to review Evaluation concepts the first week of January, Treatment Planning (Domain 2) the second week of January, and so forth. Design your study plan to meet your needs. Set target dates that are realistic and attainable.

Once your planning is complete, it is time for the studying to begin. Start with the area listed as "D4" (high priority for review) and work your way through to the last "D." Once this is finished, continue with the "C," "B," and "A" items. When you have reviewed all areas, you may choose to begin again at D4, or to reset priorities for your studying needs.

The *Occupation Therapy Examination Review Guide* **DavisPlus Online Testing Website,** for which an access code is included on the front cover of this book, offers you a particular advantage in preparing for the NBCOT exam. It is available to you at any time during the process of reviewing, or when your have completed your review, and provides you with the opportunity to practice taking full-length simulated exams. It also provides you with the option of selecting the specific kinds of questions you would like to practice. You may select questions that reflect the exam domains of evaluation, treatment planning, intervention, or management/professional practice. Or you may select practice questions according to the content areas of physical dysfunction, mental health/cognition, or pediatrics. The flexibility of question selection offered by the DavisPlus website allows you to target the high-priority areas you have identified in your study plan. Taking both the full-length exams (which include 170 multiple-choice questions and three clinical simulation tests) and the selected sections of the exams can be very useful in measuring the effectiveness of your review as well as building your confidence.

The easiest part of this task will be defining the time frame in which to study specific topics. The toughest challenge will be implementing the examination review plan!

Table 1	PERSONAL STUDY PLAN: Evaluation Questions						
Specific task areas		Self-rating of knowledge in each area of practice					
Questions test ability to acquire and analyze information about factors that impact patients'/clients' occupational performance, including performance skills, client factors, environment/context, and needs.		Pediatrics		Phys Dys		MH/Cognition	
		ABCD	1234	ABCD	1234	ABCD	1234
1. Interviewing skills							
2. Observation skills							
3. Applying theory, frames of reference, and evidence to the assessment process							
4. Screening methods							
5. Choosing appropriate assessments							
6. Administering/scoring standardized instruments							
7. Administering/scoring nonstandardized tools and methods							
8. Analyzing/interpreting findings							
9. Developing conclusions from assessment data for the basis of intervention							
10. Documenting assessment results professionally							
11. Modifying the assessment process based on client response or performance							

Background knowledge to review for the EVALUATION category

- Pathological conditions and resulting diagnoses, disabilities, injuries, and conditions; ways they affect performance of occupations and development
- Influence of contextual factors (such as physical and social environments) that can affect how people perform occupations
- Normal and abnormal human development in sensorimotor, neuromusculoskeletal, and cognitive and psychosocial development
- Progression of skill development in performance areas of ADL, work and productive activities, and play and leisure
- Impact of disability and injury in terms of the individual's roles and occupational performance
- Interviewing and observation techniques
- Selecting evaluations that are client-centered and appropriate for obtaining relevant evaluation findings
- Methods of performing and scoring screens, standardized and nonstandardized assessments
- Knowing a range of types of assessments that are suitable for a variety of needs
- Clinical reasoning used in interpreting evaluation results for intervention, including knowledge of likely outcomes
- Effects of medications and other interventions they may affect; occupational performance and occupational therapy
- Establishing an occupational profile
- Writing of assessment/evaluation reports

Exam 1. Evaluation score ____/35	Exam 2. Evaluation score ____/35	Exam 3. Evaluation score ____/35

Table 2	PERSONAL STUDY PLAN: Intervention Planning Questions

Specific task areas	Self-rating of knowledge in each area of practice					
Questions test ability to apply OT knowledge to the skills and tasks related to establishing treatment priorities and planning intervention	Pediatrics		Phys Dys		MH/Cognition	
	ABCD	1234	ABCD	1234	ABCD	1234
1. Analyzing and interpreting assessment results						
2. Client-centered goal setting and prioritization						
3. Determining intervention approaches to restore skills						
4. Selecting intervention methods and activities to meet goals						
5. Selecting environments that maximize abilities to achieve goals						
6. Identifying needed frequency and length of OT services						
7. Referring clients to other services						
8. Documenting the plan						

Background knowledge to review for the INTERVENTION PLANNING category

- Elements of an intervention plan
- Construction of long- and short-term goals based on effective OT interventions and methods for anticipated outcomes
- Issues related to developing client-centered, culturally appropriate intervention plans collaboratively, using appropriate communication skills
- Models of practice, theories, and frames of reference underlying intervention
- Principles of clinical reasoning for selection of intervention approaches to achieve goals
- Range of intervention methods for various pathological conditions and resulting diagnoses, disabilities, injuries, and conditions
- Selection of occupation-based interventions
- Impact of environments on performance
- Timing factors in intervention planning; estimating how long therapy should continue and how frequently therapy should occur to reach goals in relation to discharge process
- Prioritizing goals based on occupational profile
- Documenting intervention plans

Exam 1. Treatment planning score ____/55	Exam 2. Treatment planning score ____/55	Exam 3. Treatment planning score ____/55

Table 3	PERSONAL STUDY PLAN: Intervention Implementation Questions						
Specific task areas		**Self-rating of background knowledge in each area of practice**					
Questions test ability to apply OT knowledge to skills and tasks related to providing and monitoring intervention		Pediatrics		Phys Dys		MH/Cognition	
		ABCD	1234	ABCD	1234	ABCD	1234
1. Collaboratively selecting intervention option							
2. Proving intervention within optimal environments, settings, and times							
3. Adapting and grading techniques							
4. Adapting the environment to enhance participation and/or occupational performance							
5. Selecting therapeutic equipment, tools, objects, and assistive technology							
6. Adapting and grading therapeutic equipment, tools, objects, and assistive technology							
7. Teaching safe use of therapeutic equipment, tools, objects, and assistive technology							
8. Educating about health, wellness, and prevention							
9. Instructing in home programs							
10. Recommending equipment, strategies, and services							
11. Monitoring intervention process							
12. Modifying the response plan as needed, based on monitoring							
13. Documenting response to intervention and progress							
14. Assisting transition by recommending postintervention services							

Background knowledge to review for the INTERVENTION category

- Therapeutic use of self
- Principles of client-centered intervention, collaborative strategies, and culturally sensitive care
- The impact of various physical, cognitive, and psychosocial disabilities on development and occupational performance
- Influence of environmental factors on development and occupational performance
- The use of activity analysis in implementing and grading interventions
- Frames of reference, theories, and evidence used to guide intervention and select interventions and related occupation-based activities and environment-based interventions
- Specific approaches and techniques to enhance motor and sensory skills such as use of orthoses and orthotics, therapeutic exercise program and manual techniques, sensory reeducation desensitization and sensory processing techniques, motor learning, and neurodevelopmental approaches
- Specific approaches and techniques to enhance process and cognitive skills such as cognitive rehabilitation techniques, training techniques and methods of assisting and cuing, compensatory methods used in dementia such as task breakdown, Allen's Cognitive Disabilities approach, and perceptual rehabilitation techniques
- Specific approaches and techniques to enhance social/communication skills and psychosocial performance such as strategies for dealing with behavioral issues; interventions that address living skills, coping skills, and stress management; prevocational exploration; symptom management; and relapse prevention

(Continued on following page)

Table 3	PERSONAL STUDY PLAN: Intervention Implementation Questions *(Continued)*

- Interventions for limitations in areas of occupational performance in ADL, work, education, play and leisure, and social interaction
- Principles and application of compensatory strategies including the selection, use, and adaptation of assistive technologies, assistive and adaptive devices, environmental modification, and assistance from others
- Activity and environmental adaptation principles and methods
- Typical and atypical reactions that can be expected in response to intervention methods
- Clinical problem-solving related to individual client/patient response to intervention, reassessment of progress, and methods for adjusting intervention.
- Training, teaching, and educational methods for use with adults and children of varying developmental and cognitive abilities and for caregivers and supervised personnel
- Group interventions and underlying group dynamics and strategies for use of group process to enhance performance and goal attainment; intervention techniques based on application of group process
- Precautions associated with various conditions and contraindications for intervention; principles of safety during various intervention methods and in use of equipment
- Knowledge of intervention possibilities in various settings and service delivery models, resources in the community, and strategies and services that would support occupational performance relative to transition to other settings
- Techniques and methods for recording of treatment process, documentation of progress and outcomes, discharge planning, and recommendations

| Exam 1. Intervention score ____ /87 | Exam 2. Intervention score ____ /87 | Exam 3. Intervention score ____ /87 |

Table 4	PERSONAL STUDY PLAN: Service Management and Professional Practice Questions

Specific task areas	Self-rating of knowledge in service management and professional practice	
Questions test ability to apply OT knowledge to skills and tasks related to service management and professional practice		
	ABCD	1234
1. Coordinating for quality care		
2. Documenting of services according to institutional, regulatory, and funding guidelines		
3. Participating in team meeting processes and outcomes		
4. Complying with regulations, laws, codes, policies, and procedures		
5. Engaging in professional development activities to maintain ongoing service competency		
6. Applying content from professional activities to practice		
7. Promoting and informing others about value of OT practice		
8. Utilizing evidence to promote best practice		
9. Incorporating risk management and safety procedures in practice		
10. Incorporating continuous quality improvement processes and outcomes measures		
11. Supervising OT and non-OT personnel		

Background knowledge to review for the SERVICE MANAGEMENT category

- Collaboration methods and strategies for service management
- Knowledge of practice scope for OT and OTA
- Role of the OT practitioners and other disciplines working in teams
- Use and coordination of supplies, equipment, and time
- Cultural awareness concepts
- Relevant guidelines, standards, regulations, and laws that guide and regulate professional practice and how they are applied in practice situations
- OT Code of Ethics and how to apply it to practice situations
- Safety issues in occupational therapy services and how to manage related liabilities
- Methods for effectively supervising staff

Exam 1. PP/SM score ____/23   Exam 2. PP/SM score ____/23   Exam 3. PP/SM score ____/23

ADDITIONAL INFORMATION ABOUT THE EXAM

Basing the Certification Exam on the *Practice Analysis* ensures that exam questions accurately test the candidate's knowledge of frames of reference, evaluation, and intervention methods that are currently used within the practice of occupational therapy. The following data from the *2012 Practice Analysis* indicates the most frequently reported responses by therapists in certain categories and should be carefully reviewed. Rare or uncommon conditions are not likely to appear on the exam.

Most Frequently Seen Diagnoses

Neurological disorders
Cerebral vascular accident
Dementia
Traumatic brain injury
Parkinson disease
Cerebral palsy
Peripheral neuropathy
Low vision
Spinal cord injury

Developmental disorders
Developmental delay
Sensory integrative disorder
Intellectual disability
Learning disorder
Visual processing deficit
Congenital anomalies

Musculoskeletal/Orthopedic disorders
Fractures
Joint replacements
Osteoarthritis
Amputations

Cardiopulmonary disorders
Chronic obstructive pulmonary disease
Congestive heart failure
Myocardial infarction

Psychosocial dysfunction
Anxiety disorders
Autism spectrum disorders
Behavior disorders
ADHD
Mood disorders
Substance abuse
Schizophrenia

General Medical disorders
General deconditioning
Diabetes
Cancer
Rheumatoid arthritis
Open wounds/decubitis

Most Frequently Mentioned Frames of Reference

Biomechanical
Neurodevelopment approach
Sensory integration
Model of Human Occupation
Rehabilitation frames of reference

Most Frequently Identified Assessment Methods

Peabody scale
Goniometer/range of motion
Manual muscle testing
Sensory testing
Bruininks-Oseretsky Test of Motor Proficiency
Visual-motor

TEST-TAKING TIPS

■ Test-Taking Tip 1

Visit the NBCOT website periodically. You can access the vital information about the exam on the NBCOT website (**www.nbcot.org**). It is essential that you read the information thoroughly and *more than once*—you'll pick up something new each time. This website has the most current information regarding testing and scoring dates and locations and is updated frequently. It also has details about how the exam is developed and how it is scored.

■ Test-Taking Tip 2

Be prepared. The more prepared you are prior to the examination, the more comfortable you will feel during the actual examination. Preparation includes studying the knowledge base of occupational therapy, getting a good night's sleep, and arriving prepared to take the exam. According to the NBCOT website (www.nbcot.org), items such as headphones, tissues, and an erasable board and marking pen are available at the test site. Test candidates are permitted to use approved earplugs and reading glasses during the exam but are not permitted to bring snacks, cell phones, or any electronic devices into the exam room.

Although the exam is computerized, candidates do not necessarily need to have good computer skills. However, we have learned from NBCOT that students tend to do better if they *take the tutorial* offered at the beginning of the exam. When your studying is done, most of your preparation is complete. However, when asked to identify the single most important element in preparing for the examination, one graduating class of students all agreed that the answer was getting a good night's sleep.

It is also a good idea to have directions to the test center location ready prior to your departure date, and remember to bring along two forms of personal identification, one being a government-issued photo identification. Also, plan to arrive at the test site at least 30 minutes before the examination. Doing so will give you time to register, use the restroom, and become acclimated to your surroundings.

■ Test-Taking Tip 3

Prepare your body as well as your mind! Eating a well-balanced breakfast can actually help your performance on the examination. A breakfast high in carbohydrates and low in fat will increase your energy and not produce a sluggish feeling. Avoid caffeine, because its ultimate effect will be to leave you tired and drowsy in the middle of the examination. Dress appropriately, as you will not be allowed to put on or take of clothing once you enter the exam room. No beverages or snacks are allowed in the testing area. However, you may keep items in the lockers provided.

It is also important to be emotionally prepared for the exam. As a form of relaxation, try slow, deep breathing as well as sitting in an upright position during the exam. Try to decrease any anxiety you might have by reminding yourself that you arrived at this day as a result of your hard work (passing fieldwork and coursework) and it is one of the last steps you must take on the road to working as an occupational therapy practitioner!

■ Test-Taking Tip 4

Pace yourself. The test is to be completed within 4 hours. Within this time frame, you have to answer 170 multiple-choice questions and three clinical simulation tests. Begin by familiarizing yourself with the computer test program and reading all of the instructions carefully. One technique for pacing the examination is to divide the test into four sections. *You should not spend more than 30 minutes on the clinical simulation questions.* Then you will have about 1 minute to spend on each of the remaining 170 questions. It is not uncommon for people to slow down toward the end of a long exam like this, so it may help you to try to work more quickly at the beginning. Remember, take the tutorials—they do not count against your time. Understanding the format of the test and budgeting your time will help you work through the questions more efficiently and in the allotted time.

Another pacing technique is to use the clock provided by the computer test program. At the end of every few pages of questions, briefly glance at the time to maintain a sense of your pace. If questions remain incomplete within the last 10 minutes of the examination, select one letter and fill in all of the remaining questions with that letter. *Remember, there is no penalty for guessing—only for leaving questions unanswered!* If you find the computer test program clock too distracting, you have the option of turning it off. It is also important to remain calm if others complete the exam before you do. You do not need to leave the testing room until you have used all of the allotted examination time. If for any reason you experience problems during the exam, remain calm—a test center administrator will be available to assist you.

■ Test-Taking Tip 5

Use key techniques to help select the correct answer.

1. *Follow your instincts when answering questions.* The first answer chosen is usually the correct one. Change an answer only if you later realize that your new answer is absolutely correct.
2. *Ask, "What is this question about?"* Try to decipher what the question is testing by selecting the key terms in the questions and not being distracted by peripheral information. By sorting through the information provided to identify what the question is testing, you may be more likely to select the correct answer.
3. *Anticipate the answer.* Many times, you may anticipate an answer while reading a question. If so, look for the anticipated answer among the options. However, it is important to read and consider all of the options to verify that the anticipated answer is the correct answer.
4. *Use logical reasoning.* A commonly used technique is the process of deduction—eliminating answers that are incorrect. Doing this allows you to concentrate on the options that remain.

As you complete the questions on the exam, remember these techniques and practice using them when you have difficulty answering a question.

■ Test-Taking Tip 6

There are no trick questions.   Questions are designed to test entry-level, not advanced, knowledge and reasoning. Be careful not to read too much into the questions. However, most questions will have two answers that appear viable. Many questions will ask for the "FIRST" action the therapist should take or the "BEST" or "MOST appropriate" choice. Make sure to note the qualifiers to help you determine the "best" answer. Also, remember that all NBCOT test questions are in randomized order. Do not look for patterns in the answers.

■ Test-Taking Tip 7

Use the DavisPlus Online Testing Website to your advantage.   The online test program allows you to "flag" a question, similar to the format of the NBCOT exam so that you can go back to it later. It also allows you to identify unanswered questions and to change answers right up to the time you finally submit the test. The online practice examinations available from NBCOT are similar to those on our DavisPlus practice examinations. As stated previously (please refer to "How to Use the DavisPlus Online Testing Website"), you can select questions from specific content areas such as pediatrics, mental health/cognition, and physical disabilities. Specific Domains can also be selected in areas such as evaluation, treatment planning, intervention, and management/professional practice to create a personalized quiz or to simulate a full exam. And you can immerse yourself in an exam experience by taking our three preset examinations, which offer both multiple-choice questions and clinical simulation tests.

Simulation Examination 1

Directions: Circle the correct answer to the following questions. When you have completed this examination, check your answers against the answer key that follows. As you will see, an explanation is given for each answer along with a reference for further study. The book author is listed as well as the chapter author. See the bibliography for complete references. Study the areas in which your comprehension was low then test yourself again by taking Simulation Examination 2.

EVALUATION

1. An OT is preparing to evaluate a toddler who has upper extremity orthopedic concerns. How will the OT MOST likely obtain the majority of initial assessment data?

- A. Measurement tools that assess visual-motor skills.
- B. Dynamometer and pinch meter readings.
- C. Observation of child during activities in the child-care center.
- D. Functional independence measures.

2. During an initial evaluation, the OT suspects that a child has somatodyspraxia. In what area should the OT focus the evaluation?

- A. Ability to print or write.
- B. Reading competency.
- C. Math calculations.
- D. New motor task planning.

3. An OT working in a long-term care facility needs to evaluate the long-term memory of a resident. Which of the following methods is BEST for evaluating memory of personally experienced events (declarative memory)?

- A. Show the person a series of objects and ask him to recall the objects within 60 seconds.
- B. Ask the individual how he spent New Year's.
- C. Have the individual state the place, date, and time.
- D. Ask the client to remember to bring a specific item to the next therapy session.

4. A child avoids playground equipment that requires her feet to be off the ground. What does this behavior MOST likely indicate?

- A. Difficulty modulating proprioception.
- B. Somatodyspraxia.
- C. Gravitational insecurity.
- D. Bilateral integration/sequencing deficit.

5. When the OT suspects tactile defensiveness as a rationale for a child's challenges, in what area of participation should the OT focus on FIRST?

- A. Play behavior.
- B. Dressing habits.
- C. Social skills.
- D. Leisure interests.

6. An OT is working with an individual with schizophrenia who is in the process of preparing to move from a state hospital to a group home. During a baking group, the client becomes agitated and leaves the room when another client uses the electric hand mixer to mix the cake batter, and again when two clients begin to argue loudly about which type of icing to use. How would the OT BEST describe the behavior?

- A. Low registration.
- B. Sensory avoiding.
- C. Sensation seeking.
- D. A hearing impairment.

7. During a self-care evaluation of an individual who recently sustained a brain injury, the OT instructs the individual to comb his hair immediately after he washes his face. The individual washes his face quickly, but then the therapist must give him several reminders to comb his hair. The OT is MOST likely to identify this as a deficit in what area?

- A. Working memory.
- B. Judgment.
- C. Hearing.
- D. Abstraction.

8. **A supermarket employee with obsessive-compulsive disorder takes an hour to stock 24 soup cans on the shelf because once he has placed the cans on the shelf, he removes them and starts over, stating that "all the labels were not lined up exactly in the same direction." Which of the following methods would MOST effectively evaluate this individual's work performance?**

    A. On-site observation of performance skills.

    B. Formal cognitive assessment.

    C. Verbal interview focusing on the requirements of the job.

    D. Task evaluation using a "clean" medium such as a puzzle.

9. **An OT has been working with an individual who is recovering from a TBI. A standard pivot transfer has been successfully demonstrated in the gym. The MOST appropriate way to assess generalization of this new learning would be to have the patient perform which activity?**

    A. Identify potential hazards in the patient's bathroom at home that could make transferring unsafe.

    B. Select an appropriate tub bench and nonskid mat for the patient's bathroom at home.

    C. Attempt a standard pivot transfer from wheelchair to bed in the patient's hospital room.

    D. Attempt a sliding board transfer from wheelchair to tub.

10. **An OT is working with an individual with depression who is cognitively intact but demonstrating difficulty carrying out self-care and other ADL tasks. The OT, who has no advanced certifications, would like to identify a standardized assessment to measure ADL performance. Which is the MOST appropriate tool for this purpose?**

    A. Bay Area Functional Performance Evaluation.

    B. Routine Task Inventory-Expanded.

    C. Kohlman Evaluation of Living Skills.

    D. Assessment of Motor and Process Skills.

11. **An OT is conducting a perceptual function screening with an individual who has had a CVA. Which of the following informal screening activities would the therapist ask the individual to perform in order to identify the presence of agnosia?**

    A. Demonstrate common gestures such as waving.

    B. Name objects through touch only.

    C. Identify or demonstrate the use of common household objects.

    D. Read a paragraph and explain its meaning.

12. **An individual with an L4 spinal cord injury wishes to become independent in driving an automobile. The MOST appropriate piece of adaptive equipment for this individual is:**

    A. a palmar cuff for the steering wheel.

    B. a spinner knob on the steering wheel.

    C. pedal extensions for acceleration and braking.

    D. hand controls for acceleration and braking.

13. **What is the MOST important aspect of administering and scoring a standardized test?**

    A. Judgment to determine how best to administer the test.

    B. Previous experience as a way to gauge test results.

    C. Adherence to specific instructions for administration and scoring.

    D. Practice in administering the test items.

14. **During an initial interview, parents describe their child as having difficulty communicating and interacting with others. The OT observes him repeatedly gazing upward and scanning the ceiling or quickly patting his hip. The behaviors described are MOST likely to be associated with what disorder?**

    A. Attention deficit-hyperactivity.

    B. Childhood conduct.

    C. Obsessive-compulsive.

    D. Autism spectrum disorder.

15. **A toddler with spina bifida has been referred for assessment. When collecting the initial data during interview with the child's parent, what should the OT focus on PRIMARILY?**

    A. Parent's concerns and goals for the child.

    B. Child's medical management.

    C. Equipment needs.

    D. Physical layout of the home.

16. **When evaluating an individual with coronary artery disease for controllable risk factors, what is MOST important for the OT to include as part of the assessment?**

    A. Determine the individual's age and gender.

    B. Assess the individual's lifestyle and dietary habits.

    C. Observe the individual for obesity and cholesterol levels.

    D. Determine whether the individual has a family history of heart disease.

17. The OT has been working with an individual with deficits in the area of executive functioning postsurgery. When the OT asks about scheduling therapy appointments after discharge and transportation to the outpatient clinic, the client is unable to identify how to obtain the clinic's phone number or where to park. When the OT points out these missing areas, the client appears perplexed, then laughs if off, stating that someone else would be calling to schedule appointments and providing transportation. Attempting to subtly hint about cognitive deficits is no longer working, and the OT is concerned because despite repeated efforts, the individual is not retaining safety precautions. This patient's behavior indicates a problem in what area?

A. Denial.
B. Self-awareness.
C. Emotional regulation.
D. Sequencing.

18. An OT is evaluating two-point discrimination in an individual who sustained a median nerve injury. What is the BEST way to administer this test?

A. Apply the stimuli beginning at the little finger and progress toward the thumb.
B. Start with the thumb area first, then progress toward the little finger.
C. Present stimuli in an organized pattern to improve reliability during retesting.
D. Allow the individual unlimited time to respond.

19. An OT is initiating an evaluation of a preschool child diagnosed with autism spectrum disorder. What is the OT MOST likely to include in the evaluation process?

A. One-to-one interview with the child.
B. Observation of the child in a social, gross motor, and self-feeding task.
C. The Peabody Developmental Motor Scales-2.
D. Assessment of the child's performance skills while outside on the playground.

20. A high school teacher diagnosed with a right-hemisphere CVA is given a paper with letters of the alphabet displayed in random order across the page and is instructed to cross out every "M." The individual misses half of the "M"s in a random pattern. What type of deficit would cause such a response?

A. A left visual field cut.
B. A right visual field cut.
C. Functional illiteracy.
D. Decreased attention.

21. A college student with a history of substance abuse has been admitted to the hospital following an accidental overdose at a party. He states his goal is to return to school as soon as possible so that his GPA does not drop below a 3.0. What is the MOST important area for the OT evaluation to focus on?

A. Leisure skills.
B. Activities of daily living.
C. Academic/study skills.
D. Family education.

22. What are the MOST important items to assess when evaluating motor control after a traumatic injury?

A. Developmental factors and primitive reflexes.
B. Muscle tone, postural tone, reflexes, and coordination.
C. Blood pressure, heart rate, endurance, and confusion.
D. Self-concept and self-awareness.

23. A new parent recently returned to work and reports difficulty concentrating at work because of thoughts about the baby. When at home, the individual feels distracted by thoughts about work. This MOST likely suggests the need to help this individual in what area?

A. Parenting skills.
B. Attention span.
C. Assertiveness.
D. Role performance.

24. An OT is beginning to work with individuals in recovery in a community-based program. The OT needs an evaluation tool that can be administered in less than 20 minutes, identifies occupational performance limitations, can be used to establish goals based on client priorities, and measure outcomes. Which is the BEST tool for this purpose?

A. Occupational Performance History Interview-II.
B. Role Checklist.
C. Canadian Occupational Performance Measure (COPM).
D. Occupational Self-Assessment.

25. While making brownies, an individual is able to obtain all the supplies from the cabinet and check the oven temperature periodically. However, when the TV is turned on halfway through the activity, she becomes involved with the program and burns the brownies. This individual is showing signs of a deficit in which area?

    A. Sustained attention.
    B. Detecting and reacting.
    C. Shifting of attention.
    D. Mental tracking.

26. In preparation for an annual Individualized Family Service Plan (IFSP) meeting, the OT is developing ideas for intervention to develop a child's fine motor performance for independent play participation. To match the principles of Part C Early Intervention programs, what would be the OT's BEST recommendation?

    A. Family encouragement of the child to engage in play with toys he has at home, without concern for normal development.
    B. A periodic reassessment using Peabody Developmental Motor Scales, 2nd edition, fine motor subtest to measure progress in fine motor skill achievement.
    C. Home visit, during which OT will identify and encourage opportunities for fine motor practice within the family's preferred routines.
    D. Increased weekly home visits so OT can implement therapy activities to promote child's fine motor skill development, using a remedial approach.

27. An adolescent with a history of shoplifting and gang violence has been hospitalized with a diagnosis of conduct disorder. During a task group, what are the MOST important performance skills for the OT to evaluate?

    A. Perceptual-motor performance.
    B. Leisure and vocational interests.
    C. Attention span and social interaction skills.
    D. Interest in performing and ability to perform multiple roles.

28. An OT is evaluating an individual who has undergone a total hip replacement to determine awareness and adherence to hip precautions prior to discharge. What can the OT conclude when the individual is observed leaning forward and stopping at 90 degrees of hip flexion to use the long-handled shoehorn while donning shoes?

    A. Demonstrates independence with precautions.
    B. Requires verbal cuing to observe precautions.
    C. Needs a longer assistive device.
    D. Demonstrates cognitive deficits.

29. A client sustained a hand injury months ago while at work. The individual is now diagnosed with complex regional pain syndrome and is experiencing pain that interferes with work and self-care. Which of the following would be the best pain management modality option to discuss with the client?

    A. Hot packs.
    B. Cold packs.
    C. Fluidotherapy.
    D. Transcutaneous electrical nerve stimulation.

30. A child has considerable difficulty with problem-solving when playing with interlocking blocks, becomes frustrated, and gives up easily. An OT would MOST likely suspect a problem in what area?

    A. Sensorimotor play.
    B. Pretend play.
    C. Constructional play.
    D. Play with rules.

31. The OT is making recommendations to a community living site for a 13-year-old child with moderate intellectual disabilities. Which statement MOST accurately describes the functional ability of this child?

    A. The child requires nursing care for basic survival skills.
    B. The child can usually handle routine daily functions in a supervised home.
    C. The child requires supervision to accomplish productive, nonroutine work.
    D. The child is able to learn academic skills at the third- to seventh-grade level.

32. An individual with borderline personality disorder has been referred to occupational therapy. Which of the following would be MOST important to evaluate?

    A. Activities of daily living.
    B. Instrumental ADLs.
    C. Interpersonal skills.
    D. Sensorimotor skills.

33. An OT performing a motor skills evaluation observes that a child is awkward at many gross motor tasks. Though able to skip rope forward, the child is unable to skip rope backward, even after several attempts. This information would lead the therapist to be particularly observant for which additional signs?

    A. Delayed reflex integration.
    B. Inadequate bilateral integration.
    C. Developmental dyspraxia.
    D. General incoordination.

34. A preteen with spastic cerebral palsy wants to use a computer. Prior to evaluating computer needs, what should the OT learn about FIRST?

    A. The student's and family's goals for the device use.

    B. The family's ability to afford a computer and its upgrades.

    C. Computer learning programs to facilitate student's participation in the classroom.

    D. The student's physical and cognitive capacities to determine appropriate keyboard and screen options.

TREATMENT PLANNING

35. An OT has been asked to develop a stress management program for clients with eating disorders. For this population in particular, which is the MOST important strategy to include?

    A. A physical activity such as yoga or tai chi.

    B. Diaphragmatic breathing or progressive relaxation techniques.

    C. Training to acknowledge feeling and express emotions.

    D. Role-playing stressful situations.

36. The office doorway of an individual using a wheelchair has a clear opening of 28 inches. According to ADA guidelines, which of the following recommendations would be the MOST appropriate to facilitate clear passage of the wheelchair through the doorway?

    A. The doorway width needs to be expanded to have a minimum clearance of 32 inches.

    B. The client needs to obtain a wheelchair narrower than 28 inches.

    C. The doorway width needs to be expanded to have a minimum clear opening of 45 inches.

    D. The doorway width is satisfactory and needs no modification.

37. An individual is about to be discharged from outpatient OT after rehabilitation for a hand injury. The individual has not been able to work for 3 months and is unable to perform all of the job requirements as a truck driver. Which of the following should the OT practitioner recommend at discharge?

    A. A home exercise program.

    B. Home health OT.

    C. Work hardening.

    D. No further OT services.

38. An older adult has been hospitalized with a diagnosis of major depressive disorder following an overdose of sleeping pills. In obtaining an occupational profile, the OT discovers the patient has knitted and crocheted and enjoyed cooking. What activity should the OT practitioner recommend FIRST to achieve the goals of increasing a sense of confidence?

    A. Crocheting a sweater for her teenage granddaughter.

    B. Making spaghetti and garlic bread for her husband.

    C. Knitting a small hat for her newborn grandson.

    D. Planning meals for the week in anticipation of discharge.

39. A child demonstrates aggressive and disruptive behavior in school as a result of a low sensory threshold. Which suggestions would be MOST useful to discuss with the teacher regarding an upcoming class bus trip to the zoo?

    A. Review the bus rules with the child and apply consequences consistently.

    B. Seat child at the front of the bus and use earmuffs to dampen noise.

    C. Have child monitor classmates as "bus patrol" and report behavior.

    D. Let the child set the criteria for a successful trip, and provide a reward if the criteria are met.

40. As the school team meets to develop the IEP for a third-grade student with autism spectrum disorder, the OT helps to project longer-term academic and functional performance outcomes for the student in middle school and high school. What is the MOST significant benefit of this approach for program planning?

    A. Assurance that services will be available for the student in future years.

    B. Likelihood for optimal progress toward relevant post-high school goals.

    C. Current services that focus on steps to achieve targeted long-range outcomes.

    D. Avoidance of unnecessary duplication of services from year to year.

41. A preschooler is having difficulty performing tasks requiring eye-hand coordination as a result of poor visual tracking skills. What activity should the OT use FIRST to promote visual tracking skills?

    A. Tossing and catching a water balloon.

    B. Catching and bursting soap bubbles.

    C. Throwing and catching a beach ball.

    D. Playing softball.

42. A homemaker with weak grip strength wishes to prepare a muffin mix but cannot open the bag. Which of the following would the OT MOST likely recommend?

A. A hand-powered mixer.
B. Looped handle scissors.
C. An electric knife.
D. Prepare slice cookies instead of muffins.

43. An individual's family wants to build a ramp to the primary entrance of the home. What is the maximum slope that the OT should recommend to the family?

A. 1 inch of ramp for every foot of rise in height.
B. 1 foot of ramp for every inch of rise in height.
C. 10 inches of ramp for every 2 inches in height.
D. 1 foot of ramp for every foot of rise in height.

44. In establishing long-term goals for an individual with complete T4 paraplegia in a rehabilitation setting, the OT would MOST likely predict that the patient will attain what level of independence with bathing, dressing, and transfers?

A. Complete independence with self-care and modified independence with transfers.
B. Independence with self-care and minimal assistance with transfers.
C. Minimal assistance with self-care and moderate assistance with transfers.
D. Dependence with both self-care and transfers.

45. When planning acute treatment for a patient who has recently experienced a traumatic amputation of his right upper extremity at the below-elbow level, which of the following areas of patient education would the OT address FIRST?

A. Teaching to put on and take off a prosthesis.
B. Training in residual limb wrapping.
C. Practicing grasp and prehension functions.
D. Simulation to resume vocational activities.

46. An OT is working with an individual who is experiencing a manic episode and is highly excitable. Given that this individual has expressed interest in all kinds of craft activities, which type of craft activity would the OT be MOST likely to select to provide external structure for the client?

A. Doing a detailed needlepoint project requiring fine stitches.
B. Using clay to shape an object of one's choice.
C. Doing a watercolor paint-by-numbers project.
D. Finishing a prefabricated wood birdhouse from a kit.

47. An OT in the hospital outpatient department meets with the parents of a 7-year-old boy with developmental coordination disorder (DCD). The OT believes his performance challenges his participation in school and brings this up. What is the MOST appropriate way for the OT to address the parents?

A. Request permission to send progress report to the school district.
B. Ask parent for permission to call the school district's OT to learn about the IEP referral process.
C. Suggest that the school district pay for the child's outpatient therapy, as it likely relates to the child's school performance.
D. Ask whether the school district has addressed his coordination difficulties and if not, discuss further whether the parent wishes to raise this issue with the child's teacher.

48. An individual with complete C4 tetraplegia is able to independently use a mouth stick to strike keys on a computer keyboard for 3 minutes. To upgrade this activity, the OT practitioner should:

A. provide a heavier mouth stick.
B. have the individual work at the keyboard for 5 minutes.
C. progress the individual to a typing device that inserts into a wrist support.
D. teach the individual how to correctly instruct a caregiver in use of the keyboard.

49. An individual who is considered modified independent for functional mobility consistently leaves her cane in another room. When asked where the cane is, the client replies, "Oh, that cane—it's just so ugly." Which of the following actions is MOST appropriate to take?

A. Discuss issues related to self-concept with the individual.
B. Evaluate the individual's short-term memory.
C. Assess the individual's long-term memory.
D. Devise strategies to address time management.

50. What is the PRIMARY goal for providing a hand orthosis to a child with active juvenile rheumatoid arthritis?

A. Inhibit hypertonus.
B. Increase range of motion.
C. Prevent deformity.
D. Correct deformity.

51. Which of the following actions should the OT practitioner instruct a patient to perform FIRST when initiating a safe wheelchair transfer?

    A. Have the patient scoot forward to the front of the seat.

    B. Position foot plates in the up position.

    C. Swing away the leg rests.

    D. Lock the brakes.

52. An OT is treating a child with autism spectrum disorder. To maximize the child's benefit from intervention using Ayres Sensory Integration®, what does the therapist need to ensure?

    A. Sensory strategies are provided to enable child to process proprioceptive and tactile stimuli.

    B. Only one option for activity is available at a time, to encourage focus.

    C. Active participation and self-direction in activities matched to identified needs.

    D. Highly structured session, facilitating step by step learning.

53. An individual with ALS and mild dysphagia becomes extremely fatigued at meals. Which is the FIRST intervention the OT practitioner should consider recommending?

    A. Speak with the physician about tube feedings.

    B. Sit in a semireclined position during meals.

    C. Eat six small meals a day.

    D. Substitute pureed foods for liquids.

54. An OT has developed a work conditioning program for men and women who were previously homeless and exhibit generally decreased endurance. What is the FIRST part of a work conditioning program?

    A. Work activities adapted to the level of their ability.

    B. Exercise and limited work task simulation.

    C. Work tasks specific to the jobs they will be getting.

    D. A full day of on-the-job training.

55. A sales executive being treated for anxiety is participating in OT to develop time management skills. Which of the following would be the expected outcome for the individual?

    A. To control anxiety when arriving late for a meeting.

    B. To take responsibility when late with reports.

    C. To cope with feelings of inadequacy when missing a deadline.

    D. To eliminate late arrival to work.

56. An individual has been instructed to place towels, one at a time, on a high shelf to improve shoulder function. The individual is able to easily place 10 towels. Which of the following modifications would MOST effectively improve endurance in the shoulder flexors?

    A. Place the towels on a higher shelf.

    B. Increase the number of towels from 10 to 20.

    C. Place the towels on a lower shelf.

    D. Add a 1-pound weight to each arm.

57. The OT is planning intervention for a 10-year-old child with learning disabilities and significant difficulties accomplishing writing and drawing tasks, secondary to perceptual-motor dysfunction. When selecting a service delivery approach, which is the BEST choice?

    A. Consultation with classroom teacher so student stays in least restrictive environment.

    B. 1:1 intervention from the OT to focus on student's skill development before middle school.

    C. Intervention from the OT in a small group with other students having similar needs.

    D. A combination of service delivery models so that the OT can address student, teacher, and task needs.

58. A person with a long history of Parkinson's disease is experiencing considerable fatigue during the day. The BEST way to enable the individual to maintain his level of function is to teach him how to:

    A. work through the fatigue.

    B. perform desired activities in a simplified manner to conserve energy.

    C. employ pursed-lips breathing.

    D. eliminate activities or reduce activity level as much as possible.

59. A child with behavioral problems has difficulty with peer interactions. The OT's intervention plan is MOST likely based on which approach?

    A. Provide small group occupation-based activities in an authoritarian environment with clear expectations.

    B. Begin with 1:1 occupation-based activities to develop child's social skills, then introduce group activities.

    C. Provide small group occupation-based activities that encourage exploration and interaction.

    D. Provide small group occupation-based activities with rules to define acceptable play guidelines.

60. An OT is developing a measurement plan to track changes in social participation of several students with autism spectrum disorder. Which is the MOST likely measurement strategy the OT selects?

    A. School Function Assessment.

    B. Documentation of change in narrative progress notes.

    C. Photographs taken over a 2-month period during recess.

    D. Goal Attainment Scaling.

61. An individual with Guillain-Barré acute syndrome demonstrates poor to fair strength throughout the upper extremities. Which is the most appropriate approach for the OT practitioner to use when planning treatment for the EARLY stages?

    A. Gentle, nonresistive activities.

    B. Progressive resistive exercise.

    C. Fine motor activities.

    D. Active range of motion against moderate resistance.

62. A child with underreactive sensory processing has been referred to occupational therapy. Based on a sensory integration frame of reference, intervention activities should have which facilitatory characteristics?

    A. Arrhythmic and unexpected.

    B. Arrhythmic and slow.

    C. Sustained and slow.

    D. Unexpected and rhythmic.

63. A child with cerebral palsy and limited postural stability is developmentally ready for toileting. Which element of the treatment plan should be considered FIRST?

    A. Training in management of fasteners.

    B. Utilization of foot supports.

    C. Provision of a seat belt.

    D. Training in climbing onto the toilet.

64. The mother of a 3-year-old with spastic quadriplegia wants her son to walk independently around the house. The child is not yet ready to achieve this goal; however, his mobility would be helpful to the mother who is finding her child difficult to lift. What is the BEST way to assist in the development of family-centered intervention?

    A. Support and work on the parent's goal as she has stated it.

    B. Suggest an alternate goal of improving sitting balance for playing.

    C. Propose a modified goal that still meets the parent's needs.

    D. Include the child in the goal-setting process.

65. Following radiation therapy for breast cancer, an individual develops lymphedema in the right (dominant) upper extremity. She is experiencing functional deficits and is referred to occupational therapy. Treatment to reduce the swelling will begin with:

    A. change of dominance training.

    B. RUE exercise using isometric contractions.

    C. fitting of compression garments.

    D. a heat modality, such as warm compresses.

66. An OT is planning intervention with a young teenager following second-degree skin burns on her hands and face. What other tool would add important information to what the therapist has already learned from the medical record, evaluation of child's physical, and sensory function and ADL performance?

    A. School record, including past grades and extracurricular activities.

    B. Canadian Occupational Performance Measure (COPM).

    C. Jacob's Prevocational Assessment (JPVA).

    D. Ranchos Los Amigos Levels of Cognitive Functioning.

67. An OT practitioner is designing a stress management series using a cognitive-behavioral treatment approach for individuals who have chronic fatigue syndrome. What should the FIRST module in the series include?

    A. Teaching time management techniques.

    B. Identifying thoughts and beliefs that contribute to negative feelings.

    C. Providing aerobic exercise.

    D. Teaching how to perform progressive resistive exercise.

68. An OT is designing a series of group sessions for adolescents with eating disorders. What is the long-term goal for the group?

A. Develop healthy eating behaviors and meal preparation skills.

B. Improve school performance.

C. Develop independence in menu planning and awareness of portion size.

D. Promote communication skills and assertiveness.

69. An individual with a complete high-level tetraplegia spinal cord injury is returning home. Which type of adaptive technology would the individual MOST likely require to ensure safety in the home?

A. A simple electronic aid to daily living (EADL).

B. A second generation EADL device with speakerphone.

C. A remote control power door opener.

D. An electric page turner.

70. What should an OT do to promote playfulness and self-expression in a young child with mild intellectual disability?

A. Model imagination, and use playful facial expressions and voice.

B. Ask child to demonstrate his favorite things to do during playtime.

C. Provide child with toys that are familiar and played with frequently.

D. Provide activities with a means of release, such as leather tooling.

71. As the OT plans intervention for a parent with a mild intellectual disability who has returned home from the NICU with her daughter who was born 6 weeks prematurely, the therapist considers ways to help this mother develop positive parenting skills during feeding and dressing activities. Which is MOST likely going to help this parent?

A. Provide handouts that picture the sequence of steps required to prepare the baby's formula and launder clothes in the washing machine.

B. Encourage problem-solving about how she will respond when the baby is fussy during feeding and diaper changes.

C. Consult with the service coordinator to ensure that caretaking supports are available for the mother.

D. Practice preparing formula and washing clothes and include multiple opportunities for repetition.

72. An OT is working with an individual with Alzheimer's disease who demonstrates mild to moderate decline. She lives with her husband, who works during the day. The OT should initially focus intervention on which one of the following areas?

A. Ability to chew and swallow.

B. Kitchen safety.

C. Anger management.

D. Recognition of family members.

73. When providing caregiver training to the spouse of an individual diagnosed with early-stage dementia, the OT will MOST likely need to instruct the caregiver in strategies to compensate for what deficits?

A. Short-term memory.

B. Fine and gross motor skills.

C. Social skills.

D. Dressing skills.

74. To develop the MOST relevant goals for a student's school-based occupational therapy program, what should the OT focus on?

A. Teacher's perspective about why the student struggles in the classroom.

B. Student's ability to access and participate in the curriculum.

C. Family's priorities for their child.

D. Areas of delay identified in the occupational therapy evaluation.

75. An OT practitioner is planning a meal preparation activity for an individual with cognitive deficits in the areas of attentional and organizational skills. What is the most appropriate activity to use FIRST in addressing sequencing skills?

A. Setting the table.

B. Planning a meal.

C. Baking cookies following a recipe.

D. Preparing a shopping list.

76. An OT practitioner is working with an individual in a work program setting. What is the FIRST step to achieving the program objective of preventing reinjury?

A. Performing a prework screening.

B. Learning proper body mechanics.

C. Participating in work hardening.

D. Engaging in vocational counseling.

77. An individual was unable to achieve the following goal: "The client will initiate two requests to other group members for sharing materials within a 1-week period." What would be the BEST revised goal for this client?

A. Initiate two requests to other group members for sharing group materials within a 2-week period.

B. Initiate one request to one other group member for sharing group materials within a 1-week period.

C. Greet the other group members at the start of each group session.

D. Greet the group leader at the start of each group session.

78. A child with autism spectrum disorder demonstrates inadequate playground skills. She plays alone, generally repeating the same play each day. Which approach will the OT MOST likely select to promote her skills?

A. OT joins group on playground, facilitating child's play and including other children.

B. OT works with child on the playground when other students are not using the playground.

C. Recommend the parent enroll the child in ballet lessons after school.

D. Ask the physical education teacher to include her in small groups during gross motor activity.

79. A child with learning disabilities resulting in low frustration tolerance and poor self-esteem is learning how to tie shoelaces. Which method is the MOST appropriate for the OT to introduce to this child?

A. Physical guidance.

B. Verbal cues.

C. Backward chaining.

D. Forward chaining.

80. When an individual with neurological deficits sits down to read a magazine in the living room of her group home, she becomes distracted by the conversations of her housemates. Which of the following activities BEST addresses the underlying cognitive problem?

A. Playing a simple, repetitive card game in a quiet environment.

B. Measuring ingredients for a recipe while there is music playing.

C. Referring to a catalog and filling out a catalog form.

D. Walking and bouncing a ball simultaneously.

81. An OT is planning intervention for a student who has difficulty manipulating her pencil to erase errors on her papers. What activities should be included to improve her in-hand manipulation?

A. Finger-to-palm translation.

B. Palm-to-finger translation.

C. Simple rotation.

D. Complex rotation.

82. An OT practitioner is planning a vocational intervention program to assist an individual in a community mental health day program develop skills needed for obtaining employment. Which of the following would be the MOST relevant intervention to include?

A. Self-assessment of work habits and personality characteristics.

B. Activities focused on time and stress management skills as well as practice of job-seeking strategies.

C. Educating the work supervisors about the individual's needs and offering environmental modifications to maximize performance.

D. Expressive activities such as making a collage with pictures of different types of jobs.

83. An individual with Guillain-Barré acute syndrome was recently admitted to a rehabilitation unit and is expected to remain for 3 to 4 weeks. At what point in the rehabilitative process should the OT order adaptive equipment for this individual?

A. After the patient and family have accepted the individual's disability.

B. As soon as the insurance provider approves it.

C. Within the first week of therapy.

D. Just before discharge.

84. An individual diagnosed with cancer has developed chemotherapy-induced neuropathy, resulting in wristdrop and decreased sensation in the RUE. The individual is right-handed. Which treatment approach is MOST appropriate for optimizing UE functional performance?

A. Meaningful activities to improve right-hand pinch and grasp.

B. RUE sensory reeducation.

C. Use of orthosis to provide support until wrist strength returns.

D. Change of dominance training.

85. An OT is planning a group program in an acute care psychiatry setting for severely mentally ill individuals who display disorganized thinking and difficulty functioning in many areas. What is the MOST appropriate type of group to use with these patients?

    A. Activity.
    B. Psychoeducational.
    C. Neurodevelopmental.
    D. Directive.

86. An OT is concerned about a child's inability to control flexion and extension of the arm when reaching for toys. He flexes or extends the arm too much, making accurate placement of the hand very difficult. When developing goals, what area is MOST likely in need of development?

    A. Ability to isolate movement.
    B. Ability to grade movement.
    C. Ability to control how fast movement occurs.
    D. Bilateral integration of arm movements.

87. While evaluating an individual with arthritis, the OT observes PIP joint hyperextension and DIP joint flexion in the digits. The OT will MOST LIKELY document this as a:

    A. boutonniere deformity.
    B. mallet finger deformity.
    C. congenital deformity.
    D. swan neck deformity.

88. An OT is helping the parent of a 4-year-old with autism spectrum disorder to identify strategies to support grooming and hygiene. They are focused on ways to overcome difficulties during toothbrushing routines. What should the OT recommend?

    A. Advise that many children with autism spectrum disorder outgrow difficulties with toothbrushing.
    B. Identify and trial several different strategies, such as various toothpaste flavors, use of electric toothbrush, pictures to show steps.
    C. Give the child a choice between brushing his teeth and another, less-preferred activity.
    D. Vary the schedule so the child doesn't begin to associate negative activities with bedtime.

89. The goal for an individual in the later stages of Parkinson's disease is to dress independently. The BEST adaptation to compensate for this person's physical deficits would be:

    A. hook and loop closures on front-opening clothing.
    B. large buttons on front-opening clothing.
    C. larger clothing slipped on over the head with no fasteners.
    D. stretchy fabric clothing with tie closures in the back.

INTERVENTION

90. A patient with poor visual acuity is about to be discharged after completing a rehabilitation program following a total hip replacement. The MOST appropriate environmental adaptation to ensure that the individual can go up and down stairs safely is:

    A. installing a stair glide.
    B. mounting handrails on both sides of the steps.
    C. marking the end of each step with high-contrast tape.
    D. instructing the patient to take only one step at a time when going up or down.

91. A 7-year-old child with limited pincer grasp wants to zip his own pants in school because he gets embarrassed when he has to ask his teacher for assistance after using the bathroom. Which should the OT recommend the child try FIRST?

    A. Large key ring.
    B. Oversized fasteners.
    C. Colored zippers.
    D. Hook and loop fasteners.

92. An elderly individual who was hospitalized for a right CVA with left upper extremity flaccidity and decreased sensation is beginning to experience sensory return in the left upper extremity. What intervention strategies should now be included in the treatment plan?

    A. Remedial treatment, such as rubbing or stroking the involved extremity.
    B. Remedial treatment, such as the use of hot mitts to avoid burns.
    C. Compensatory treatment, such as testing bathwater with the uninvolved extremity.
    D. Compensatory treatment, such as using a one-handed cutting board to avoid cutting the insensate hand.

93. A client arrives to exercise group wearing traditional garments consistent with religious practices that cover the body from head to toe, restricting movement while exercising. The OT observes the individual's discomfort and is concerned about participation, but also wants the client to be comfortable in an environment that is obviously culturally different for her. What is the BEST action for the OT to take, demonstrating cultural competence in this situation?

    A. When the opportunity arises, discreetly explain to her that dressing more appropriately for the group will allow for better participation.

    B. Comment on the beauty of the clothes, asking for affirmation from the rest of the group.

    C. Gently suggest that next time the client wear loose-fitting clothing that will be comfortable to exercise in.

    D. Ask the individual if there are cultural guidelines for how to dress for exercise group.

94. An OT is running a group for women with eating disorders. The activity is to create a gift box with a message inside about what they appreciate about another individual in the group. After accidentally tearing the side of her gift box, one client looks very distressed and stops participating. Which response is BEST for the OT to enable the client to continue working on her goal of self-acceptance?

    A. Set up a time to work with her one-on-one.

    B. Take the box, make the necessary repairs, and encourage her to continue writing her message.

    C. Discuss the symbolism of how we all experience breaking and healing.

    D. Bring her the supplies to start over again, and leave out the message part of the activity.

95. An OT has been asked to design a health promotion group for individuals with cognitive impairment functioning at a parallel task group level. What is the MOST appropriate activity for the OT to use?

    A. Planning a dinner party.

    B. A "Healthy Eating" board game.

    C. A Weight Watchers support group.

    D. A therapist-led aerobics class.

96. The OT is treating a child with an above-elbow amputation who is experiencing hypersensitivity of the residual limb. The therapist would MOST likely perform which intervention in the preprosthetic phase of treatment?

    A. Engage the child in play activities that strengthen bilateral upper extremities.

    B. Include activities to increase the range of motion in the shoulder on the affected side.

    C. Encourage play activities that incorporate tapping, application of textures, and weight-bearing to the residual limb.

    D. Practice dressing activities that include putting on and taking off the UE prosthesis.

97. An OT is assessing an individual with dysphagia. Which of the following should the OT address FIRST?

    A. Jaw pain and tooth-grinding habits.

    B. Cranial nerve function assessment.

    C. Mental status, oral structures, and motor control of head.

    D. Muscle length control via finger-to-nose tests.

98. A flight attendant with a low back injury is participating in a work-hardening program. The individual can successfully simulate distributing magazines to all passengers in a plane using proper body mechanics. To upgrade the program gradually, what should the OT NEXT request that the individual simulate?

    A. Serving from the beverage cart.

    B. Issuing blankets and pillows.

    C. Distributing magazines to half of the passengers.

    D. Putting luggage in the overhead compartments.

99. An OT is fabricating an orthotic for an individual who presents with a low ulnar nerve injury lesion. The orthosis MOST appropriate for this individual is one that includes which components?

    A. Prevents hyperextension of the PIP joints and allows PIP flexion.

    B. Prevents hyperextension of the MCP joints and allows MCP flexion.

    C. Allows hyperextension of the MCP joints and prevents MCP flexion.

    D. Allows flexion and hyperextension of the MCP joints.

100. An OT is seeing an individual with Stage IV cancer for palliative care. What will the emphasis of intervention be for this individual?

    A. Emphasizing quality of life and engagement in meaningful activity.

    B. Improving strength and endurance and managing pain.

    C. Maximizing independence in perineal activities.

    D. Dealing with the psychological issues associated with preparing for death.

101. An elderly individual who ambulates with a walker in the home states he does not like sponge baths and would prefer to resume taking showers but is afraid of falling. Which of the following should the therapist do FIRST?

    A. Suggest bathtub bathing instead of showering.

    B. Encourage the client to purchase a shower chair.

    C. Demonstrate how using a shower chair improves safety.

    D. Explain that therapy will boost his confidence level when showering.

102. An OT is treating a restaurant worker with pain resulting from a cumulative trauma disorder. The OT suggested using elastic taping to decrease pain in the UE while working. In addition to decreasing pain, this type of taping can also assist with:

    A. decreasing inflammation and edema.

    B. potentially increasing muscle fatigue.

    C. limiting ROM and strength.

    D. desensitizing the UE.

103. An OT has provided a cup with a cutout area at the rim to a 6-year-old child with dysphagia. What is the BEST way to explain the purpose of the cutout in the cup to the family?

    A. Slow the drinking process.

    B. Allow the chin to remain tucked when drinking.

    C. Allow the caregiver to control the flow of liquid.

    D. Minimize biting reflexes when the cup is placed in the mouth.

104. A 6-year-old received OT for dressing skill development and is now independent. At discharge, what is the BEST advice for the OT to give the child's parents to maintain the child's independence in dressing at home?

    A. Give assistance when the child asks for it to provide a successful experience.

    B. Provide praise for completed dressing; do not help the child get dressed.

    C. Supply oversized clothing with hook and loop closures and large snaps.

    D. Use verbal prompts when needed and help with closures only.

105. Which leisure activity BEST suits a sixth-grade student with juvenile rheumatoid arthritis to help him maintain range of motion?

    A. Swimming.

    B. Basketball.

    C. Soccer.

    D. Aerobics.

106. The OT has determined that progressive muscle relaxation training would benefit an individual who has anxiety and a limited attention span. What is the FIRST step in the training program?

    A. Make a fist, and then gradually relax it.

    B. Focus on a rhythmic, repetitive word.

    C. Walk until an increased heart rate is achieved.

    D. Deeply inhale and slowly exhale.

107. An OT is working with an individual with amyotrophic lateral sclerosis who developed a sacral decubiti and has recently become too weak to turn himself in bed. What should the OT plan to do NEXT in regard to client/caregiver instruction?

    A. Begin a strengthening program.

    B. Suggest that client and caregiver begin a wheelchair education program.

    C. Teach the caregiver how to position the client safely.

    D. Provide an environmental control unit to the client.

108. A hospital-based OT is working on discharge plans for a 2-year-old child with paraplegic spina bifida who has just started using a power wheelchair. Which community resource recommendation is the MOST critical for this child?

    A. Social service agency.

    B. Wheelchair equipment vendor.

    C. Family physician.

    D. Early intervention program.

109. A client presents with chronic, poststroke upper extremity edema of the right arm and hand. Which of the following would the OT most likely suggest to manage the edema?

    A. Manual edema mobilization.

    B. Hot pack applications.

    C. Paraffin treatments.

    D. Sensory reeducation.

110. An individual with left upper extremity flaccidity is observed sitting at a table in his wheelchair at lunchtime with his left arm dangling over the side. The FIRST positioning strategy the OT should introduce to the individual is:

    A. positioning the UE on the tabletop surface with Dycem™.

    B. repositioning the arm back on to the wheelchair armrest.

    C. using an arm sling.

    D. attaching a lap tray.

111. An OT is discharging a 4-year-old child with cerebral palsy from a rehabilitation setting to home. What are the MOST appropriate instructions for the OT to provide to the family for maintaining correct jaw control while feeding the child from the side?

    A. Jaw opening and closing are controlled with your index and middle fingers; place your thumb on the child's cheek.

    B. Jaw opening and closing are controlled with your index and middle fingers; place your thumb on the child's larynx for stability.

    C. Jaw opening and closing are controlled with the palm of your hand on the child's jaw cupping it gently.

    D. Jaw opening and closing are controlled with your index and middle fingers; place your thumb on the child's ear for stability.

112. Individuals in a mental health clubhouse program are participating in a social skills training group focused on learning skills for meeting someone for the first time. The participants have completed the step in which they performed the role-play as it most recently occurred, without trying to use the most effective social skills. What is the NEXT action the OT should take when using a responsive social skills training protocol?

    A. Give a homework assignment focusing on meeting someone for the first time.

    B. Provide positive and constructive feedback about performance in the role-play.

    C. Discuss how to carry out strategies when meeting someone for the first time.

    D. Run the role-play again, this time using effective social skills for the same situation.

113. The BEST way for an individual with hemiparesis and mild perceptual deficits to button a shirt is to:

    A. button all the buttons before putting the shirt on.

    B. get the shirt all the way on, then line up the buttons and holes, and begin buttoning from the top.

    C. get the shirt all the way on, then line up the buttons and holes, and begin buttoning from the bottom.

    D. use a buttonhook with a built-up handle.

114. An OT practitioner wants to provide functional activities as part of an individual's hand rehabilitation program. Which of the following activities are appropriate?

    A. Active and self-care range-of-motion techniques.

    B. Crafts, games, and self-care tasks.

    C. Cone stacking, pegs, and pulleys.

    D. Mild, moderate, and resistive Thera-Band™ exercises.

115. The OT is observing a worker with an intellectual disability perform a packaging task requiring assembly of a game box by placing first a pad of paper, then a pencil, then a plastic game piece into a box. The OT realizes the client is having difficulty utilizing the correct assembly sequence. The OT decides that backward chaining would be the most effective technique for training this worker. How can the OT BEST introduce this technique?

A. Instructing the worker to reverse the packaging sequence, placing the plastic game piece in first.
B. Prompting the worker to use the correct sequence with each item, then gradually eliminating prompts beginning with elimination of the prompt for the plastic piece.
C. Having the worker master the first step, putting the pad into the game package, then passing the package on to another worker to insert the pencil and the plastic piece.
D. Demonstrating and repeating the correct sequence before each of the worker's attempts to package all three items.

116. The OT is working with the parents of a 4-year-old boy who demonstrates a strong tonic bite reflex when eating. What type of utensils will the OT MOST likely recommend to the child's parents?

A. Weighted universal grips.
B. Curved utensils.
C. Swivel utensils.
D. Rubber-coated spoons.

117. Participants from a partial hospitalization program are taking an outing into the community. One program member complains of shortness of breath. The OT practitioner determines the individual's resting heart rate is 128 bpm, and blood pressure is 230/180 mm Hg. What is the MOST appropriate action for the OT to take?

A. Continue the community re-entry outing, watching to see if additional symptoms emerge.
B. Immediately return the rest of the clients to the day program.
C. Help the patient lie down and wait until his vital signs return to normal.
D. Activate the emergency response by calling 911.

118. Which of the following activities would BEST represent an expected outcome for an individual who completes an energy-conservation program?

A. Getting dressed without becoming fatigued.
B. Lifting heavy cookware without pain.
C. Doing handicrafts without damaging his or her joints.
D. Dusting and vacuuming more quickly.

119. An OT is working with an individual who is s/p RUE shoulder replacement. The client is right-hand dominant and an avid woodworker. Currently, limited RUE ROM prevents participation in woodworking, which requires at least 120 degrees of shoulder flexion. The OT and the patient collaboratively develop a plan that incorporates woodworking to increase RUE ROM. After establishing the "just right challenge" at 40 degrees of shoulder flexion for sanding the pieces of a wood project, how should the OT progress the patient in order to achieve his goal?

A. Progress him to the use of power tools.
B. Apply increasingly heavier wrist weights during sanding and staining activities.
C. Provide him with tasks that require bilateral coordination.
D. Involve him in sanding and staining increasingly larger pieces.

120. The OT has been working with a group of individuals with co-occurring mental illness and substance abuse in a clubhouse model for several months. The group is functioning at a mature level. Which is the BEST way for the OT to be involved in this group?

A. Functioning as a peer in the group.
B. Functioning as group leader.
C. Functioning as group advisor.
D. Functioning as group facilitator.

121. A man with arthritis in his hands is attending outpatient OT to learn joint protection techniques. He wants to continue his hobby of needlepoint, which he does every day during his train commute to and from work. What advice should the OT give him regarding his hobby?

A. Provide him with needlepoint designs that have a low level of complexity.

B. Teach him to take breaks frequently when doing needlepoint and to respect pain.

C. Encourage him to take up a different hobby that does not require him to hold small items, such as a needle.

D. Recommend he do only small needlepoint projects that can be completed in less than an hour.

122. A child with developmental delay in a kindergarten class has just developed the strength and stability in his right hand to hold scissors properly and make snips in paper. Which activity would help the child to develop the next level of scissor skills?

A. Cut cloth and cardboard.

B. Cut along curved lines.

C. Cut along straight lines to cut out a triangle.

D. Cut the paper in two following a straight line.

123. The OT fitted a 6-year-old child with an adapted seat to use during mealtime and other tabletop activities at home. What information is MOST appropriate to convey to the parents?

A. Use the seat as the child is willing.

B. Bring the seat in for each weekly therapy session.

C. Bring the seat in for reevaluation in 4 to 6 months.

D. Keep the seat until the end of the IEP.

124. An individual preparing for discharge following a brief inpatient hospitalization for depression describes to the OT the type of services she would like to be involved in postdischarge. She is interested in structuring her day around work but does not feel she is ready for paid employment. She enjoys being in the company of others and does not feel she will need the support of professional mental health providers. Which setting best meets her criteria?

A. Transitional employment.

B. Clubhouse model.

C. Partial hospitalization.

D. Group home.

125. During a task group, an individual diagnosed with borderline personality disorder tells one group member that their project "looks like it was made by a little kid" and tells another group member that their project "looks stupid" and tosses the project across the room. Which is the BEST approach for the OT to take with the person who is displaying this behavior?

A. Ban the individual from group activities until her behavior improves.

B. Tell the individual how disappointed you are in her behavior.

C. Work with the individual on appropriate communication skills.

D. Ask the individual how she thinks the other group members felt when she did that.

126. When instructing the parents of a toddler in the use and care of a hand orthosis, on which instruction should the OT place the MOST emphasis?

A. Checking for irritation and pressure problems.

B. Avoiding excessive heat exposure.

C. Cleansing the orthosis regularly.

D. Adhering strictly to the wearing schedule.

127. A 7-year-old child with cerebral palsy demonstrates fair sitting stability and good head control with fluctuating lower extremity extensor tone. What position device would the OT MOST likely use during feeding?

A. Prone stander with lateral trunk supports.

B. Rifton child's chair with footrest and padded abductor post.

C. Caregiver's lap, with one arm stabilizing his trunk.

D. Beanbag chair for full sitting support.

128. An OT is preparing to do a parachute activity as part of a sensory integration program. Because several of the patients in the group are taking antipsychotic medications, the OT should be alert for which possible side effect that could occur as a result of this activity?

A. Orthostatic hypotension.

B. Photosensitivity

C. Excessive thirst.

D. Blurred vision.

129. A very confused long-term care facility resident is frequently found in the rooms of other residents in the middle of the night. Which of the following environmental adaptations would MOST effectively prevent wandering?

    A. Apply wrist restraints after the client has fallen asleep.

    B. Keep hallways clear of obstructions to prevent injury.

    C. Install an alarm on the client's door.

    D. Move the individual's room close to the nurses' station.

130. An OT has been hired by a community residence for women with mental health issues as a consultant to address the problem of low motivation and low activity levels in the areas of activities of daily living and instrumental activities of daily living. What approach is MOST appropriate?

    A. Provide occupational therapy treatment to increase occupational performance in the areas identified.

    B. Develop a plan with staff to change the social environment to one that will enhance motivation and activity levels.

    C. Design a range of living skills groups so that every resident will be included.

    D. Help the residents to achieve personal goals, make decisions, or change behaviors.

131. An OT is working with a 6-year-old child who occasionally drops his utensils when eating because of a slight decrease in hand range of motion/grasp limitation. Which piece of equipment would the OT MOST likely recommend FIRST?

    A. Swivel utensils.

    B. Pediatric universal holders.

    C. Foam tubing around the utensils.

    D. Weighted utensils.

132. During an infant's OT session, the mother reports she has observed that her baby has difficulty with swallowing and frequently chokes. To reduce the risk of aspiration and facilitate swallowing, the OT should keep the head in what position?

    A. Neutral position.

    B. Slightly flexed.

    C. Slightly extended.

    D. Rotated toward the feeder.

133. A 60-year-old auto mechanic with diabetes and impaired sensation in the residual lower limb has been referred to OT for prosthetic training following an above-knee amputation. The FIRST item the OT practitioner should address is:

    A. skin inspection.

    B. grooming techniques.

    C. retirement planning.

    D. returning to work.

134. The OT and client have agreed on a baking activity to work on decision-making skills, but when the time comes, the individual is reluctant to participate. Which of the following approaches would be MOST appropriate?

    A. Premeasure all the dry and liquid ingredients.

    B. Use a recipe with no more than three steps.

    C. Offer a choice of slice-and-bake cookies or a cake mix.

    D. Create a checklist to use as each ingredient is added.

135. A client who presents with little to no active range of motion in the left shoulder after a CVA requires the OT to perform passive range of motion. How would the OT proceed?

    A. Teaching the client to utilize a wall-mounted shoulder wheel.

    B. Having the OT move the shoulder joint through its full range of motion.

    C. Using an overhead pulley system.

    D. Training with an arm ergometer.

136. An individual with bipolar disorder demonstrates frequent verbal outbursts and has been referred to occupational therapy to work on developing social skills. When using a Dialectical Behavior Therapy approach, what is the MOST appropriate format to use?

    A. Individual treatment sessions in a quiet place such as the individual's room.

    B. A group format following a specified protocol.

    C. Individual treatment sessions that allow for flexibility within each session.

    D. A group format that alternates leadership opportunities between group members.

137. An OT is applying PNF techniques for weight shifting during an activity that requires an individual to use the right hand to remove groceries from a bag on the floor to the right. The MOST benefit would be gained from this activity by then placing the groceries:

    A. on the counter directly in front.
    B. on the counter to the left side.
    C. in the upper cabinet to the right side.
    D. in the upper cabinet to the left side.

138. A student is learning to activate a switch for a communications device. Although the switch is mounted on the wheelchair tray, the student continues to have difficulty operating it because of excessive muscle tone. Despite practicing for extended periods of time, the student is not making any progress. What should the OT do NEXT?

    A. Reposition the switch to facilitate easy access and adjust further as needed.
    B. Passively stretch the student's upper extremity to increase range of motion.
    C. Use a brightly colored switch to increase visibility.
    D. Use systematic behavioral reinforcement through shaping.

139. To develop a preschool child's letter recognition skills, what would the OT MOST likely encourage the child to do?

    A. Use flashcards with bright colors.
    B. Form letters out of clay.
    C. Match cut-out letters to a sample.
    D. Color large letter outlines.

140. To improve written communication, an OT practitioner would be MOST likely to recommend a large keyboard to enhance computer access when an individual:

    A. has limited UE range of motion, but adequate fine coordination.
    B. fatigues rapidly when reaching for the keys.
    C. uses only one hand to access the keyboard.
    D. has good UE range of motion, but difficulty accessing small targets.

141. An older adult day-care facility has contracted an OT practitioner to develop programming for its clients at risk for falls. The BEST type of program to provide regular group physical activity and enhance balance would be:

    A. safe-transfer training.
    B. walking.
    C. tai chi.
    D. gardening.

142. In order for an individual sitting in a wheelchair to achieve maximal postural positioning, the OT should position the individual's pelvis in what position?

    A. Moderate posterior tilt.
    B. Neutral.
    C. Slight anterior tilt.
    D. Slight posterior tilt.

143. An OT practitioner is working in a sheltered workshop with adults with intellectual disabilities functioning at Allen's Cognitive Level 4. The upcoming job requires an assembly-line approach. Which of the following is the BEST method for introducing an assembly activity to this population?

    A. Provide simple, repetitive tasks.
    B. Visually and verbally demonstrate a two- or three-step activity.
    C. Provide one-step directions and samples for individuals to duplicate.
    D. Provide written directions for individuals to follow.

144. What would an OT who is fitting a first-grade child for a desk and chair recommend to promote optimal hand function during classroom seat work?

    A. Placing the writing surface at a level slightly below the child's elbow.
    B. Providing a wrist weight for writing activities.
    C. Placing the writing surface at a level slightly above the child's elbow.
    D. Stabilizing the child's trunk against the seat back.

145. A 9-year-old child with intellectual disabilities has received OT to become independent in dressing and feeding. He is now dressing himself and is ready for discharge. What is the BEST approach for the OT to take when developing home program recommendations?

    A. Schedule a session with his parent to demonstrate specific therapeutic strategies for their use.
    B. Discuss daily routines with his parent and explain how they can reinforce independence within those routines.
    C. Recommend his parent purchase oversized clothing with hook and loop closures and large snaps.
    D. Advise his parent to give child verbal prompts when he is dressing and help with closures only.

146. When the OT implements intervention to support a child with neuromotor disorder to increase her participation in home and community activities, what approach should be the PRIMARY focus?

    A. Securing assistive technology devices that promote participation in everyday activity, followed by training to develop her competent use of the AT.

    B. Developmental approaches that maximize skill development and prevent further range-of-motion limitations.

    C. Assurance that a peer buddy is available in all contexts and settings to provide assistance with unanticipated needs.

    D. Knowing the child and family's priorities, modifying contexts to promote participation, enhancing performance, and educating family.

147. An individual with cognitive deficits exhibits little transfer of skills from one activity to the next. Which intervention would be BEST to assist this individual in performing the steps of doing laundry?

    A. Performing memory drills of the steps involved in doing a laundry activity.

    B. Placing serial pictures of a laundry activity in sequence.

    C. Consulting a checklist of steps while doing laundry in context.

    D. Reading a story about a person doing laundry with the individual and then discussing the story.

148. A young child with developmental delay has just learned to sit independently on the floor. To facilitate the NEXT step toward refining postural reactions in sitting, what should the OT encourage the child to do?

    A. Sit straddling a bolster with both feet on the floor.

    B. Maintain sitting balance on a scooter while being pulled.

    C. Bounce on a ball with a handle without falling off.

    D. Maintain floor-sitting position with the therapist providing pelvic support.

149. The teacher notes that a student with quadriplegia frequently slumps to the side when sitting in a wheelchair. What would the OT MOST likely recommend to enable the child to maintain optimal wheelchair positioning for seat work?

    A. A reclining wheelchair.

    B. An arm trough.

    C. Lateral trunk supports.

    D. Lateral pelvic supports.

150. An OT working with a group of children who have behavioral challenges is planning activities to develop their play patterns and interaction skills. Which activity will MOST effectively address this aim?

    A. Have children paint pictures during "free time."

    B. Organize a game of soccer during recess with the group of children.

    C. Recommend the teacher include additional "game" software in the classroom library.

    D. Suggest the teacher include age-appropriate jigsaw puzzles in the classroom's game center.

151. The OT has completed an evaluation on an individual with serious and persistent mental illness observed during a music therapy group. The individual actively engaged with other group members and was able to problem solve with other group members when they were asked to select their instruments. It was clear the individual was interested in participating in a performance scheduled for a week later. However, some assistance was needed to sustain appropriate social interaction and for setting limits. Which group level would BEST enable social participation for this individual?

    A. Parallel.

    B. Associative.

    C. Cooperative.

    D. Mature.

152. An individual diagnosed with chronic obstructive pulmonary disease is participating in a pulmonary rehabilitation program. Which of the following will the OT MOST likely recommend?

    A. Perform pursed-lip breathing when doing activities.

    B. Use a long-handled sponge while in the shower.

    C. Take hot showers to reduce congestion.

    D. Avoid air-conditioned rooms during warm months.

153. An OT is fabricating a resting hand orthotic device for an individual with extremely fragile skin. Which of the following areas will the OT have to inspect MOST carefully for signs of skin breakdown?
   A. Metacarpal heads, pisiform, and, trapezium.
   B. Volar PIP joints, medial fifth digit, and thumb MP joint.
   C. Ulnar styloid, distal head of radius, and thumb CMC joint.
   D. Thumb PIP joint, pisiform, and hamate.

154. A first-grade child has difficulty with mature pincer grasp and handwriting. The MOST appropriate activity the outpatient OT would recommend to the parent to complete at home would be:
   A. crayon drawing on sandpaper.
   B. copying shapes from the blackboard.
   C. rolling out clay with a rolling pin.
   D. picking up raisins with a pair of tweezers.

155. Which of the following are the MOST appropriate interventions for the OT to plan in treating a person following a total knee replacement?
   A. Using range-of-motion and strengthening activities for the upper extremities.
   B. Providing range-of-motion and strengthening activities for the lower extremities.
   C. Providing ADL training in use of adaptive techniques for LE dressing and transfers.
   D. Administering an evaluation of homemaking activities.

156. While working with an OT on bed mobility, a patient being seen for home health OT following spinal surgery complains of constant fatigue and difficulty getting a good night's sleep. Which suggestion is MOST appropriate for addressing this individual's sleep concerns from the perspective of habits and routines?
   A. Avoid caffeine and get into bed only when ready to go to sleep.
   B. Use a white-noise machine.
   C. Make sure the room is dark and quiet.
   D. Exercise and take a warm bath prior to bedtime.

157. An 8-year-old boy with conduct disorder is disruptive, uncooperative, and occasionally combative during therapy. From a behavioral point of view, what is the MOST appropriate strategy to use to address the child's behavior?
   A. Allow the child to express his anger without restraint for a short period to vent his frustration.
   B. Ignore the behavior and continue with therapy with or without the child's cooperation.
   C. Attempt to reason with the child to get his cooperation.
   D. Set clear expectations for behavior and enforce consequences.

158. An OT practitioner is addressing concerns about sexual activity with a person who has left-sided hemiplegia with spasticity. The BEST recommendation for positioning during sexual intercourse for this person would be:
   A. lying on the left side, propped up with pillows.
   B. lying on the right side, propped up with pillows.
   C. lying in a supine position.
   D. lying in a prone position.

159. An OT is educating the family of an individual admitted to the ICU after sustaining full-thickness dorsal hand burns. Which of the following MOST accurately explains the purpose of burn hand orthoses?
   A. Decrease pain and allow for active range of motion.
   B. Minimizes hypertrophic scarring.
   C. Diminishes the need for skin grafting.
   D. Prevents stress on the extensor tendons and ligaments while decreasing edema.

160. What type of interactive play would an OT MOST likely recommend to a mother of a 5-year-old child?
   A. Coloring on paper.
   B. Playing a simple board game.
   C. Looking at picture books.
   D. Participating in a reading club.

161. An OTA and OT are planning to discharge a child from an early intervention program. What advice to the parents will MOST likely promote parents' ability to support their young child's continued development?

    A. Set aside a certain time daily to focus on developmental stimulation activities.

    B. Incorporate developmental stimulation activities into family routines.

    C. Provide therapeutic activities on an as-needed basis.

    D. Do therapeutic activities daily, but vary the time of day.

162. Individuals with schizophrenia living in a supported housing apartment have expressed an interest in having more control over what they do on weekends. In response, the OT began offering a leisure skills group; however, attendance has been poor. What action should the OT take FIRST to improve group attendance?

    A. Provide a desirable snack for those who attend.

    B. Ask the program manager to make attendance mandatory for all residents.

    C. Break down the activities into smaller steps.

    D. Provide positive feedback and avoid criticism.

163. During a home visit with a parent and her 11-month-old infant who was born 4 weeks prematurely, the OT observes the child assume a quadruped position and rock back and forth momentarily. What does this behavior MOST likely indicate?

    A. Perseverative behavior.

    B. Expected development.

    C. Low muscle tone.

    D. Delayed development.

164. When evaluating self-care performance with an individual with functional limitations in shoulder abduction and external rotation, which of the following is MOST essential for the OT practitioner to assess?

    A. Buttoning a shirt.

    B. Combing the hair.

    C. Tucking in a shirt in the back.

    D. Tying a shoe.

165. An individual with a C6 spinal cord injury has been referred to OT 2 days postinjury. Immobilized with a halo brace, the individual demonstrates fair plus wrist extension and poor minus finger flexion. Which of the following interventions should be implemented FIRST?

    A. Volar resting hand orthoses to prevent flexion contractures.

    B. Wrist support with universal cuff to promote independence.

    C. Wrist orthoses to promote development of tenodesis.

    D. Instruction in bed mobility techniques to prevent decubiti.

166. An individual with multiple sclerosis reports exhaustion after cleaning the house but cannot afford a house cleaner. Which of the following strategies is MOST appropriate to recommend to this individual?

    A. Suggest that the client hire outside help with the financial support of family members.

    B. Prescribe activities that will increase strength.

    C. Use the largest joints available for the task.

    D. Alternate tasks that require standing with those that can be performed sitting.

167. An individual is having difficulty getting around her home as a result of low vision. What is the MOST appropriate strategy the OT practitioner can recommend to improve accessibility?

    A. Instruct the individual to sit while performing ADLs.

    B. Provide strong color contrast at key areas to identify steps, pathways, etc.

    C. Arrange for another person to provide assistance when moving within the home.

    D. Recommend training in white cane use for identifying obstacles in the home.

168. An OT is reviewing bathing skills with a 13-year-old boy when the teen asks questions regarding his sexuality. What should the OT do FIRST?

    A. Refer the teenager to someone who has increased knowledge regarding the subject of sexuality, such as a psychologist.

    B. Tell the client that you don't mind discussing sexuality-related questions as long as his parents are comfortable with the idea.

    C. Attempt to change the subject because the child is too young to be educated on this topic.

    D. Try openly and honestly to address the client's questions to the best of your knowledge.

169. An individual with mental illness has accepted a secretarial position but is concerned that her high levels of distractibility may interfere with concentration and job performance. Which of the following interventions is MOST appropriate for this individual?

    A. Arrange for the individual to have a job coach.

    B. Suggest that the employer provide more frequent breaks.

    C. Explain the problem of distractibility to the employer.

    D. Ask the employer to provide an isolated cubicle as the work space.

170. An individual arrives late to the morning social skills group, sits slumped in a chair, and appears to have trouble staying alert and engaged. The OT notices the same is true for several other individuals. Which preparatory activity would be MOST effective in promoting the client's engagement with the group?

    A. Slowly rocking in a rocking chair.

    B. Listening to a CD of ocean sounds.

    C. Wrapping themselves up in heavy, warm blankets.

    D. Dancing to a strong, fast beat.

171. During a discharge-planning group, one individual states that she may as well stay in the hospital because she is such a burden to her family, even though they say they want her home with them. Using a cognitive-behavioral approach, which response should the OT give to promote cognitive restructuring?

    A. "What might someone who disagrees say?"

    B. "I'm sure your family wants you home with them very much."

    C. "How about writing a poem that expresses your feelings?"

    D. "Take 15 minutes to do some mindfulness meditation."

172. While performing endurance training activities, an individual on a cardiac rehabilitation unit begins to slow down, using progressively smaller movements to perform the activity. Which of the following is the MOST appropriate action for the OT practitioner to take?

    A. Stop the activity immediately.

    B. Upgrade the activity for the next session.

    C. Reassess the patient's vital signs and consider modifying the activity to make it less challenging.

    D. Replace the activity with isometric exercises.

173. An OT who works in an outpatient facility frequently recommends that individuals with Parkinson's disease consider taking part in a community-based therapeutic group. What is the PRIMARY reason for recommending group treatment?

    A. Is more effective in preventing motor problems associated with Parkinson's disease.

    B. Provides social interaction and support, as well as activity.

    C. Is an effective way to present therapeutic exercise activities.

    D. Requires less therapist time because the therapist can leave once the group has started.

174. The mother of an 18-month-old child with hypertonia reports that dressing is extremely difficult. When teaching the parent how to put on the toddler's shoes and socks, what should the OT suggest to the mother FIRST?

    A. Flex the child's hips.

    B. Flex the child's knees.

    C. Flex the child's neck.

    D. Flex the child's shoulders.

175. Which is the BEST position to promote isolated head control in a child with very limited postural control and significant upper and lower extremity weakness while participating in a fine motor activity?

    A. Standing in a standing frame with knee and hip support.

    B. Quadruped with chest supported in a sling.

    C. Prone over a wedge with toys in front.

    D. Side-lying with suspended toys nearby.

176. An individual with amyotrophic lateral sclerosis is no longer able to ambulate for kitchen or home management activities. Which of the following interventions BEST addresses the goals of independence in meal preparation for this individual?

    A. Teaching wheelchair-level techniques.

    B. Training in the use of adapted equipment.

    C. Standing at the counter for gradually increasing amounts of time.

    D. Beginning with cold meals and progressing to hot meals.

177. An OT is implementing a self-feeding session with an individual with a C5 spinal cord injury. Which piece of feeding equipment would be MOST appropriate for the OT to introduce?

    A. A wrist-driven flexor hinge orthotic device.

    B. A mobile arm support.

    C. An electric self-feeder.

    D. Built-up utensils.

SERVICE MANAGEMENT AND PROFESSIONAL PRACTICE

178. Prevention of cumulative trauma disorders (CTDs) in the workplace is the primary focus of an OT working as an industry consultant. What suggestions should the OT make that would have the greatest impact to reduce the risk of CTD in an industry in which there is heavy keyboard use?

- A. Teach employees to identify the early symptoms.
- B. Educate employees about ergonomic adaptations.
- C. Provide inexpensive resting orthoses to employees.
- D. Instruct employees in exercise routines to increase strength in weak upper extremities.

179. The OT who provides information and resources that are helpful to the family of a young child with multiple disabilities MOST likely includes what type of information?

- A. Updates about their child's developmental age according to standardized test results.
- B. Explanation of how occupational therapy services differ from those provided by other team members.
- C. Suggestions for activities in which parents can engage with their child to help the child practice developing skills.
- D. Reports of the child's behavior during therapist-implemented interventions.

180. The OT researcher would like to strengthen a study related to a constraint-induced movement (CIMT) protocol. The research committee recommended learning more about experimental design, as their current methodology is quasi-experimental. One of the PRIMARY differences between an experimental design and a quasi-experimental design relates to:

- A. dependent variable(s).
- B. control group.
- C. manipulation.
- D. randomization.

181. An OT received the following information: 6-27-15: ADL evaluation and treatment for diagnosis of RCVA: Three times a week for 1 month. Signed, L. Martelli, MD. What did the OT just receive?

- A. Referral.
- B. Screening.
- C. Goal setting.
- D. Treatment planning.

182. An OT performs an initial evaluation on an individual who requires moderate assistance for upper body and lower body dressing. The OT expects the individual to achieve independence in dressing, with occasional assistance for small fastener, by discharge in 2 weeks. The initial G-code and severity modifier are determined to be G8987-CK. How should the self-care goal status be identified?

- A. G8987-CI.
- B. G8987-CN.
- C. G8988-CI.
- D. G8988-CN.

183. An OT is working with his first level I fieldwork student. What should the focus of this experience be?

- A. Facilitating clinical reasoning.
- B. Achieving entry-level competence.
- C. Assisting the student in developing a general understanding of client needs.
- D. Encouraging the student to partake in ethical and reflective practice.

184. An OT practitioner wishes to assess outcomes for life skills training services provided to individuals at a shelter for women who experienced domestic violence. Which of the following methods would be the MOST comprehensive method for obtaining this information?

- A. Final evaluation of each client involved.
- B. Client satisfaction survey.
- C. Program evaluation.
- D. Utilization review.

185. An OTA frequently administers the Allen Cognitive Level Test and then discusses it with the supervising OT. Which of the following MOST accurately describes the OT's role during these discussions?

- A. Determine the OTA's service competency.
- B. Collect data on the patient's performance.
- C. Interpret the results based on data collected.
- D. Develop the treatment plan.

186. An instructor from a local nursing school has asked an OT to speak about OT to a class of first-year nursing students. The practitioner feels uncertain about giving the lecture because of a lack of resources. What is the MOST appropriate action to take?

- A. Recommend that the nursing course instructor call AOTA and obtain information to share.
- B. Decline to do the lecture but send information to the instructor.
- C. Decline to do the lecture and try to find another OT to present the lecture.
- D. Use the AOTA website to obtain resources about occupational therapy.

187. When an OT selects a standardized test to assess a child, what can the therapist OT assume about the test?

- A. It is valid.
- B. It has normative data.
- C. It has a standard format.
- D. It is reliable.

188. An OT has been hired as a program manager to develop a community-based program for individuals with severe and persistent mental illness. What is the FIRST step in the process that the OT must complete?

- A. Program planning.
- B. Program implementation.
- C. Needs assessment.
- D. Program evaluation.

189. While preparing a presentation for a professional conference, an OT planned to copy and distribute an article but realizes the name of the author is missing. Which of the following is the MOST appropriate action for the OT to take?

- A. Distribute the handout and apologize for not having the author's name.
- B. Show the handout with an overhead projector and apologize for not having the author's name.
- C. Use the handout only as a resource while developing the presentation.
- D. Use the article without mentioning the author.

190. What is the NEXT step for an OT to follow after initial evaluation of a 1-year-old child requiring early intervention services?

- A. Independently develop an IEP.
- B. Collaboratively develop an IEP.
- C. Independently develop an IFSP.
- D. Collaboratively develop an IFSP.

191. Which of the following is the BEST example of the plan section of a discharge summary when using the SOAP note format?

- A. The patient reports intentions to continue to practice proper body mechanics at work.
- B. The patient demonstrates independence in performing the home exercise program.
- C. The patient expressed a desire to return to work but does not yet demonstrate the capacity for the required sitting tolerance.
- D. The OT recommends the use of lumbar support and regular performance of home program.

192. A rehabilitation manager is attempting to find a way to have financial success in the department while ensuring patient satisfaction. Which of the following is MOST likely to be implemented to assess patient flow, develop critical pathways, and cut costs?

- A. Quality improvement.
- B. Peer review teams.
- C. Cost accounting.
- D. Cross training.

193. Which BEST depicts the recommended service approach when the IEP team has included occupational therapy services to support the student's participation in the school curriculum?

- A. The OT engages the student in activities outside of the classroom to avoid distraction from peers.
- B. The OT works with the student in the back of the classroom when all students are completing seat work.
- C. The OT arranges to work with the student in the classroom during after-school hours, when other students are not present.
- D. The OT recommends strategies that are easily embedded within the student's activities and routines in the curriculum and promote his or her participation.

194. An OT has been working with an individual with schizophrenia who has been living in a homeless shelter. The individual has been consistent about taking medication and his symptoms are currently well controlled. The individual has expressed an interest in renting an apartment in the community, where he can have responsibility for his own meals and housekeeping, develop social and leisure activities, and still receive necessary social and rehabilitation services. Which type of housing should the OT recommend in order to BEST meet this individual's preferences?

    A. Partial hospitalization.
    B. Assisted living.
    C. Custodial housing.
    D. Supportive housing.

195. An OT completing a home assessment has recommended a hospital bed, lightweight wheelchair, bedside commode, reachers, long-handled sponge, shower chair, and hand-held shower. The family states they can only afford the items that can be billed as durable medical equipment. What should the OT do NEXT?

    A. Order all of the equipment.
    B. Order the reacher and long-handled sponge.
    C. Order the shower chair and hand-held shower.
    D. Order the lightweight wheelchair and hospital bed.

196. The administrator of a long-term care facility asks the OT who works there to help develop a job description so he may hire a second OT. What would an OT job description MOST likely contain?

    A. Previously established mutual goals, quality of patient care, achievement of predicted outcomes, and evidence of relationship building.
    B. A summary of primary and secondary job functions, references, and physical exertion requirements.
    C. Organizational relationships, personality characteristics, and accomplishments desired in a candidate.
    D. Job title, employer's expectations, productivity expectations, and how performance will be measured.

197. An OT is considering the use of an electronic documentation system within a private practice setting. Some of the advantages to electronic health records are increased legibility, speed of documentation, and improved organization. What are the disadvantages of such a system?

    A. Issues related to storage capacity.
    B. Retrieval of information.
    C. Confidentiality, time, and money.
    D. Determining a system for remote site access.

198. A hand therapy research group is attempting to determine whether the experiment caused a change in the dependent variable in a study that used orthoses as the OT intervention in relation to contracture prevention, or whether issues related to the actual passage of time and/or accuracy of the tool used to measure the contractures were responsible for the results. The research group is looking at which of the following?

    A. Study biases.
    B. External validity.
    C. Internal validity.
    D. Context specificity.

199. A school-age child with fine motor skill difficulties is ready for discharge from outpatient OT services. What is the MOST important information to include in the discharge summary that will go to his school?

    A. Child's interests and hobbies.
    B. Child's writing, dressing, and self-feeding performance.
    C. Child's academic achievement.
    D. Recommendations for the child to return to the clinic for follow-up services.

200. An OT is offered a job upon completion of fieldwork and accepts the position even though she had not yet applied for her license. The employer wants her to start working immediately. What would be the BEST action for this therapist to take under the circumstances?

    A. Schedule an immediate start date and send for a license, hoping it will arrive in time.
    B. Confide in the rehabilitation director and follow her recommendation to start as scheduled.
    C. Ask whether the company can delay the start date until her license arrives.
    D. Start the job knowing that no one with the company will ask to see her license.

Answers for Simulation Examination 1

1. (C) Observation of child during activities in the child-care center. Through observation of the child during child-care center activities (answer C), the OT can collect information about the child's motor performance skills and participation in activities that require upper extremity/hand skill. Naturalistic observation is a method of ecologic assessment, which is "a primary mechanism for obtaining data relevant to the child's performance context.... Skilled observation of a child performing a functional task offers...important information about the child's performance" (p. 207). Answers A, B, and D are all appropriate choices after the child is old enough for these assessments. See Reference: Case-Smith & O'Brien. (2010). Stewart, K.B.: Purposes, processes, and methods of evaluation.

2. (D) New motor task planning. Answer D, new motor task planning, is correct. "Somatodyspraxia is described as a deficit in learning new motor skills, planning new motor actions, and generalizing motor plans" (p. 140). Inability to print or write (answer A) is termed "dysgraphia." The term "dyslexia" (answer B) means dysfunction in reading. Inability to perform mathematics (answer C) is known as "dyscalculia." See Reference: Hinojosa & Kramer. (2009). Schaaf, R.C., Schoen, S.A., Smith Roley, S., Lane, S.J., Koomar, J., & May-Benson, T.A.: A frame of reference for sensory integration.

3. (B) Ask the individual how he spent New Year's. "Declarative memory is one aspect of long term memory and includes conscious memory for events, knowledge or facts" (p. 802). It is commonly assessed through verbal interviews and informal testing such as asking a question about an individual's recall of personal events (answer B). Working memory refers to "the temporary storage of information while one is working with it or attending to it" (answer A). "Prospective memory involves the ability to remember intentions or activities that will be required in the future" (answer D) (p. 802). Knowing the date, place, and time is indicative of orientation (answer C). See Reference: Schell, Gillen, & Scaffa. (2014). Toglia, J.P., Golisz, K.M., & Goverover, Y.: Cognition, perception, and occupational performance.

4. (C) Gravitational insecurity. Gravitational insecurity is described as "fear response to movement" (p. 161). The child easily experiences a fear of falling and prefers to keep her feet firmly on the ground. Tactile defensiveness (answer A) is a term used to describe discomfort with various textures and with unexpected touch. Somatodyspraxia (answer B) has its

"foundation in somatosensory (e.g., primarily tactile but also proprioceptive) discrimination deficits, which interfere with the development of body scheme and awareness" (p. 124). Bilateral integration and sequencing deficits are related to "poor vestibular-proprioceptive discrimination, which interferes with the ability to coordinate, sequence, and execute motor actions quickly and efficiently" (p. 124). See Reference: Hinojosa and Kramer, 2009. Schaaf, R.C., Schoen, S.A., Smith Roley, S., Lane, S.J., Koomar, J., & May-Benson, T.A.: A frame of reference for sensory integration; Kaplan, M.: A frame of reference for motor skill acquisition.

5. (B) Dressing habits. Answer B, dressing habits, is correct. Children with tactile defensiveness are "bothered by tactile aspects of daily living activities...specific types of clothing...specific textured materials" (p. 135t). The child may be bothered by certain textures or avoid wearing turtlenecks, socks, or shoes. Conversely, some children may never take off their shoes to avoid tactile stimulation. Play behavior (answer A), social skills (answer C), and the choice of hobbies (answer D) could be affected secondarily, as a result of intolerance to certain textures or human touch. Knowledge of the child's dressing habits will give the OT key information at the start of the evaluation process. See Reference: Hinojosa & Kramer. (2009). Schaaf, R.C., Schoen, S.A., Smith Roley, S., Lane, S.J., Koomar, J., & May-Benson, T.A.: A frame of reference for sensory integration.

6. (B) Sensory avoiding. The individual's actions are indicative of sensory avoiding behavior, characterized by a low threshold to stimuli perceived as noxious, followed by an active response such as leaving the room. Individuals with sensory avoiding behavior may "become distressed in situations in which they cannot control the environment" and "do well in low stimulus situations or settings that others find dull" (p. 292). An individual with low registration (answer A), sensory seeking behavior (answer C), or a hearing impairment (answer D) would not have difficulty with the auditory stimulation caused by the roar of the mixer or loud voices. See Reference: Brown & Stoffel. (2011). Brown, C. & Nicholson, R.: Sensory skills.

7. (A) Working memory. "Working memory is the temporary storage of information while one is working with it or attending to it. It includes the ability to recall information immediately after exposure. It allows one to focus conscious attention and keeps track of information as one is performing an activity" (p. 802). This individual's inability to comb his hair without reminders suggests a deficit in working memory (answer A). Judgment (answer B), the ability to make realistic and safe decisions based on available environmental information, would not be needed for this task. Because the person performed the first request, hearing (answer C) would seem to be intact. Abstraction (answer D) is the ability to extrapolate information from an idea to generalize to another situation and would not be needed to follow this direction. See Reference: Schell, Gillen & Scaffa. (2014). Toglia, J.P. et al: Cognition, perception, and occupational performance.

8. (A) On-site observation of performance skills. Individuals with obsessive-compulsive disorder often experience difficulties with work. Observation in a situational context (answer A) is "likely to be more useful in fully understanding their behavioral success" and is "the preferred approach for assessing work function of persons with psychiatric disabilities" (p. 701). There is nothing to suggest the individual has a cognitive deficit or a need for cognitive assessment (answer B). Interview (answer C) is most useful for assessing an individual's readiness for work, occupational development, and interests. Task evaluation with a "clean" medium (answer D) may be indicated for individuals with OCD of the washing type. However, this individual has OCD of the checking type. See Reference: Brown & Stoffel. (2011). Pitts, D.B.: Work as occupation.

9. (C) Attempt a standard pivot transfer from wheelchair to bed in the patient's hospital room. Giving the individual a functional task, then changing it, and observing the response will tell the therapist how well the individual can transfer learning to new situations. "Transfer of learning, or generalization of skill, is seen when the learner is able to spontaneously perform the task in different environments" (p. 109). If the individual cannot perform the activity when it is changed slightly, then there may be difficulty transferring learning. If the patient can perform the activity with many changes and in a different setting, it suggests a greater aptitude for transfer of learning to new situations. None of the other answers assesses the ability to transfer learning. See Reference: Pedretti. (2013). Richardson, P.: Teaching activities in occupational therapy.

10. (C) Kohlman Evaluation of Living Skills. The Kohlman Evaluation of Living Skills (answer C) "combines interview items with simulated performance" to obtain information about "(s)eventeen living skills, in the areas of self-care, safety and health, money management, transportation and telephone, and work and leisure" (p. 666). The Assessment of

Motor and Process Skills (answer D) assesses an individual's motor and process skills, sometimes embedding a task that is an ADL category. In order to administer the AMPS, one must have special training, so the OT could not begin using it immediately. The Routine Task Inventory (answer B) uses observation to assess 14 different areas of ADL and is based on the cognitive disabilities model, which would not be appropriate for this client. The Bay Area Functional Performance Evaluation (answer A) was designed to measure performance skills such as memory, organization, attention span, test completion, motivation, and frustration tolerance. It also includes a social interaction scale that assesses verbal and nonverbal social interaction behaviors. Although it can help the OT develop conclusions about ADL performance, it is not actually an ADL evaluation tool. See Reference: Brown & Stoffel. (2011). Brown, C.: Activities of daily living and instrumental activities of daily living.

11. (C) Identify or demonstrate the use of common household objects. Answer C is correct because visual agnosia is the inability to recognize common objects and demonstrate their use in an activity. Asking the individual to demonstrate common gestures such as waving (answer A) is a technique to screen for apraxia or the inability to perform purposeful movement on command. Answer B, asking the individual to identify objects through touch only, would be used to evaluate stereognosis, which is the ability to identify an object by manipulating it with the fingers without seeing it. Asking the individual to read a paragraph and explain its meaning (answer D) would be a screening method for alexia, or the inability to understand written language. See Reference: Pedretti. (2013). Phipps, S.C.: Assessment and intervention for perceptual dysfunction.

12. (D) hand controls for acceleration and braking. An L4 spinal cord injury would result in paraplegia. Hand controls use hand motions to control the accelerator and brake mechanisms, eliminating the need for any lower extremity function. The palmar cuff and spinner knob (answers A and B) are steering options for individuals who need to steer single-handed and allow constant contact with the steering wheel. Pedal extensions (answer C) can be installed on accelerator and brake pedal for individuals with limited lower extremity reach. See Reference: Pedretti. (2013). Bolding, D., Adler, C., Tipton-Burton, M., Verran, A., & Lillie, S.M.: Mobility.

13. (C) Adherence to specific instructions for administration and scoring. Answer C is correct. In standardized assessments, the instructions to the examiner are detailed and fixed so that procedures are followed consistently each time the test is administered (p. 206). Following these instructions assures the highest level of reliability and validity possible. Subjective judgment (answer A) and previous experience (answer B) may be factors in administration of nonstandardized tests, which depend on the skill and judgment of the OT administering them, but not in the administration and scoring of standardized tests. Although practice of a test (answer D) can help to develop competence in the use of the test, it would not influence how to administer and score the test. See Reference: Case-Smith & O'Brien. (2010). Richardson, P.K.: Use of standardized tests in pediatric practice.

14. (D) Autism spectrum disorder. Autism (answer D) is "characterized by severe and complex impairments in reciprocal social interaction and communication skills, and by the presence of stereotypical behavior, interest and activities." (p. 170). Children with ADHD (answer A) display behaviors of "inattention, hyperactivity, and impulsivity" (p.172). Children with childhood conduct disorder (answer B) display "severe forms of chronic misbehavior such as physical aggression towards property, animals, or people, theft, and/or lying" (p. 414). Obsessive-compulsive disorder (answer C) is characterized by "intrusive thoughts and repetitive behaviors that have little or no functional purpose beyond decreasing tension" (p. 413), such as repeated hand washing. See Reference: Case-Smith & O'Brien. (2010). Rogers, S.L.: Common conditions that influence children's participation; Davidson, D.A.: Psychosocial issues affecting social participation.

15. (A) Parent's concerns and goals for the child. The caregiver's concerns and goals (answer A) is correct. Interviews enable the OT and parent to develop rapport and "provide a unique opportunity for parents, children and adolescents to identify and discuss issues that are important to them" (p. 208). The child's medical management (answer B), equipment needs (answer C), and the physical layout of the home (answer D) are important issues as well, but can be addressed at a later time. See Reference: Case-Smith & O'Brien. (2010). Stewart, K.B.: Purposes, processes, and methods of evaluation.

16. (B) Assess the individual's lifestyle and dietary habits. Controllable risk factors include smoking, cholesterol level, hypertension, sedentary lifestyle, obesity, diabetes, and psychological stress. OT practitioners have expertise in working with individuals to address goals associated with lifestyle performance and dietary habits (answer B) that can help to prevent heart disease. Whereas obesity can be observed, cholesterol levels cannot (answer C). Age, gender, and family history (answers A and D) are all uncontrollable risk factors associated with heart disease. See Reference: Trombly. (2008). Huntley, N.: Cardiac and pulmonary diseases.

17. (B) Self-awareness. Problems that contribute to deficits and self-awareness (answer B) include not recognizing errors, inability to use feedback, and false beliefs about capabilities. Whereas an individual who lacks self-awareness may be "perplexed and surprised or confused when given feedback regarding limitations," an individual who is in denial (answer A) may "demonstrate resistance or anger when given feedback regarding [his] limitations" (p. 68). Deficits in the area of emotional regulation (answer C) may be characterized by uncontrolled anger, laughter, or crying. Deficits in the area of sequencing (answer D) may be characterized by difficulty planning or enacting the steps of an activity. See Reference: Gillen. (2009). Self-awareness and insight: Foundations for intervention.

18. (A) Apply the stimuli beginning at the little finger and progress toward the thumb. "The principles of sensory testing optimize the reliability of the testing results.... The purpose of these principles is to eliminate non-tactile cues and to ensure that the responses from the patient accurately reflect actual sensation.... Choosing an environment with minimal distractions, ensure the patient is comfortable and relaxed,...state the instructions,...occlude the patient's vision,...[and] apply stimuli at irregular intervals" (p. 219). The general guidelines for sensation testing are that an individual's vision should be occluded, the stimuli should be randomly applied with intermingled false stimuli (opposite of answer C), a practice trial should be performed before the test, and the unaffected side or area should be tested before the affected side or area (opposite of answer B). With a median nerve injury, the ulnar side of the hand is the uninvolved side, and should be tested first. Also, the tested individual should be given a specified amount of time in which to respond; therefore, answer D is incorrect. See Reference: Trombly. (2008). Bentzel, K.: Assessing abilities and capacities: Sensation.

19. (B) Observation of the child in a social, gross motor, and self-feeding task. Answer B, observation of the child's social play, motor processes, and self-feeding skills, is correct. Recommended practices suggest that "occupational therapists conduct observations of clients with an ASD before selecting and administering formal assessment tools because of the wealth of knowledge that is gained through the observation process" (p. 290). Answer A, relying on a one-on-one interview, would not be the most valuable choice, as communication difficulties are a core feature of ASDs. It would be more helpful to combine an interview of the child in conjunction with a parent-teacher interview. Answer C, the Peabody Developmental Motor Scales-2, may be something the therapist administers based on recommendations following review of observation data. Answer D, observation of the child on the playground, is something the OT might consider, but a more comprehensive picture can be drawn from a combined observation of the child's social, motor, and feeding skills. See Reference: Kuhanek & Watling. (2010). Watling, R.: Occupational therapy evaluation for individuals with an autism spectrum disorder.

20. (D) Decreased attention. "Selective Attention: The ability to attend to relevant stimuli while inhibiting distractions and irrelevant information" (p. 794). Having an individual cross out a specific letter (M) every time she sees it, then observing her randomly missing the letter in no apparent pattern is an example of impaired selective attention (answer D). Because the errors were random does not reflect a visual field cut. A visual field cut (answers A and B) is evidenced by missed letters appearing close together in one area, on either the left or right side of the page. Illiteracy (answer C) is unlikely because the individual is a high school teacher. See Reference: Schell, Gillen, & Scaffa. (2014). Toglia, J.P., Golisz, K.M., & Goverover, Y.: Cognition, perception, and occupational performance.

21. (A) Leisure skills. In this situation, the college student appears to be having more difficulty with healthy use of leisure time (answer A) than with academic skills (answer C). In this case, it is particularly evident that "leisure is affected, with the individual's primary leisure activity being substance ingestion.... Individuals who are dependent on the substances spend much of their leisure time obtaining and using the substance.... Routines involve drinking with friends.... The skills required to accomplish activities/instrumental activities of daily living [answer B] are rarely severely impaired" (pp. 108–109). Family education (answer D) is an important element; however, it would not be a focus of evaluation. See Reference: Bonder. (2010). Substance-related disorders.

22. (B) Muscle tone, postural tone, reflexes, and coordination. "After observing functional performance, the OT usually will find it necessary to assess the performance components that underlie motor control: muscle tone (normal/abnormal), the postural mechanism, muscle tone assessment/reflexes, sensation, and coordination" (p. 467, answer B). Answer C, evaluation of vital signs, endurance, and confusion, is associated with evaluation of cardiopulmonary function. Answer D, assessment of self-concept and self-awareness, is related to the psychological impact of trauma. Answer A, developmental factors, pertains to an individual's life experiences and how those experiences relate to coping with the musculoskeletal disorder. See Reference: Pedretti. (2013). Preston, L.A.: Evaluation of motor control.

23. (D) Role performance. Role performance (answer D) involves identifying, maintaining, and balancing functions one assumes or acquires in society. Changes in important roles may result in "feelings of anger, frustration, apprehension, confusion, boredom, and fear.... Occupational therapists help people to construct or reconstruct their roles when they have experienced a lack of engagement in desired roles or an unexpected/undesired loss or change in roles" (p. 164). This individual is having difficulty balancing the roles of worker and mother and is feeling stressed and conflicted. This stress may result in difficulty maintaining attention (answer B); however, the larger issue is related to role performance/identification. Evaluation by an OT could include assessment of parenting and assertiveness skills (answers A and C) to determine whether these are areas of need, and if so, interventions could be designed to address these areas to support successful role performance. However, these have not been identified as areas of need. See Reference: Schell, Gillen, & Scaffa. (2014). Matuska, K. & Barrett, K.: Patterns of occupation.

24. (D) Occupational Self-Assessment. The Occupational Self-Assessment is a "self-report measure...that identifies clients' problem areas in occupations, their competence in the occupation, and the level of importance they assign to them" (p. 853). It takes 10 to 20 minutes to administer, and goals can be set based on the results. It can also be used as an outcome measure. The Occupational Performance History Interview II (answer A) is a "semistructured interview focused on occupational adaptation in three areas: occupational identity, occupational competence, and impact of occupational behavior environment" (p. 852). It takes about an hour to complete, generates a narrative of the individual's life history, and allows the therapist to compare performance over time. The Role Checklist (answer B) takes approximately 15 minutes to complete and identifies roles in which the individual has participated in the past, currently participate in, or hopes to in the future. It does not provide a way to measure occupational performance. The Canadian Occupational Performance Measure (answer C) takes about 30 to 40 minutes to complete. It is a "semistructured interview in three areas: self-care, productivity, and leisure. Client scores their performance and satisfaction with identified occupational performance challenges" (p. 852). It is also useful for goal setting, intervention planning, and measuring outcomes, but takes longer to administer than the Occupational Self-Assessment. See Reference: Cara & MacRae. (2013). Hoppes, S., Bryce, H.R., & Peloquin, S.M.: Substance abuse and occupational therapy.

25. (D) Mental tracking. Mental tracking (answer D) is "the ability to simultaneously keep track of two or more stimuli, during ongoing activity," such as cooking and watching television at the same time. Sustained attention (answer A) is "the ability to consistently engage in an activity over time." Detecting and reacting (answer B) is "the ability to detect and react to gross changes in the environment such as a telephone ringing, a name being called, or a ball that is thrown" (p. 795). Shifting of attention (answer C) is "the ability to shift or alternate attention between tasks with different cognitive and or motor requirements" (p. 794). See Reference: Schell, Gillen, & Scaffa. (2014). Toglia, J.P., Golisz, K.M., & Goverover, Y.: Cognition, perception, and occupational performance.

26. (C) Home visit, during which OT will identify and encourage opportunities for fine motor practice within the family's preferred routines. Answer C is correct as it reflects use of "natural environments." "Ecocultural theory suggests that working within the culture of the family, and by extension within the natural environments of children, supports the development of meaningful and sustainable routines" (p. 53). Answer A is vague and does not help the parent identify toys most matched to child's specific fine motor skill needs. Answer B is incorrect as it describes an evaluation, rather than intervention approach. Answer D is incorrect as it is counter to the principles of Part C Early Intervention programs designed to support learning and development within the context of children's and families' everyday activities and routines. See Reference: Lane & Bundy, 2012. Morrison, C.D.: Early Intervention.

27. (C) Attention span and social interaction skills. Conduct disorders often involve aggression toward people or animals and destruction of property. The individual with conduct disorder "violates rules, age appropriate norms, or the rights of others, evidenced by aggression against people or animals, property destruction, lying or theft, or seriously violating rules. The symptoms cause impairment in job, school, or social life" (p. 432). When working with this population, OT typically addresses the areas of attention span, impulse control, age-appropriate social role performance, and social skills (answer C). Children with developmental delays typically require intervention for perceptual-motor skills (answer A). Multiple role performance (answer D) is more developmentally relevant to adulthood than it is to adolescence. Although leisure and vocational interests (answer B) may be relevant to the adolescent population, the issues of attention span and social interaction would be more significant for an individual with conduct disorder. See Reference: Cara & MacRae. (2013). Lambert, W.L. & Carley, E.: Mental health of adolescents.

28. (A) Demonstrates independence with precautions. Precautions following total hip replacement include no hip flexion past 90 degrees, no internal rotation, and no adduction past midline. Flexing the hip to 90 degrees (answer A) is acceptable. Individuals with poor short-term memory, impulsivity, or poor judgment may require verbal cuing (answers B and D) to remember hip precautions. A longer shoehorn (answer C) may be necessary for an individual who is not able to put on shoes safely with the shorter shoehorn. See Reference: Trombly. (2008). Maher, C. & Bear-Lehman, J.: Orthopaedic conditions.

29. (D) Transcutaneous electrical nerve stimulation. "TENS is an intervention technique that is thought to stimulate the afferent A nerve fibers in the high-frequency mode and stimulate the release of morphine-like neural hormones, the enkephalins, in the low-frequency mode. Its efficacy as an intervention for pain control is well documented in medical literature" (answer D, p. 1063). Answers A, B, and C may assist more with joint stiffness and cumulative trauma disorders, but not necessarily for the pain experienced with complex regional pain syndrome. See Reference: Pedretti. (2013). Kasch, M.C., & Walsh, J.M.: Hand and upper extremity injuries.

30. (C) Constructional play. Answer C is correct. Constructive play is described as "manipulation of objects to construct or to 'create' something" (p. 416). Sensorimotor play (answer A) is sensory exploration and is "characterized by practice and repetition" (p. 416). Pretend play (answer B) involves manipulating people and objects "to create situations; ...objects take on new purposes" (p. 417). Game play (answer D) involves the "acceptance of prearranged rules and adjustment to these rules" (p. 416). See Reference: Parham & Fazio. (2007). Lane, S. & Mistrett, S.: Facilitating play in early intervention.

31. (B) The child can usually handle routine daily functions in supervised home. Answer B is correct because "children with moderate ID have an IQ range of approximately 40 to 55.... [They] can usually handle routine daily functions and do unskilled or semiskilled work" (p. 169). This child would most likely be able to complete ADLs and live in a group home setting. Answer A describes a child with profound ID (IQ below 25), answer C describes a child with ID (IQ range 25 to 40), and answer D describes a child with mild ID (IQ 55 to 70). See Reference: Case-Smith & O'Brien. (2010). Rogers, S.L.: Common conditions that influence children's participation.

32. (C) Interpersonal skills. "The most common area of difficulty across all personality disorders, is in interpersonal skills" (p. 152). Specific personality disorder categories indicate that there is some variation among the types of relationships that are impacted. For example, authority relationships seem particularly dysfunctional in those with antisocial personality disorders, and difficulty in establishing relationships is linked to avoidant personality disorders. ADLs and IADLs (answers A and B) are often problems for individuals with mood and thought disorders. Sensorimotor deficits (answer D) are more likely to be observed in individuals with schizophrenia. See Reference: Brown & Stoffel. (2011). Urish, C.: Personality Disorders.

33. (C) Developmental dyspraxia. Answer C is correct. Dyspraxia is a "deficit in learning new motor skills, planning new motor actions, and generalizing motor plans" (p. 140). Children with dyspraxia often learn tasks such as jumping rope with great difficulty, effort, and considerable practice. However, when the task is altered, such as in this case by asking the child to skip backward, the child is unable to adapt the task for a long period. Answer A is incorrect because there is no description to suggest reflex activity affects posture and movement. Answer B is incorrect because the child coordinates the two sides of his body to skip rope forward (p. 142). Answer D also is incorrect because general incoordination would likely affect performance during both forward and backward rope jumping. See Reference: Hinojosa & Kramer. (2009). Schaaf, R.C., Schoen, S.A., Smith Roley, S., Lane, S.J., Koomar, J., & May-Benson, T.A.: A frame of reference for sensory integration.

34. (A) The student's and family's goals for the device use. Answer A is correct. "Prior to the AT assessment, the team needs to understand the consumer's goals related to roles and the performance of activities to support roles" (p. 516). Although answers B, C, and D do address other relevant factors regarding computer use, they need to be considered in relation to the overall goals the AT is intended to achieve. See Reference: Radomski & Trombly. (2008). Buning, M.E.: High-technology adaptations to compensate for disability.

35. (C) Training to acknowledge feeling and express emotions. Training individuals with eating disorders "to acknowledge feelings and express emotions [answer C] promotes the development of better coping strategies, decreases inner conflicts, and limits the disordered eating habits and their impact on occupational performance" (p. 135), which is particularly important to this population. Answers A, B, and D are also effective stress management techniques. Other techniques include healthy eating; assertiveness skills; changing attitudes; and balancing work, rest, and leisure. See Reference: Cottrell. (2000). Mueller, S. & Suto, M.: Starting a stress management program.

36. (A) The doorway width needs to be expanded to have a minimum clearance of 32 inches. According to the ADA accessibility guidelines, a doorway needs to have a minimum clear opening of 32 inches with the door open 90 degrees, measured between the face of the door and the opposite stop, answer A. In an environmental evaluation process, according to ADA guidelines, the doorway rather than the individual's wheelchair (answer B) needs to be adapted. See Reference: Pedretti. (2013). Kornblau, B.L.: American with Disabilities Act and related laws that promote participation in work, leisure, and activities of daily living.

37. (C) Work hardening. Work-hardening programs (answer C) are designed to include and/or simulate job-related tasks that gradually progress the individual to obtain the skills that meet the actual demands of a job. Continuing to perform a home exercise program and discontinuing OT services (answers A and D) would probably not enable the individual to return to the workforce after a 3-month absence. Home health OT (answer B) is only appropriate for individuals who are unable to leave their homes to attend outpatient occupational therapy. See Reference: Pedretti. (2013). Haruko Ha, D., Page, J.J., & Wietlisbach, C.M.: Work evaluation and work programs.

38. (C) Knitting a small hat for her newborn grandson. The "therapist's focus is on providing structure and meeting demands. Interventions should be concrete and tangible, and activities should be short term, simple, and success enhancing" (p. 238). In addition, decision-making should be kept to a minimum. All of the choices are client centered and could contribute to a sense of self-esteem and a positive outlook toward the future. However, the small knitted hat (answer C) is the simplest and most short-term activities listed. It will not require new learning and the outcome is very predictable, making it the most appropriate activity at this point in her hospitalization. All of the other activities could be appropriate as the patient's symptoms lessen and she gets closer to discharge. See Reference: Cara & MacRae. (2013). Cara, E.: Mood disorders.

39. (B) Seat child at the front of the bus and use earmuffs to dampen noise. Answer B is correct as it reduces sensory stimulation present on the bus ride. A child with low sensory threshold overresponds and is "overwhelmed by ordinary sensory input and reacts defensively to it, often with strong negative emotion and activation of the sympathetic nervous system" (p. 346). When seated at the front of the bus, the child will experience less jostling by peers, resulting in less tactile and visual stimulation. The earphones will reduce auditory overload. Answers A, C, and D are behavioral management techniques that do not take the child's hypersensitivity into account. See Reference: Case-Smith & O'Brien. (2010). Parham, D. & Mailloux, Z.: Sensory integration.

40. (C) Current services that focus on steps to achieve targeted long-range outcomes. Answer C, related to designing the current service plan, is correct. "Projecting outcomes...provides clarity about what might be appropriate or inappropriate for current intervention plans" (p. 143). Whereas IDEA requires transition planning be included in the IEP by the student's 16th birthday, earlier planning sets expectations and guides the team toward that vision. Answers A and B are incorrect, as targeting future outcomes does not ensure services are available or goals are achieved. Service duplication (answer D) is avoided by effective collaboration and consideration of services in the student's IEP and not through targeting future outcomes, so this response is incorrect. See Reference: Dunn. (2011). Dunn, W.: Developing intervention plans that reflect best practice.

41. (B) Catching and bursting soap bubbles. This activity involves visually tracking a slow-moving target and requires minimal fine motor precision to accomplish a successful "hit." Answers A, C, and D also require visual tracking and eye-hand coordination, but they involve faster-moving targets that require immediate, more precise movement. These activities can be used to promote advanced skills as the child's visual tracking ability improves. See Reference: Case-Smith & O'Brien. (2010). Exner, C.: Evaluation and intervention to develop hand skills.

42. (B) Looped handle scissors. To open a plastic muffin mix bag, the OT would most likely recommend that the homemaker use looped handle scissors (answer B). This device would be much safer than the use of an electric knife, answer C, while compensating for the limited grip strength. Answer A, using a hand-powered mixer, does not address how the homemaker will open the muffin bag, whereas answer D does not coincide with the client's desire to make muffins rather than prepared slice cookies. See Reference: Trombly. (2008). Fasoli, S.E.: Restoring competence for homemaker and parent roles.

43. (B) 1 foot of ramp for every inch of rise in height. According to the ADA Accessibility Guidelines for Buildings and Facilities, the maximum slope for a ramp should be 1:12. A foot of ramp for every inch of rise in height would be the maximum amount of incline to allow for independent and safe navigation by an individual using a wheelchair (answer B). "Slope is given as ratio of the height to the length. 1:12 means for every 12 inches along the base of the ramp, the height increases one inch. For a 1:12 maximum slope, at least one foot of ramp

length is needed for each inch of height" (p. 314). Answers A, C, and D would all make extremely short and steep ramps, which would be either unsuitable or unsafe for an individual independently entering or exiting a home. See Reference: Trombly. (2008). Rigby, P., Lowe, M., Letts, L., & Stewart, D.: Assessing environment: Home, community, and workplace access.

44. (A) Complete independence with self-care and modified independence with transfers. An individual with T4 paraplegia will have sufficient trunk balance, upper extremity strength, and coordination to complete self-care and transfers independently to moderate independently (answer A). Individuals with high cervical injuries are likely to be dependent in self-care and transfers (answer D). Individuals with low cervical and high thoracic injuries require assistance with transfers and some self-care (answers B and C). See Reference: Pedretti. (2013). Adler, C.: Spinal cord injury.

45. (B) Training in residual limb wrapping. "Shrinking and shaping the residual limb are necessary to form a tapered limb that will tolerate a snug-fitting socket. Compression using an elastic bandage, a tubular bandage, or a shrinker sock applied to the residual limb aids in the shrinking and shaping process" (p. 1163). Training in how to put on and take off the prosthesis (answer A), and activities to improve grasp and prehension (answer C), come later (postacutely) in the intervention process when the prosthesis has been selected, prescribed, and fitted. Training to resume vocational activities (answer D) also would normally occur later in rehabilitation process after the patient has mastered the basics of prosthetic use. See Reference: Pedreitti, 2013. Keenan, D.D. & Glover, J.S.: Amputations and prosthetics.

46. (D) Finishing a prefabricated wood birdhouse from a kit. "An individual who is manic rarely completes projects; attention is fragmented.... [H]eightened activity, difficulty concentrating and attending to tasks, distractibility, and intrusiveness often make individuals experiencing a manic episode candidates for individual treatment with engagement in simple concrete tasks or movement" (p. 231). "Interventions should be concrete and tangible, and activities should be short term, simple and success enhancing" (p. 238). A person experiencing a manic episode is likely to exhibit high energy levels, short attention span, poor frustration tolerance, difficulty delaying gratification, and difficulty making decisions. Finishing a prefabricated wood birdhouse (answer D) would be the most appropriate activity because it is a short-term, concrete, predictable activity with a few steps that provides high likelihood of success. It also can be carried with the person if he or she needs to get up and move around during the activity. A needlepoint project (answer A) would require too much attention to detail for guaranteed success. Making a clay object (answer B) uses an unpredictable material and requires creative decisions, both of which are qualities that should be avoided. Watercolor painting (answer C) would not be a good choice because it is an unfocused activity involving artistic skill performance that could lead to frustration. See Reference: Cara & MacRae. (2013). Cara, E.: Mood disorders.

47. (D) Ask whether the school district has addressed his coordination difficulties and if not, discuss further whether the parent wishes to raise this issue with the child's teacher. Answer D is correct, as the OT raises the issues and provides the opportunity for the parent to learn about the OT's concerns and make decisions about the next steps. This response encourages further communication that is fundamental in best practice approaches (p. 86). Answers A, B, and C are incorrect as they do not respect the collaborative team process embraced in contemporary occupational therapy. Clinic-based OT programs and school-based OT services address different needs presented by families and their children. As they have "different purposes,...there is ample possibility for either conflict or fractionation of services.... Therapists who work with the same children and families from different agencies need to prioritize the families' needs and find ways to communicate in a collaborative way" (p. 85). See Reference: Dunn. (2011). Dunn, W.: Structure of best practice programs.

48. (B) have the individual work at the keyboard for 5 minutes. Increasing the duration the individual is able to tolerate working on the computer is the most appropriate way to progress this individual (answer B). A heavier mouth stick (answer A) would make the task more difficult than it already is and yield no benefit. An individual with C4 tetraplegia would not have the potential to use a typing device that inserts into a wrist support (answer C). Teaching the individual how to correctly instruct a caregiver in use of the keyboard (answer D) would be downgrading the activity. See Reference: Trombly. (2008). Atkins, M.S.: Spinal cord injury.

49. (A) Discuss issues related to self-concept with the individual. This individual has demonstrated competence in using the cane, but does not seem to desire to use it (answer A). Her response most likely indicates her discomfort with the cane that is related to how it looks, or, more likely, how it makes her look. The image of a woman with a cane may not be consistent with her self-concept. Discussion about how she feels about using the cane may

enable the individual to integrate it more successfully into her self-concept. "People who acquire disability share the common experience of feelings of shame and inferiority, along with avoidance of being identified as a person with a disability" (p. 85). Memory and time management (answers B, C, and D) appear to be intact, as indicated by her ability to arrive for therapy on time each day. See Reference: Pedretti. (2013). Burnett, S.E.: Personal and social contexts of disability: Implications for occupational therapists.

50. (C) Prevent deformity. Answer C is correct; hand orthoses are provided for a child with juvenile rheumatoid arthritis to prevent deformity (p. 154). Hypertonus (answer A) is not a characteristic of this condition. Owing to the active nature of the child's condition, increasing range of motion (answer B) may be contraindicated. The correction of deformity (answer D) also may be contraindicated with this child owing to the active nature of the disease. See Reference: Case-Smith & O'Brien. (2010). Rogers, S.L.: Common conditions that influence children's participation.

51. (D) Lock the brakes. Brakes should be locked first to stabilize the wheelchair. Answers A, B, and C involve movements that could cause loss of balance or wheelchair movement unless the brakes are locked. See Reference: Pedretti. (2013). Bolding, D., Adler, C., Tipton-Burton, M., Verran, A., & Lillie, S.M.: Mobility.

52. (C) Active participation and self-direction in activities matched to identified needs. Answer C is correct. Intervention based on Ayres Sensory Integration™ includes unique guiding principles. Key features include an emphasis on the child's inner drive and active participation. "Self-direction on the part of the child is encouraged because therapeutic gains are maximized if the child is fully invested as an active participant.... Because the brain responds differently when the child is actively involved in a task rather than merely receiving passive stimulation, it is considered optimal for a child to be an active participant" (p. 358). Answers A, B, and D are incorrect, as they create an intervention context that is counter to essential characteristics of Ayres Sensory Integration™. See Reference: Case-Smith & O'Brien. (2010). Parham, D. & Mailloux, Z.: Sensory integration.

53. (C) Eat six small meals a day. An individual with ALS who becomes fatigued eating three full meals a day should attempt eating six smaller meals a day before resorting to tube feedings or pureed diets (answers A and D). Eating regular food is usually more enjoyable, and therefore is likely to enhance the quality of life. An upright position is optimal when feeding individuals with dysphagia. A semireclined position (answer B) can make swallowing more difficult or dangerous. See Reference: Pedretti. (2013). Schultz-Krohn, W., Foti, D., & Glogoski, C.: Degenerative diseases of the central nervous system.

54. (B) Exercise and limited work task simulation. "Work conditioning programs emphasize physical conditioning, which addresses issues of strength, endurance, flexibility, motor control, and cardiopulmonary function. They...use exercise, aerobic conditioning, education and limited work task simulation.... Work conditioning programs...are usually half-day programs" (p. 687). Nonspecific job-simulated work tasks such as carrying, pushing, and pulling are appropriate examples of work conditioning that will improve skills needed for a variety of physical labor jobs and also increase physical endurance. Job-specific work tasks (answer C) are tasks that relate to developing skills to prepare for a determined job and are representative of a work-hardening program. Performing adapted work activities (answer A) is an example of work hardening that is implemented after the clients achieve work-conditioning goals. On-the-job training (answer D) would also occur after a work conditioning program has been completed. See Reference: Schell, Gillen, & Scaffa. (2014). King, P.M. & Olson, D.L.: Work.

55. (D) To eliminate late arrival to work. "Learning effective time management techniques is a useful strategy for people with anxiety disorders.... For example the occupational therapist can teach how to prioritize tasks and break them down into manageable and attainable steps" (p. 291). The focus of time management training is to provide individuals with strategies in order to manage their time appropriately so that they are able to live successful and productive lives. In this case, time management training would train the individual in developing strategies in order to consistently show up to work on time. Answers A, B, and C are ways of coping with being late, not strategies for the time management goal of being on time. See Reference: Cara & MacRae. (2013). Cara, E.: Anxiety disorders.

56. (B) Increase the number of towels from 10 to 20. Endurance is improved by increasing the number of repetitions so the muscle has to work over a longer period of time. Placing towels on a higher shelf (answer A) would help to increase range of motion. Placing towels on a lower shelf (answer C) decreases the difficulty of the activity and does not lengthen the period of time needed to improve endurance by providing more repetitions. The arm could be strengthened by adding a 1-pound weight (answer D), but that would not increase the repetitions needed to improve endurance. See Reference:

Pedretti. (2013). Phillips Killingsworth, A., Pedretti Williams, L., & Pendleton McHugh, H.: Evaluation of muscle strength.

57. (D) A combination of service delivery models so that the OT can address student, teacher, and task needs. Answer D is correct. As the aim of pediatric OT services is to "increase the child's participation in important childhood occupations,... [therapists] often choose multiple ways of delivering services for any one child" (p. 605). Service delivery in the schools relies on multiple models to meet students' needs across activities and routines. For example, an OT may work together with the student in the classroom during seat work, work with the teacher to modify ways that math worksheets are set so that the student receives needed visual cues and supports, and co-lead groups with the teacher during art class. Answers A, B, and C are incorrect as they each offer only one service delivery model, therefore limiting the OT's ability to support the student in various ways, according to different needs that arise across instructional settings. See Reference: Lane & Bundy. (2012). Bundy, A.: Reflections of pediatric practice.

58. (B) perform desired activities in a simplified manner to conserve energy. One method used to extend an individual's occupational performance as Parkinson's disease progresses is to introduce task simplification. This allows conservation of energy, which can then be expended on desired activities (answer B). In a person with long-standing Parkinson's disease, encouragement to "work through" fatigue (answer A) would further deplete available energy. Using pursed-lips breathing is recommended for individuals with pulmonary diagnoses such as COPD (answer C). Recommendations to decrease activity level as much as possible (answer D) also would be detrimental to maintaining occupational performance levels. See Reference: Pedretti. (2013). Schultz-Krohn, W., Foti, D., & Glogoski, C.: Degenerative diseases of the central nervous system.

59. (C) Provide small group occupation-based activities that encourage exploration and interaction. Answer C is correct, as recommended approaches point out that "(e)ven when the therapist wants to teach a specific task...after initial practice of the skill, the opportunity to use the skill by exploring and playing will enhance skill development" (p. 338). "Children can learn and immediately apply strategies for emotional regulation as well as specific social skills to activity participation with a peer group. Over time, regular positive peer interaction within the context of shared occupation will support the development of friendship. Activity groups operate under the premise that children are intrinsically interested in play and peer acceptance" (p. 335). It is unlikely that the child will initiate and develop social interaction in an environment that inhibits independence, interaction, and exploration (answers A and D). Answer B, intervention provided in the therapist-student dyad, is incorrect as explained above. See Reference: Hinojosa & Kramer. (2009). Olson, L.J.: A frame of reference to enhance social participation.

60. (D) Goal Attainment Scaling. Answer D is correct. Goal Attainment Scaling "can be effective for both developing and measuring progress toward social skills goals" (p. 336). These can be highly individualized and used systematically to measure progress over time. Narrative notes (answer B) represent the therapist's report of activities and outcomes and are not a systematic measurement approach. Photographs (answer C) may contribute to measuring changes; however, because they represent a moment in time, the quality and extent of students' social interaction is not captured. The School Function Assessment (answer A) does include items that measure aspects of social function; however, it is not a comprehensive assessment, and it may not include items that reflect priority areas for each student. See Reference: Kuhanek & Watling. (2010). Hilton, C.L.: Social skills for children with an autism spectrum disorder.

61. (A) Gentle, nonresistive activities. The initial phase of treatment for the individual with Guillain-Barré acute syndrome includes PROM and use of orthosis, and positioning to protect weak muscles and prevent contractures. This should be followed by gentle, nonresistive activities and light ADL, as tolerated. Resistive exercises and activities (answers B and D) should be implemented after strength begins to improve. Activities within later treatment sessions should alternate between gross and fine motor (unlike answer C) and resistive and nonresistive types to avoid fatigue. See Reference: Pedretti. (2013). Southam, M., Schmidt, A., & George, A.H.: Disorders of the motor unit.

62. (A) Arrhythmic and unexpected. Answer A is correct. "For children with low arousal in the vestibular system, the therapist would use fast, irregular, and rotational movement" (p. 161). Answer B is incorrect because, although arrhythmic input is excitatory, slow sensory input is inhibitory. Sustained and slow sensory input (answer C) is inhibitory, not facilitatory. Answer D is incorrect because, although facilitatory input is unexpected, rhythmic input is inhibitory. Sensory integration treatment is complex and highly individualized and must be monitored carefully to observe the effects of sensory input of varying types on the individual. See Reference: Hinojosa & Kramer. (2009). Schaaf, R.C., Schoen, S.A., Smith Roley, S., Lane, S.J., Koomar, J., & May-Benson, T.A.: A frame of reference for sensory integration.

63. (B) Utilization of foot supports. Adequate foot support (answer B) is correct. This is the practitioner's first concern so that the child feels secure and "when the feet rest firmly on the floor, the abdominal muscles that aid in defecation effectively fulfill their function." (p. 500). Answer A is incorrect because management of fasteners requires hand skills that depend on stable posture and balance. Answer C is incorrect because provision of a seat belt may not be necessary if foot support (or back support) is provided. Answer D is incorrect because climbing onto the toilet independently may be developed later (as occurs with normal developmental progression). See Reference: Case-Smith & O'Brien. (2010). Shepherd, J.: Activities of daily living.

64. (C) Propose a modified goal that still meets the parent's needs. Developing an alternate goal that meets the family's needs (answer C) is correct. In family-centered intervention, "families deserve to have control and make choices regarding the care their child receives" (p. 682). Proposing a modified goal of functional mobility with an adaptive mobility device would best address both the parent's need for decreased carrying and the child's need to improve functional mobility within the environment. Agreeing to work on a goal that is likely unachievable in the near future (answer A) would not meet the child's needs for developmentally appropriate intervention. Answer B, offering an alternative goal, and Answer D, encouraging the child to help set goals, are not responsive to the concerns identified by the family. See Reference: Case-Smith & O'Brien. (2010). Myers, C.T., Stephens, L., & Tauber, S.: Early intervention.

65. (C) fitting of compression garments. Lymphedema results in swelling that can be painful and stigmatizing. Treatment begins with the fitting of a "compression garment [answer C] or wrap" (p. 1225). Manual lymphatic therapy/massage can also help to lessen the swelling. Change of dominance (answer A) is not usually necessary for individuals with lymphedema. Neither isometric exercise (answer B) nor heat modalities (answer D) would be useful. See Reference: Pedretti. (2013). Burkhardt, A. & Schultz-Krohn, W.: Oncology.

66. (B) Canadian Occupational Performance Measure (COPM). The Canadian Occupational Performance Measure (answer B) allows the OT to gather information concerning the teen's perception about the importance of various daily occupations, together with her rating of satisfaction with current levels of performance. Following burn injury, the "child is an invaluable source of information" (p. 576). The COPM also establishes a baseline that can be referenced over time to contribute to the plan to document intervention outcomes. Answer A is incorrect, as this information is not a priority to help the OT plan intervention early in the course of burn recovery. Answers C and D suggest other potential assessments, yet these are incorrect as neither provides important information for planning at this stage in the rehabilitation process. See Reference: Lane & Bundy. (2012). Tomcheck, S. & Aberli, L.: Multitraumatic injuries.

67. (B) Identifying thoughts and beliefs that contribute to negative feelings. Guided self-assessment (answer B) of each individual's stressors and stress reactions is the first step in a stress management program. The goal of CBT for this population is on "helping a client become aware of his/her thought process to identify and change negative beliefs, behaviors, and emotions to become more functional by managing activity levels, stress, and symptoms" (p. 1133). Time management techniques (answer A), which help individuals schedule, prioritize, and develop appropriate attitudes about daily task requirements, may comprise one of the following sessions. Aerobic exercise (answer C) is an appropriate method for reducing stress in individuals with CFS but care should be taken in designing a program that will not lead to overexertion. Progressive relaxation exercises (answer D) involve systematic tensing and relaxing of muscles and are not appropriate for individuals with hypertension, cardiac disease, upper motor neuron lesions, or spasticity. See Reference: Schell, Gillen, & Scaffa. (2014). Vaughn, P.: Appendix I: Common conditions, resources, and evidence.

68. (A) Develop healthy eating behaviors and meal preparation skills. "Occupational therapists can enable individuals with eating disorders to eat, participate in adaptive activity, communicate, and manage stress effectively.... The literature suggests that enabling clients to eat effectively is essential" (pp. 135–136). The overarching goals of healthy eating and meal preparation (answer A) are essential to the health and safety of individuals (p. 135). Menu planning and awareness of portion size (answer C) along with food shopping, cooking, and eating at a normal speed are all aspects of healthy eating and meal preparation. Although academic performance can be affected (answer B), it is of secondary importance because it does not result in the same level of risk to the individual as dangerous eating behaviors. "Communication and assertion training [answer D] is widely cited as helpful" (p 135), but is, again, secondary to healthy eating. See Reference: Brown & Stoffel. (2011). Lock, L.C. & Pepin, G.: Eating disorders.

69. (B) A second generation EADL device with speakerphone. "Second generation EADL (Electronic Aids to Daily Living) systems [answer B] use various remote control technologies to remotely switch power to electrical devices in the environment. These strategies include the use of ultrasonic pulses (e.g., TASH Ultra 4), infrared light (e.g., infrared remote control), and electrical signals propagated through the electrical circuitry of the home (e.g., X-10). All these switching technologies remain in use, and some are used for much more elaborate control systems" (p. 431). "Because the target consumers for an EADL will often have severe restrictions in mobility, the manufacturers of many of these systems believe that a significant portion of the customer's day will be spent in bed and thus include some sort of control system for standard hospital beds.... Many EADL systems include a speakerphone, which will allow the user to originate and answer telephone calls by using the electronics of the EADL as the telephone" (p. 433). The simplest EADL (answer A) does allow independence in operating appliances, lights, and so on through the use of switches or voice control, but would not be a necessity for safety. A remote control power door opener that would allow a caretaker to enter would be useless if the individual is unable to call for assistance. An electric page turner (answer D) is useless without the ability to call for someone to position or replace reading material. See Reference: Pedretti. (2013). Anson, D.: Assistive technology.

70. (A) Model imagination, and use playful facial expressions and voice. Answer A, modeling playful behavior, expressions, and voice, is correct. Strategies to "create a playful atmosphere [suggest the OT]...express a playful attitude through speech, body language, and facial expressions...[and] must know how to play and model play for the child" (p. 550). Asking the child to demonstrate favorite play (answer B) and using familiar toys (answer C) may provide insight into the child's current play, yet these approaches do not help to expand the child's current play behavior to become more playful. Answer D, leather tooling, requires a structure and focus on sequential steps and these generally do not promote imagination, pleasure, and playfulness. See Reference: Case-Smith & O'Brien. (2010). Knox, S.H.: Play.

71. (B) Encourage problem-solving about how she will respond when the baby is fussy during feeding and diaper changes. Answer B, helping the parent problem-solve, is correct. OTs should "focus on helping parents with intellectual or mental health problems build problem-solving skills. Everyday care for children requires constant problem-solving" (p. 135). Answers A and D do not include problem-solving by the parent and "[w]hen others direct parents, they become more dependent" (p. 135). Answer C is incorrect, as there is no evidence in this question that the parent needs additional support for her own caretaking. See Reference: Case-Smith & O'Brien. (2010). Jaffe, L., Humphry, R., & Case-Smith, J: Working with families.

72. (B) Kitchen safety. Short-term memory loss is one of the earliest symptoms of Alzheimer's disease. This individual would demonstrate moderate memory loss, decreased concentration, and difficulty with problem-solving. Intervention would focus on analyzing and adapting "meaningful leisure, home management, and other productive activities to allow the client to safely participate and exert initiation, independence, and control" (p. 926). Because her husband is still working, this individual may want to continue preparing meals. Kitchen safety issues (answer B), such as remembering to turn off the stove, would be the most important of the options listed to evaluate. The awareness of declining abilities may be very frustrating for some individuals, leading to anger, social withdrawal, and depression. There may be a need for anger management strategies (answer C), but this issue is a secondary concern to safety. Difficulty with motor abilities develop as the disease progresses, and the ability to chew and swallow (answer A) may need to be evaluated in the later stages. Severe memory loss (answer D), inability to process information, and loss of communication skills would also develop in the later stages of the disease. See Reference: Pedretti. (2013). Schultz-Krohn, W. et al: Degenerative diseases of the central nervous system.

73. (A) Short-term memory. The earliest symptoms of Alzheimer disease involve "mild memory deficits [answer A] particularly short-term memory (forgetting appointments, recent conversations, dates)" (p. 1099). The onset of most dementias is slow and progressive. Sensorimotor abilities used in functional activities, such as dressing (answer D), tend to follow. Motor skills (answer B) become involved in the later stages, and changes can be seen in tone, reaction time, movement time, and gait. Superficial social abilities (answer C) are often preserved until the last stages of dementia and may often hide the earlier cognitive changes. See Reference: Schell, Gillen, & Scaffa. (2014). Appendix 1: Common conditions, resources, and evidence.

74. (B) Student's ability to access and participate in the curriculum. Answer B is correct. Promoting the student's participation in activities and routines within the curriculum so he/she is able to benefit from education is a priority for OTs working in the education system. School-based OTs work together with other team members to develop "measurable annual goals (both academic and functional) designed to enable the student to have access to and make progress in the general education curriculum

and meet the child's other education needs that result from the child's disability." (p. 724). The Individualized Education Program (IEP) process is designed to incorporate contribution from all team members (p. 723). One person's perspective is not intended to drive the process so Answers A and C are incorrect. The IEP process includes steps to learn about the teacher's perspective and the family's priorities for their child and these become part of the data the team uses in its decision-making. Answer D is incorrect as the difficulties established in the occupational therapy evaluation are not the only basis for developing the student's IEP goals. See Reference: Case-Smith & O'Brien. (2010). Bazyk, S. & Case-Smith, J.: School-based occupational therapy.

75. (C) Baking cookies following a recipe. Baking cookies (answer C) is a well-delineated meal preparation activity that provides structure with a specific sequence of tasks. "Planning involves the ability to efficiently organize the steps or elements of a behavior or activity and includes the ability to look ahead, anticipate consequences, weigh and make choices, conceive of alternatives, sustain attention, and sequence the activity" (p. 804). The above skills will all be addressed when following a recipe in order to make a batch of cookies. Setting a table or preparing a shopping list (answers A and D) do not necessarily require sequencing of tasks. Planning a meal (answer B) involves a great deal of organizational ability, and would not be an appropriate choice for an initial activity to address goals relating to sequencing tasks. See Reference: Schell, Gillen, & Scaffa. (2014). Toglia, J.P., Golisz, K.M., & Goverover, Y.: Cognition, perception, and occupational performance.

76. (B) Learning proper body mechanics. Learning proper body mechanics, answer B (along with achieving a good fitness level), is one of the first steps to reducing the risk of reinjury in a work program. Answer C, work hardening, is appropriate to implement after the physical demands of the job's specific tasks are achieved. Answer D, engaging in vocational counseling, is appropriate after it is determined that a client cannot return to the same job or employer. Answer A, a prework screening, is typically completed by the practitioner before the employer offers the new employee a job. See Reference: Pedretti. (2013). Haruko Ha, D., Page, J.J., & Wietlisbach, C.M.: Work evaluation and work programs.

77. (B) Initiate one request to one other group member for sharing group materials within a 1-week period. Occupational therapists may "downgrade the demands so that the task can be achieved despite a client's limitations" (p. 323). Reducing the number of requests and the variety or number of individuals with whom the client is expected to interact (answer B) is the best way to simplify the initial goal, giving the client an opportunity to master the task at a lower level before progressing him/her. Extending the amount of time to accomplish the goal (answer A) does not make the goal easier to achieve. Increasing the number of individuals (answer C), and subsequently the number of requests, also makes the goal more difficult to achieve. Changing interactions to those with the group leader (answer D) moves the goal away from the original problem area of peer social conversation to authority conversations. See Reference: Schell, Gillen, & Scaffa. (2014). Gillen, G.: Occupational therapy interventions for individuals.

78. (A) OT joins group on playground, facilitating child's play and including other children. The correct response is answer A. Using the natural setting enables the OT to observe the child's typical behavior as well as the supports and challenges that characterize the recess period. In working with children with autism, "adults in the child's environment have a critical role...in facilitating play as partners who are able to shape or scaffold the play of children with autism" (p. 499). Additionally, research has suggested that "(p)eers...support the play of children with ASD on the playground, with adequate training and supervision" (p. 499). Answer B does not represent characteristics in the typical recess period and it does not support the child to generalize behaviors learned in this isolated experience. Answer C is not appropriate as a primary approach to address the need identified in the question; however, ballet may be something the parent and child have interest in pursuing outside of school. Answer D is incorrect, as there are no individualized supports included to adapt the context, instructions, or supports in the physical education class and if the existing conditions were sufficient to support her performance, one can expect the child would already participate in these activities. See Reference: Lane & Bundy. (2012). Rodger, S. & Ziviani, S.: Autism spectrum disorders.

79. (C) Backward chaining. Backward chaining (answer C) is correct. In this method, the OT completes all of the steps of a task except the last one. As the child becomes competent, the OT completes all but the last two steps, and so on, until the child is able to perform the entire activity. This method "is particularly helpful for children with a low frustration tolerance or poor self-esteem because it gives immediate success" (p. 486). Physical guidance (answer A) requires the least amount of cognitive ability and provides the child the opportunity to learn through a sensory motor experience. Verbal cues (answer B) may be perceived as intrusive and critical by children with low self-esteem. Forward chaining (answer D) begins with the child completing the first step and the practitioner completing the rest. When competent, the child progressively takes on more of the steps. This method is "helpful for children who have difficulty with sequencing and generalizing skills" (p. 486). See Reference: Case-Smith & O'Brien. (2010). Shepherd, J.: Activities of daily living.

80. (B) Measuring ingredients for a recipe while there is music playing. The client demonstrated difficulty in attending to the activity because the presence of other environmental stimuli was distracting. This suggests a deficit in selective attention. "Selective attention occurs when an individual concentrates on one set of stimuli while ignoring competing stimuli, as when the cook ignores the noise from the television while measuring or counting ingredients" (p. 262). Answer B, measuring ingredients for a recipe while there is music playing, is correct because it would provide the needed practice in concentrating on one set of stimuli while ignoring competing stimuli to improve selective attention. Playing a repetitive card game (answer A) provides practice in maintaining sustained attention. Referring to a catalog while filling out a catalog form (answer C) would require the person to alternate attention from the catalog to the form. Playing a game in which the person must walk and bounce a ball simultaneously (answer D) provides practice in dividing attention between to two activities at the same time. See Reference: Trombly. (2008). Radomski, M.V.: Assessing abilities and capacities: Cognition.

81. (D) Complex rotation. Complex rotation (answer D) is correct. This skill "involves the rotation of an object 180° to 360° once or repetitively" (p. 285). Answers A, B, and C are incorrect. Finger-to-palm translation is described as "grasping the object with the pads of the fingers and thumb and moving it into the palm.... Palm-to-finger translation is the reverse.... Shift involves linear movement of an object on the finger surface to allow for repositioning of the object on the pads of the fingers.... The object is usually held solely on the radial side of the hand" (p. 284). See Reference: Case-Smith & O'Brien. (2010). Exner, C.: Evaluation and intervention to develop hand skills.

82. (B) Activities focused on time and stress management skills as well as practice of job-seeking strategies. There are several aspects and phases to vocational programming but answer B, activities focused on time and stress management skills, are relevant activities for building job hunting skills at the level of the community mental health setting. "Skills training can include finding and keeping a job, problem solving, and managing work-related social interactions..... Service options can include job-seeking skills groups, time management and stress management skills training" (pp. 816, 824). Answer A, self-assessment of work habits and personality characteristics, is a prevocational evaluation method used to help determine the individual's potential for work readiness rather than develop skills. Answer C, educating the work supervisors about the individual's needs and offering environmental modifications to maximize performance, might occur after employment is obtained. Expressive activities, such as making a collage with pictures of different types of jobs, answer D, provides opportunities for exploration of ideas about job possibilities, but would not directly develop job seeking skills. See Reference: Cara & MacRae. (2013). Auerbach, E.: Vocational programming.

83. (D) Just before discharge. "An intensive interdisciplinary rehabilitation program is typically implemented during the recovery phase as the client begins to regain physical movement.... As the client's strength increases, activities promoting more resistance can be incorporated into the intervention program. Adaptive equipment...are typically necessary during this phase" (p. 988). Equipment should be ordered just before discharge to accurately determine the individual's needs (answer D). Equipment ordered during the first week of therapy, or as soon as approved (answers B and C), may not be necessary at the time the individual is discharged. Although collaborating with the patient and family on decisions about ordering equipment is essential, acceptance of the disability (answer A) may not necessarily correspond with the appropriate time for ordering equipment. See Reference: Pedretti. (2013). Southam, M., Schmidt, A., & George, A.H.: Disorders of the motor unit.

84. (C) Use of orthosis to provide support until wrist strength returns. "Chemotherapy-induced neuropathy usually causes wristdrop and footdrop, which are transient" (p. 1219). Because the condition is temporary, positioning (answer C) the wrist in a functional position is the best approach. Sensory reeducation (answer B) and change of dominance training (answer D) would be unnecessary for a temporary condition. Wristdrop is a result of radial nerve involvement, which would not affect the muscles of the hand needed for pinching and grasping (answer A). See Reference: Pedretti. (2013). Burkhardt, A. & Schultz-Krohn, W.: Oncology.

85. (D) Directive. "The directive group [answer D]...meets the needs of the most severely and acutely mentally ill and most minimally functioning patients.... The environment is actively structured in form, organization, and leadership to assure maximum participation. The directive group format is a consistent one involving orientation, introduction, a warm-up, selected activities, and a wrapup" (p. 694). Activity groups (answer A) require a higher level of

task behavior and ability to engage in occupation to enable skill development. Psychoeducation groups (answer B), which are based on cognitive-behavioral theory and focus on teaching information and techniques, require a level of learning capacity that may be impaired during acute mental illness. Neurodevelopmental groups (answer D) use gross motor activity and sensory stimulation techniques to enhance sensory integration in persons with long histories of chronic schizophrenia. See Reference: Cara & MacRae. (2013). Cara, E.: Groups.

86. (B) Ability to grade movement. Grading of movement (answer B) best addresses the child's difficulty. "Children with poorly graded movements lack the ability to use the middle ranges of movement effectively; instead, during attempts at hand use they hold one or more joins in a locked position of full flexion or full extension" (p. 291). Answer A is incorrect because this goal would be appropriate for a child who cannot break up a flexion or extension pattern during a movement. Answer C is incorrect because this goal is appropriate for a child who has difficulty with an arm or hand movement being too fast or too slow (graded movements are also too fast). Answer D is also incorrect because this goal is appropriate for a child who has difficulty bringing both arms together using them effectively in everyday activities. See Reference: Case-Smith & O'Brien. (2010). Exner, C.: Evaluation and intervention to develop hand skills.

87. (D) Swan neck deformity. A swan neck deformity (answer D) is typically characterized by PIP joint hyperextension and DIP joint flexion. Answer A, a boutonniere deformity, is characterized by PIP joint flexion and DIP joint hyperextension. Answer C is related to a deformity present at birth, and answer B, mallet deformity, is characterized by DIP joint flexion and loss of active extension. See Reference: Pedretti. (2013). Deshaies, L.: Arthritis.

88. (B) Identify and trial several different strategies, such as various toothpaste flavors, use of electric toothbrush, pictures to show steps. Answer B is correct. "Self-care can be challenging for children with ASD due to sensory, motor, and cognitive issues; however, these children can learn to become independent with the assistance of visual schedules, skills acquisition and learning techniques, and modifying the tasks and environment to support their performance" (p. 500). With this understanding, a systematic trial and assessment of specific strategies is the best option. Answer A is inappropriate as it does not provide the parent with support for current concerns. Answers C and D are incorrect as they do not establish clear expectations for desired behavior, nor do they represent the consistency that benefits many students with autism. See Reference: Lane & Bundy. (2012). Rodger, S. & Ziviani, S.: Autism spectrum disorders.

89. (A) hook and loop closures on front-opening clothing. Parkinson's disease has five stages. In stage 1, a resting tremor appears and symptoms are mild and unilateral. In stage 2, problems develop with trunk mobility and postural reflexes, and symptoms are bilateral. Stage 3 results in mild-moderate functional disability with postural instability. Difficulty with manipulation and dexterity emerges in stage 4, as disability increases. Individuals in stage 5 are confined to a wheelchair or bed. Hook and loop closures on front-opening clothing (answer A) would require the least amount of dexterity, which becomes increasingly difficult for individuals in stage 4. Large buttons on front-opening clothing (answer B) might be easier than smaller buttons, but would still require more manipulation than Velcro closures. Clothing slipped on over the head with no fasteners (answer C) would eliminate the need for dexterity, but having to raise the arms would be problematic because of the rigidity and stiffness of the limbs that typically accompanies Parkinson's disease. Although clothing that stretches freely is easier to put on than tightly constructed clothing, the need to tie the closures in the back of the garment (answer D) would be difficult for a person with upper extremity rigidity. See Reference: Trombly. (2008). Forwell, S.J., Copperman, L.F., & Hugos, L.: Neurogenerative diseases.

90. (C) marking the end of each step with high-contrast tape. Difficulty in seeing contrast and color are two forms of decreased visual acuity that cannot be addressed by corrective lenses. "Changing the background color to contrast with an object can help the client see objects more clearly.... Application of this step can be as simple as using a black cup for milk and a white cup for coffee" (p. 605). Two effective environmental adaptations to these deficits are increasing background contrast and illumination. Using tape or paint to make the edge of each step contrast sharply with the rest of the step is an inexpensive way to adapt the environment. Installing a stair glide or handrails (answers A and B) are more costly adaptations that do not address the problems of decreased visual acuity. Instructing the patient to take only one step at a time (answer D) may cause the individual to be unnecessarily slow, and does not address the problems of decreased visual acuity. See Reference: Pedretti. (2013). Warren, M.: Evaluation and treatment of visual deficits following brain injury.

91. (A) Large key ring. Answer A is correct. A large key ring attached to the zipper pull is an adaptation to enable a child with limited grasp to hold and move the zipper (p. 505). Answer B, oversized fasteners, would not address the child's need to become independent in zipping, unless all of the zippers were removed from the child's pants and replaced with fasteners. Colored zippers, answer C, would be most helpful for a child with visual discrimination problems. Hook and loop fasteners, answer D, are something the OT may recommend if the more convenient and less expensive key ring adaptation does not assist the child in meeting his goals. See Reference: Case-Smith & O'Brien. (2010). Shepherd, J.: Activities of daily living.

92. (A) Remedial treatment, such as rubbing or stroking the involved extremity. When sensation begins to return, it is appropriate to initiate remedial activities for sensory retraining. Stimulating the involved extremity by rubbing or stroking (to provide tactile input) or through weight-bearing activities (to provide proprioceptive input) are examples of remedial activities. Compensatory activities, which are essential for individuals with decreased or absent sensation, would have been part of the original treatment plan. Whereas B, C, and D are interventions to protect the client from further injury, the question implies a neuro-educational approach and how the OT should initiate return of the affected extremity. Answers B, C, and D are all examples of compensatory strategies. See Reference: Pedretti. (2013). Cooper, C. & Canyock, D.J.: Evaluation of sensation and intervention for sensory dysfunction.

93. (D) Ask the individual if there are cultural guidelines for how to dress for exercise group. Munoz describes several components necessary for effective culturally responsive interaction skills. For example, in the area of communication, it is important to identify whether an individual needs an interpreter. In the area of cultural sanctions and restrictions, it is important to identify issues related to gender, touch, and expression of emotions, and to obtain information from the individual concerning their thoughts and feelings about these areas. "The goal is to solicit detailed information in a nonthreatening manner and with an intentional culturally relevant perspective" (p. 447). Competence in this area could be demonstrated by asking the individual if there are guidelines for how women can dress for exercise group in her culture (answer D). Singling her out to comment on her clothing (answer A) could be embarrassing to her. Making suggestions about how to dress (answers B and C) without first obtaining culturally relevant information is not a culturally sensitive approach. See Reference: Brown & Stoffel. (2011). Munoz, J.P.: Mental health practice in a multicultural context.

94. (C) Discuss the symbolism of how we all experience breaking and healing. Individuals with eating disorders share several common characteristics: "1. overvaluation of weight, shape and their control; 2. mood intolerance; 3. core low self-esteem; 4. perfectionism; 5. interpersonal problems" (p. 130). OT intervention, utilizing craft activities in particular, can promote self-esteem, self-confidence, and tolerance of imperfection. The OT must be supportive and empathetic and help the individual to allow herself to make mistakes (answer C), and repairing the box (answer B) would send the wrong message. Working with her one-on-one (answer A) would remove her from the group type of intervention that is so important for this population."Within groups, activities should foster interaction, trust, and collaboration, creating opportunities for social support, unconditional acceptance, and practice of occupations perceived as risky" (p. 136). Downgrading the activity by removing the message (answer D) would remove a key element of the activity. See Reference: Brown & Stoffel. (2011). Lock, L.C. & Pepin, G.: Eating disorders.

95. (D) A therapist-led aerobics class. A parallel test group "is structured by each client having his or her own project, which encourages work in a specific spot, focuses attention on a personal project, and provides opportunities for sharing and social interaction" (pp. 970–971). An aerobics class would provide the opportunity for each client to work individually, without the need to interact with others, while providing an opportunity for sharing and social interaction if desired. These individuals would not be ready for the higher levels of interaction required by planning a dinner party (answer A), playing a board game (answer B), or participating in a support group (answer C). See Reference: Cara & MacRae. (2013). Glossary.

96. (C) Encourage play activities that incorporate tapping, application of textures, and weight-bearing to the residual limb. Answer C is correct. "Interventions to desensitize the residual limb include weight bearing on the end of limb against various surfaces, massage, tapping and rubbing, and residual limb wrapping" (p. 1268). Answers A and B will not affect hypersensitivity, and answer D is incorrect because the child is in the preprosthetic phase and does not yet have access to the prosthesis. See Reference: Radomski & Trombly. (2008). Stubblefield, K. & Armstrong, A.: Amputations and prosthetics.

97. (C) Mental status, oral structures, and motor control of head. "The clinician notes the patient's insight into his or her dysphagia and observes head, neck trunk, and limb control and endurance for being out of bed at mealtimes" (p. 1326). A dysphagia evaluation usually consists of assessing a client's mental status; oral motor structure; and head, trunk, and extremity motor functions (answer C).

Answer A is most related to an evaluation of TMJ. Answer B, a cranial nerve assessment, would typically be performed by a physiatrist and/or neurologist. Answer D, muscle length control or dysmetria (a result of overshooting or pointing past an object), is typically not included in the assessment of dysphagia. See Reference: Trombly. (2008). Avery, W.: Dysphagia.

98. (A) Serving from the beverage cart. "The demands of jobs vary considerably. Many employers now have someone on staff to assess workstations and determine whether modifications can be made. In many cases, however, it is up to the individual worker to modify his or her work situation. Many improvements can be made by simply using correct lifting techniques, using the proper equipment for the job, pacing the activity, and asking for help" (p. 1107). When distributing magazines, the flight attendant uses negligible reaching, bending, pushing, or pulling movements. Serving from the beverage cart involves pushing and pulling on a horizontal plane, and somewhat more resistive reaching and bending than that required to distribute magazines (answer A is correct). Blankets and pillows (answer B) are lightweight like magazines, and would not be considered an upgrade. Putting luggage into the overhead compartments (answer D) would be the final step in the work-hardening process, because it involves the most weight and the riskiest back position. Distributing magazines to half of the passengers (answer C) would be downgrading the activity. See Reference: Pedretti. (2013). Grangaard, L.: Low back pain.

99. (B) Prevents hyperextension of the MCP joints and allows MCP flexion. "Laceration of the ulnar nerve at the wrist level is called a low ulnar lesion. This injury results in loss of most of the hand intrinsics.... The ring and small fingers present a claw deformity, a position of MP hyperextension and PIP flexion associated with muscle imbalance in ulnar-innervated structures" (p. 1151). An ulnar nerve orthosis's primary purpose is to support the hand secondary to ulnar intrinsic muscle paralysis or weakness. This orthosis also allows for MCP flexion. Answers A, C, and D are all inappropriate techniques for fabricating an ulnar nerve orthosis. See Reference: Trombly. (2008). Cooper, C.: Hand impairments.

100. (A) Emphasizing quality of life and engagement in meaningful activity. "The palliative approach focuses on providing clients with relief from the symptoms, pain and stress of a serious illness.... The goal is to improve quality of life [answer A] for both the client and their family" (p. 334). Hospice care, unlike palliative care, is carried out only in the last weeks or months of life; therefore, a focus of hospice care is on the dying process (answer D).

Goals related to strength and endurance (answer B) and maximizing independence (answer C) are consistent with a rehabilitation approach, but not a palliative approach. See Reference: Schell, Gillen, & Scaffa. (2014). Gillen, G.: Occupational therapy interventions for individuals.

101. (C) Demonstrate how using a shower chair improves safety. Educating the client is the first response the OT practitioner should make (answer C). By describing and demonstrating the shower chair and how it makes showering safer, the therapist is conveying the concept that occupational performance is based on the interaction of performance contexts (physical environment) and performance components (the confidence to execute tasks safely). The therapist would then inquire about the client's desire to purchase a shower chair (answer B). Getting into a bathtub is even more dangerous than getting into the shower (answer A), so this is not a viable option. Answer D, explaining that the therapy will increase the client's confidence level, is a subjective belief of the therapist that may not be embraced by the client because of his very valid fear of falling. See Reference: Trombly. (2008). Goodman, G. & Bonder, B.R.: Preventing occupational dysfunction secondary to aging.

102. (A) decreasing inflammation and edema. The "goals and concepts of elastic taping include...reducing inflammation and edema by stimulating the lymphatic system" (answer A, p. 1066). Taping does not increase muscle fatigue (answer B); rather, it "normalizes muscle tone by reducing overstretching and overcontraction of muscles" and it does not decrease ROM (answer C), but potentially improves "ROM by relieving pain" (p. 1066). Answer D, taping to desensitize the UE, is not a primary function of elastic taping. See Reference: Pedretti. (2013). Kasch, M.C. & Walsh, J.M.: Hand and upper extremity injuries.

103. (B) Allow the chin to remain tucked when drinking. Answer B is correct. The cutout area surrounds the child's nose so the liquid goes into the child's mouth without extending the neck. Tucking the chin toward the chest is "recommended when the child has delayed swallow initiation" (p. 466). Methods the caregiver can use to control or slow the rate of liquid intake (answers A and C) include using a drinking spout with a small opening, pinching a straw, or using a vacuum feeding cup with a control button. Plastic cups and plastic-coated utensils are best for individuals with a bite reflex (answer D) to prevent damage to their oral structures. See Reference: Case-Smith & O'Brien. (2010). Schuberth, L.M., Amirault, L.M., & Case-Smith, J.: Feeding intervention.

104. (B) Provide praise for completed dressing; do not help the child get dressed. Answer B is correct. "The social environment, family and other caregivers...provide encouragement and support ADL independence. They also shape expectations regarding the child's ADL occupations" (p. 477). To help a child maintain his level of independence, it also is important to be aware of social, cultural, and physical routines/expectations. Since the child has achieved dressing independence, he does not need assistance (answer A), clothing adaptations (answer C), or verbal prompts (answer D) to complete the task. In fact, assisting him now may cause him to lose his independence and regress to relying on his parents again. See Reference: Case-Smith & O'Brien. (2010). Shepherd, J.: Activities of daily living.

105. (A) Swimming. Swimming (answer A) is correct, as it provides active movement through wide ranges of motion with minimal impact on the joints. The sports in answers B, C, and D involve bouncing, jumping, and kicking, which place additional stress on the joints and would be contraindicated. (p. 154). See Reference: Case-Smith & O'Brien. (2010). Rogers, S.L.: Common conditions that influence children's participation.

106. (A) Make a fist, and then gradually relax it. Progressive muscle relaxation is one of several methods OTs use for relaxation training. Making a fist and relaxing it (answer A) is an example of progressive muscle relaxation, which is optimal for this individual because of his short attention span. When teaching progressive muscle relaxation, the OT instructs clients "to tighten and release voluntary muscle groups slowly and methodically in a progressive fashion, thereby contrasting the state of tension and relaxation. This technique offers a discharge of tension as a means to achieve a state of deep relaxation, with the underlying hypothesis that relaxation of the body leads to relaxation of the mind. For clients with limited concentration, the active involvement of tensing and relaxing can be more engaging and therefore more successful than pure mental activity" (p. 286). The remaining answers represent different types of relaxation training. Deep breathing involves deeply inhaling and slowly exhaling (answer D). Meditation may take many months to learn and involves focusing on a word or phrase (answer B) to reduce stress. Walking to increase the heart rate is an example of aerobic exercise (answer C), which can reduce pain and relieve stress and involves repetitive contractions of the large muscles of the arms and legs. See Reference: Cara & MacRae. (2013). Cara, E.: Anxiety disorders.

107. (C) Teach the caregiver how to position the client safely. "The progressive nature of the disease necessitates that rehabilitation in ALS be compensatory, focusing on adapting to disability and preventing secondary complications.... As motor function declines, mobility and self-care become increasingly difficult.... The OT helps the caregiver-client team to optimize safety, assess positioning, perform safe transfers, and maintain skin integrity" (p. 1095), answer C. Answer A (strengthening program) and B (wheelchair education) would have most likely have occurred at this point in the disease process and would not address the issue of transferring and decubiti, whereas answer D (providing and environmental control unit) also would not address the ability to transfer and decubiti prevention. See Reference: Trombly. (2008). Forwell, S.J., Copperman, L.F., & Hugos, L.: Neurogenerative diseases.

108. (B) Wheelchair equipment vendor. Although any of these community resources may be helpful to a family and child with a significant physical disability, answer B is correct because of the possible breakdown of this already purchased piece of equipment. Part of the OT's responsibility in fitting a wheelchair is to ensure the consumer's satisfaction (p. 503), and access to assistance for repairs and refinements contributes to this outcome. The OT needs to consider this possible problem and provide local support for a solution. Therefore, although answers A, C, and D may serve as resources for other needs of the child, only a specialist in wheelchair equipment would be able to solve mechanical problems that arise. See Reference: Radomski & Trombly. (2008). Dudgeon, B.J. & Dietz, J.C.: Wheelchair selection.

109. (A) Manual edema mobilization. "Manual edema mobilization [answer A] is a method of edema reduction based on methods to activate the lymphatic system. These methods include the principles of manual lymph-edema treatment (MLT) massage, medical compression bandaging, exercise, and external compression adapted to meet the specific needs of subacute and chronic postsurgical and poststroke edema. The goals are to stimulate the initial lymphatics to absorb excess fluid and large molecules from the interstitium and to move this lymph centrally" (p. 1059). Answers B and C, hot packs and paraffin, can assist with soft tissue and joint mobility as well as pain, but are often contraindicated in cases in which edema is present because the direct heat source increases blood flow to the area and subsequently increases edema. Answer D, sensory reeducation, would address the client's limitations with sensation, not edema. See Reference: Pedretti. (2013). Kasch, M.C. & Walsh, J.M.: Hand and upper extremity injuries.

110. (A) positioning the UE on the tabletop surface with Dycem™. "Flaccidity stemming from upper motor neuron dysfunction (e.g., recovering from spinal or cerebral shock resulting from acute CNS insult) is treated with facilitation techniques.... The arm can be passively positioned as normally as possible during ADL tasks to provide sensory and proprioceptive feedback. When the client is eating, [have] him or her place his or her arm on the dining room table, resting on top of a piece of Dycem" (p. 483). This positioning technique (correct answer A) would keep the individual's arm in a safe and appropriate position. A lap tray (answer D) would provide support, but is more restrictive than placing the hand on a surface with Dycem, which should be attempted first. The fact that the individual's arm was seen dangling by the side of the wheelchair indicates that the wheelchair armrest alone (answer B) is inadequate. Answer C, an arm sling, would provide support for his arm, but would immobilize it in adduction and internal rotation. Current literature supports the use of slings only when necessary, such as during ambulation when a flaccid upper extremity may sublux or cause loss of balance. See Reference: Pedretti. (2013). Preston, L.A.: Evaluation of motor control.

111. (A) Jaw opening and closing are controlled with your index and middle fingers; place your thumb on the child's cheek. The correct position of the adult's hand for jaw control when the child is fed from the side is described in answer A. Answers B and D are incorrect because the thumb should be placed on the child's cheek to provide joint stability. Answer C is incorrect because controlling the child's jaw movement with the adult's whole hand provides less control of the child's jaw than the recommended method. Placing the adult's thumb on the child's ear (answer D) is also incorrect because of discomfort for the child, and because thumb placement should be near the fulcrum of jaw movement (at the temporomandibular joint). If the child is fed from the front, the adult's thumb is placed on the chin, with middle finger under the chin to control opening and closing of the jaw. The index finger then rests on the side of the child's face to provide stability. See Reference: Case-Smith & O'Brien. (2010). Schuberth, L.M., Amirault, L.M., & Case-Smith, J.: Feeding intervention.

112. (B) Provide positive and constructive feedback about performance in the role-play. Once the problem-solving sequence has been completed, the social skills training sequence moves on to the role-play. After initially performing the role-play as the situation most recently occurred, without trying to implement the most effective social skills, the OT should provide positive and constructive feedback (answer B). This is then followed up with a second role-play in which the participants practice using more effective social skills (answer D). After more feedback, the OT provides a real-life homework assignment (answer A) and closes the session by summarizing the skills covered in the session. Discussion of how to carry out the solution in a social interaction (answer C) would have occurred earlier, during the problem-solving sequence (p. 309). See Reference: Brown & Stoffel. (2011). Stoffel, V.C. & Tomlinson, J.: Communication and social skills.

113. (C) get the shirt all the way on, then line up the buttons and holes, and begin buttoning from the bottom. It is easier to see the buttons and buttonholes at the bottom of the shirt (answer C) than at the top (answer B). Therefore, beginning to button from the bottom is more likely to result in success for the individual with motor or visual-perceptual deficits. Buttoning first (answer A) may result in ripping off the buttons as the shirt is pulled over the head. A buttonhook with a built-up handle (answer D) would be more helpful for an individual with finger weakness or incoordination (e.g., quadriplegia). See Reference: Pedretti. (2013). Gillen, G.: Cerebrovascular accident/stroke.

114. (B) Crafts, games, and self-care tasks. "Purposeful and occupation-based activities are an integral part or rehabilitation of the hand. Purposeful and occupation-based activities include crafts, games, dexterity activities, ADLs, and work samples. Several studies have shown that clients are more likely to choose occupationally embedded exercise and performed better using this type of exercise over rote exercise" (p. 1067). Crafts, games, and self-care tasks can best be described as purposeful and occupation-based activities that should be a component of hand rehabilitation (answer B). Answers A, C, and D are all considered to be adjunctive activities that may be implemented as a precursor to functional activities. See Reference: Pedretti. (2013). Kasch, M.C. & Walsh, J.M.: Hand and upper extremity injuries.

115. (B) Prompting the worker to use the correct sequence with each item, then gradually eliminating prompts beginning with elimination of the prompt for the plastic piece. Backward chaining is "used to teach multistep tasks; in this approach the therapist shows or prompts all of the steps of the task. On the next trial, all of these steps except for the last one is demonstrated or prompted and the person being taught this skill must demonstrate it. After each trial prompts are withdrawn and that technique progresses until all of the steps are learned" (p. 230). Answers A, B, and C, are not examples of backward chaining. See Reference:

Gillen. (2009. Managing memory deficits to optimize function.

116. (D) Rubber-coated spoons. Children who have a strong tonic bite reflex can use rubber-coated, plastic, or rubber spoons (p. 461). This will allow the parent and/or child to more easily remove the utensil from the child's mouth. Rubber-coated spoons provide a smoother surface than that of a regular stainless-steel utensil. Answers A, B, and C would not be recommended for a child with a strong tonic reflex, but would be for other children whose feeding/eating is impacted by incoordination, tremors, and apraxia. See Reference: Case-Smith & O'Brien. (2010). Schuberth, L.M., Amirault, L.M., & Case-Smith, J.: Feeding intervention.

117. (D) Activate the emergency response by calling 911. The OT practitioner should be knowledgeable about situations that may be potentially dangerous for patients. This question requires that the practitioner be knowledgeable about the appropriate ranges for heart rate and blood pressure. Both of the measures are above safe ranges (p. 1209) and indicate that the patient is medically unstable. Therefore, immediate medical services would be necessary. Answers A, B, and C do not recognize the seriousness of the situation and could delay the necessary medical attention. See Reference: Schell, Gillen, & Scaffa. (2014). Matthews, M.M.: Cardiac and pulmonary disease.

118. (A) Getting dressed without becoming fatigued. Prevention of fatigue is the primary purpose of energy conservation. Energy conservation techniques may often result in slower, not faster (answer D), performance. Using proper body mechanics may enable an individual with back pain to lift heavy cookware without pain (answer B). Using joint protection techniques may prevent further joint damage to arthritic hands when the patient is doing handicrafts (answer C). See Reference: Pedretti. (2013). Deshaies, L.: Arthritis.

119. (D) Involve him in sanding and staining increasingly larger pieces. This individual's goal is to increase ROM in order to return to work. In woodworking, "the larger the project, the greater the movement required" (p. 81). Progression to power tools (answer A) would not necessarily promote greater ROM but might involve increasing the cognitive complexity of the task. Wrist weights (answer B) would be used to promote strengthening. Bilateral activities (answer C) could be useful for some individuals with coordination or perceptual deficits. See Reference: Tubbs & Drake. (2012). Woodworking.

120. (A) Functioning as a peer in the group. "A mature group is heterogeneous in composition and is characterized by members taking those task and so-cial emotional roles that are required for adequate group functioning.... The therapist interacts as a co-equal group member" (p. 396). The OT would func-tion as a leader in parallel, project, and egocentric-cooperative level groups. The OT would function as an advisor (answer C) or facilitator (answer D) in a cooperative level group. See Reference: Cole. (2012). Appendix B.

121. (B) Teach him to take breaks frequently when doing needlepoint and to respect pain. When doing needlepoint, individuals with arthritis should "minimize long periods of static holding. Maintaining a static grasp for an extended period of time can damage an inflamed joint.... Those with ar-thritis who desire to participate in needlework should be instructed to take frequent rest breaks and to re-spect pain [answer B]" (p. 138). Designs with a lower level of complexity (answer A) could benefit an indi-vidual with cognitive deficits. A different hobby (an-swer C) might be better for his joints in theory, but working with him to find ways that he can continue the hobby that he values is a more client-centered option. Because needlepoint can easily be stopped and started at any point, it is not necessary to limit him to short-term projects (answer D). See Refer-ence: Tubbs & Drake. (2012). Needlework.

122. (D) Cut the paper in two following a straight line. Answer D is correct. Scissor skills de-velop from first cutting snips to cutting a single straight line (p. 73). The ability to cut heavier materi-als such as cardboard and cloth (answer A) develops last in the sequence of scissor skills. The ability to cut along curved lines (answer B) develops after the abil-ity to cut a straight line. The ability to cut along straight lines with enough control to cut out a trian-gle (answer C) develops after the ability to cut a sin-gle straight line and before the ability to cut a curved line. See Reference: Case-Smith & O'Brien. (2010). Case-Smith, J.: Development of childhood occupations.

123. (C) Bring the seat in for reevaluation in 4 to 6 months. Answer C is correct, as "once a child receives a seating mobility system, the therapist should reevaluate its fit and function every 4 to 6 months" (p. 643) to account for the child's growth, changes in posture, comfort, and other factors that may affect function (p. 642). Answer A is incorrect, as a well-fitting seating system that enhances func-tion should be regularly used to enhance the child's participation in everyday activities. Weekly adjust-ment (answer B) is usually not necessary, and trans-porting the seat every week would be unnecessarily inconvenient. The end of the IEP (answer D) may be more than 6 months away and, therefore, too long to wait. See Reference: Case-Smith & O'Brien. (2010). Wright-Ott, C.: Mobility.

124. (B) Clubhouse model. The clubhouse model (answer B) operates "with a blend of staff and mem-bers to assume leadership for all clubhouse opera-tions in an egalitarian and strength-based context in which members pursue personal goals related to their recovery" (p. 559). It is centered on the "concept of the work ordered day" and "conveys the expectation that members and staff run the clubhouse, side-by-side, at least five days per week during typical work hours" (p. 561). Members are not paid. Transitional employment (answer A) may be provided by the clubhouse by contracting positions in business and industry. These positions, however, are paid a pre-vailing wage. Partial hospitalization environments (answer C) provide more structure and professional support for people who still need a higher level of care. A group home (answer D) is a type of residen-tial programming. Individuals living in group homes may opt to participate in a clubhouse during the day. See Reference: Brown & Stoffel. (2011). Stoffel, V.C.: Psychosocial clubhouses.

125. (C) Work with the individual on appropri-ate communication skills. Characteristics associ-ated with personality disorders include "excessive and unstable expression of emotions, maladapted in-terpersonal relationships, and a disregard for the needs and rights of others" (p. 145). "The general fo-cus of occupational therapy intervention...includes mood stabilization [and]...appropriate feeling expres-sion; increased self-concept, self-esteem, insight, and judgment; and the development of appropriate inter-personal relationships, effective coping strate-gies,...conflict resolution skills, social skills, and as-sertive communication [answer C]" (p. 151). Asking the individual how other people feel (answer D) re-quires empathy, for which this individual does not have the capacity. Because individuals with BPD are often manipulative and test professional boundaries, "practitioners need to be aware of these facts and monitor their own emotional state to ensure their therapeutic ability with clients who have this diagno-sis" (p. 150); therefore, expressing feelings of disap-pointment (answer B) would not be beneficial. Ban-ning the individual from group therapy sessions (answer A) would deprive her of the necessary inter-vention. See Reference: Brown & Stoffel. (2011). Ur-ish, C.: Personality disorders.

126. (A) Checking for irritation and pressure problems. Because a toddler cannot always articu-late discomfort effectively, skin irritation may go un-noticed. Therefore, a young child is at higher risk for developing skin and pressure problems than an older, more verbal one. Although answers B, C, and D describe important factors in orthosis care, primary emphasis for the young child should be placed on answer A (p. 315). See Reference: Case-Smith & O'Brien. (2010). Exner, C.: Evaluation and intervention to develop hand skills.

127. (B) Rifton child's chair with footrest and padded abductor post. Answer B is correct, as general positioning guidelines for optimal oral motor control during feeding suggest "stability in the trunk and support the child in midline orientation with the head and neck aligned in neutral or slight flexion" (p. 459). The prone stander (answer A) would place the child in a standing or extended position, which would reinforce undesirable extensor tone. A supine position (answer C) is not appropriate for eating if other positions are available. The child would not benefit from a beanbag chair (answer D) "since a beanbag is particularly inappropriate for children with extensor posturing because it does not successfully inhibit these postures" (p. 469). See Reference: Case-Smith & O'Brien. (2010). Schuberth, L.M., Amirault, L.M., & Case-Smith, J.: Feeding intervention.

128. (A) Orthostatic hypotension. A frequent side effect of antipsychotic drugs is orthostatic hypotension (answer A), a decrease in blood pressure in response to sudden movements, specifically up and down, resulting in faintness or loss of consciousness. The parachute activity involves significant up-and-down body movements, and therefore warrants the therapist's full attention with this patient population. Photosensitivity (answer B) is a common side effect of some antipsychotic drugs, and dry mouth resulting in excessive thirst (answer C) is a common side effects of some antidepressant drugs; however, these would not be of particular concern during an indoor parachute activity. Blurred vision (answer D) is a common side effect of anticonvulsant drugs, which are commonly used for the treatment of bipolar disorder (pp. 239–257). See Reference: Bonder. (2010). Howland, R.H.: Psychopharmacology.

129. (C) Install an alarm on the client's door. Installing an alarm on the client's door (answer C) would be the preferred intervention to address the issue of wandering. Additional strategies to prevent wandering include regular exercise, putting up stop signs, and diversion (p. 494). Moving the individual's room (answer D) would likely add to his/her confusion. Keeping hallways clear of obstructions (answer B) results in a safer environment for wanderers but does not prevent wandering. Modifying the environment is preferable to increasing demands on nursing staff (answer D). Applying restraints (answer A) would be the last choice for intervention because it interferes with a client's functional independence.

See Reference: Cara & MacRae. (2013). MacRae, A. & Smith, J.: Mental health of the older adult.

130. (B) Develop a plan with staff to change the social environment to one that will enhance motivation and activity levels. Consultation is providing "the best advice/plan possible to assist the organization to meet the needs of its service population and the needs of the organization.... The consultant is able to do this without becoming enmeshed in the day to day operations of the organization" (p. 169). Answer B is correct because it best reflects the scope of the consultant with populations in community-based practice, which is to provide problem-solving in the area of concern. Answer A represents direct service; answer C represents a program development approach, and answer D would be more typical of a counseling role. All of these are levels of occupational therapy intervention, not consultation. See Reference: Fazio. (2008). Staffing and personnel.

131. (C) Foam tubing around the utensils. Answer C is correct because foam tubing increases the diameter of the utensils and "larger grip diameters may help a child to self-feed more independently" (p. 451). Swivel utensils (answer A) are most appropriate for children who experience incoordination or tremors, whereas pediatric universal holders (answer B) are commonly introduced when a child has no grip at all. In this case, the cuff is directly attached to the child's hand while the utensils are inserted into the sleeve of the cuff. Weighted utensils (answer D) would not assist the child with decreased grip but may assist a child with motor incoordination. See Reference: Case-Smith & O'Brien. (2010). Schuberth, L.M., Amirault, L.M., & Case-Smith, J.: Feeding intervention.

132. (B) Slightly flexed. Answer B is correct. "A chin-tuck position may be recommended when the child has delayed swallow initiation. During a videofluoroscopic swallow study, a delay is typically seen as pooling of food or liquid in the pharyngeal space located close to the opening of the larynx. When the child is positioned with a slight chin-tuck, the laryngeal opening may become smaller, reducing the risk of aspiration or penetration" (p. 466). Positioning the infant with the head in extension (answer C) can increase the risk of choking. Rotating the head (answer D) does not facilitate swallowing. See Reference: Case-Smith & O'Brien, 2010 Schuberth, L.M., Amirault, L.M., & Case-Smith, J.: Feeding intervention.

133. (A) skin inspection. Visual inspection of an insensate area is essential for preventing pressure sores, which may develop when there are no sensory cues to alert a person to skin breakdown, answer A.

"The residual limb may have areas of absent or impaired sensation requiring education and special attention.... The person must rely on visual and proprioceptive feedback because sensation is functionally lost when the prosthesis is worn" (p. 1154). Nail trimming (answer B) is an important issue to address in individuals with diabetes, but it is secondary to skin inspection in importance. Many individuals with diabetes have abnormalities in nail growth, and instead of trimming their own nails, they have them trimmed by a podiatrist. Moreover, the nursing staff may address this issue with the patient. Retirement planning (answer C) and returning to work (answer D) are issues that may be addressed when discussing discharge plans. See Reference: Pedretti. (2013). George, A.H.: Infection control and safety issues in the clinic.

134. (C) Offer a choice of slice-and-bake cookies or a cake mix. Strategies to address impairment in decision-making skills include "limit the number of options [answer C], teach the individual about potential biases, teach the individual to step back and think through important decisions, and ask others of input when making important decisions" (p. 247). Premeasuring ingredients (answer A) could save time and be a useful strategy for an individual with a short attention span. Limiting the number of steps (answer B) and creating a checklist (answer D) could be useful strategies for individuals with memory deficits. See Reference: Brown & Stoffel. (2011). Brown, C.: Cognitive skills.

135. (B) Having the OT move the shoulder joint through its full range of motion. "A client with little or no active range of motion would require the therapist to passively move the joint through its full arc of motion, termed PROM" (p. 53, answer B). Answers A, C, and D are all representative of strategies to elicit active range of motion and/or active assisted range of motion techniques. See Reference: Meriano & Latella. (2008). Proulx-Sepelak, D.: Foundational skills for functional activities.

136. (B) A group format following a specified protocol. Dialectical Behavior Therapy (DBT) uses a protocol-based cognitive-behavioral approach to work with individuals with complex psychiatric conditions in a group format (answer B)."The skills taught in DBT include mindfulness, interpersonal effectiveness, emotional regulation, and distress tolerance. As with all group formats, consumers benefit from the interpersonal interaction, support, and modeling of other consumers. The group format also supports the therapist staying with the current training agenda and protocol even in the face of current problems or crises of the individual group members" (p. 351). Therefore, an individual format (answers A

and C) or a structure that alternates leadership (answer D) would not be appropriate. See Reference: Brown & Stoffel. (2011). Scheinholz, M.: Emotion regulation;.

137. (D) in the upper cabinet to the left side. Placing the groceries in the upper cabinet to the left side will promote the greatest degree of weight shift to the affected side. Putting groceries on the counter directly in front of the person (answer A) or in the upper cabinet to the right side (answer C) would not cause enough weight to be shifted to the affected side and would even shift weight away from that side. When placing groceries on the counter to the left side (answer B), minimal weight shift occurs. See Reference: Pedretti. (2013). Schultz-Krohn, W., Pope-Davis, S.A., Jourdan, J.M., & McLaughlin-Gray, J.: Traditional sensorimotor approaches to intervention.

138. (A) Reposition the switch to facilitate easy access and adjust further as needed. Answer A is correct as the OT determines a position in which the switch can be easily accessed to increase independence and self-efficacy of the child (p. 597). Answer B addresses a limitation in range of motion; answer C is a strategy for dealing with a visual impairment; and answer D pertains to behavioral and cognitive issues, none of which were mentioned as concerns for this child. See Reference: Case-Smith & O'Brien. (2010). Schoonover, J., Argabrite Grove, R.E., & Swinth, Y.: Influencing participation through assistive technology.

139. (B) Form letters out of clay. Answer B, form letters with clay, is correct. Preschoolers learn best using a multisensory approach and they "should be encouraged to feel shapes, letters and words through their hands and bodies.... Studies have shown that the incorporation of visuo-haptic and haptic exploration of letters in reading training programs facilitates 5-year-old children's understanding of the alphabet" (p. 391). Furthermore, recognition of letters occurs before actual letter writing-related activities and using a multisensory approach to recognition and placement of letters would be most likely recommended by OTs. Making letters out of materials such as clay, bread dough, pudding, or sandpaper uses the child's tactile, kinesthetic, and, in some cases, gustatory senses, as well as vision, reinforcing learning through a variety of sensory channels. Flash cards (answer A), matching to sample (answer C), and coloring (answer D) are methods that rely primarily on visual processing, and these approaches that tap cognitive skills are better suited for strengthening existing skills in older children. See Reference: Case-Smith & O'Brien. (2010). Schneck, C.: Visual perception.

140. (D) has good UE range of motion, but difficulty accessing small targets. A large keyboard would be best for someone who has good range of motion, but difficulty accessing small targets (answer D). A person with limited range of motion but who has adequate fine coordination (answer A) would benefit from a smaller or contracted keyboard. If someone fatigues rapidly when reaching for the keys (answer B), having to reach farther on a large keyboard would cause more fatigue. A large keyboard would be more difficult for a person using one hand (answer C), because the hand would have to move farther to complete typing, adding more work to the process. See Reference: Pedretti. (2013). Anson, D.: Assistive technology.

141. (C) tai chi. Tai chi would be the best activity because it incorporates slow stretching and provides graduated challenge to coordinated movements, which can help improve balance, answer C. "Complementary therapies, such as participation in Reiki, Tai Chi, Ai Chi, and yoga, are also being recommended to foster holistic health while also drawing exaggerated attention to the sense of body position" (p. 52). Answer A, safe transfer training, is useful to teach safety precautions but would not have as much impact on motor skills. Answer B, walking, is a good general exercise but would not provide stretching movement or challenge balance. Answer D, gardening, would not be particularly useful because it can be performed while in a stationary position. See Reference: Meriano & Latella. (2008). Proulx-Sepelak, D.: Foundational skills for functional activities.

142. (C) Slight anterior tilt. "Generally, after the acute onset of a disability or prolonged time spent in bed, clients assume a posterior pelvic tilt (i.e., a slouched position with lumbar flexion). In turn, this posture moves the center of mass back toward the buttocks. The therapist may need to verbally cue or manually assist the client into a neutral or slightly anterior pelvic tilt position to move the center of mass forward over the center of the client's body and over the feet in preparation for the transfer" (p. 254). Answers A, B, and D would not be conducive to maximal postural positioning. See Reference: Pedretti. (2013). Bolding, D., Adler, C., Tipton-Burton, M., Verran, A., & Lillie, S.M.: Mobility.

143. (C) Provide one-step directions and samples for individuals to duplicate. Individuals functioning at Allen's Cognitive Level 4 have difficulty making corrections and require "visual demonstration, limited instruction to one step at a time. Make all objects clearly visible. Provide visual comparisons so that individual knows what he or she is working toward. Situation specific training is useful" (p. 255). Providing a sample to copy (answer C) pro-

vides the visual cueing and situation-specific training that is needed at this cognitive level. Individuals functioning at Cognitive Level 3 are capable of using their hands for simple, repetitive tasks (answer A) but are unlikely to produce a consistent end product. Those functioning at Cognitive Level 5 can generally perform a task involving several familiar steps and one new one (answer B). Individuals functioning at Cognitive Level 6 can anticipate errors and plan ways to avoid them. These individuals would be capable of following written directions (answer D). See Reference: Brown & Stoffel. (2011). Brown, C.: Cognitive skills.

144. (C) Placing the writing surface at a level slightly above the child's elbow. Answer C is correct, because a position at a level higher than slightly above the child's elbows "promotes the use of abduction and internal rotation of the arms" (p. 299) and this position enables proximal and optimal positioning of the hand for skilled activity. Answer A is incorrect, as a surface lower than that of the elbow "promotes the use of body flexion" (p. 299). Answer B is incorrect as there is no indication that this child requires any external weight to optimize hand function. Stabilizing the trunk (answer D) is incorrect because unless the pelvis is stabilized, arm movements may still be compromised. Further, stabilizing the child's back against the seat limits the postural adjustments that contribute to refined hand skills. See Reference: Case-Smith & O'Brien. (2010). Exner, C.: Evaluation and intervention to develop hand skills.

145. (B) Discuss daily routines with his parent and explain how they can reinforce independence within those routines. Answer B is correct. "Before making recommendations, the therapist should ask the parents about daily routines and typical flow of family activities.... [This] enables the therapist and the parents to embed goals and activities in interactive routines, in which the therapeutic process does not diminish the value and pleasure" (p. 132). Further, this provides opportunity for the child's continued practice to sustain independence. In studies, "[m]others reported that they did not have the time, energy, or confidence to follow [home] programs" (p. 132), so suggesting a parent carry out specific procedures (answer A) is not appropriate. Clothing adaptations (answer C) or verbal prompts (answer D) to complete the task are incorrect as they provide assistance he does not need. In fact, assisting him now may cause him to lose his independence and regress to relying on his parents again. See Reference: Case-Smith & O'Brien. (2010). Jaffe, L., Humphry, R., & Case-Smith, J: Working with families.

146. (D) Knowing the child and family's priorities, modifying contexts to promote participa-

tion, enhancing performance, and educating family. Answer D is correct. Best practice approaches emphasize a multicomponent "top-down" approach. Once priorities are determined, intervention begins, "focusing on occupational performance" (p. 476). "Children with a variety of neuromotor disorders, and their families will benefit from consultation with supportive, creative therapists as they learn to problem-solve their way through daily challenges" (p. 477). Answers A and B may be part of the multicomponent program just described, yet they do not describe an adequate program approach, nor are they relevant for all children with neuromotor disorders. Answer C is incorrect as this emphasis in an OT program encourages the child to rely on others and may lead to persistent dependence and lack of progress in independent occupational performance. See Reference: Lane & Bundy. (2012). Missiuna, C., Polatajko, H., Pollock, N., & Cameron, D.: Neuromotor disorders.

147. (C) Consulting a checklist of steps while doing laundry in context. Making a checklist and having the individual use the checklist during the activity would provide an external memory aid during practice of the functional activity. "The checklist itself may be both a prompt if placed in an obtrusive location and a reinforcer as the patient checks each completed step" (p. 760). This would provide compensation for cognitive deficits during task training in the specific context where it will be performed. Answers A, B, and D are methods that require an individual to be able to transfer learning of skills from one context to another. See Reference: Trombly. (2008). Radomski, M.V. & Davis, E.S.: Optimizing cognitive abilities.

148. (A) Sit straddling a bolster with both feet on the floor. Answer A is correct as once independent postural reactions are developed on a stable surface (the floor), the child can further refine sitting skills by learning to maintain posture when placed on an unstable surface Once the child has learned to sit independently on the floor, an external stabilizing support is no longer necessary (answer D). At first, the child should be left in control of the movement on this surface, and she should have both feet on the floor for maximal stability. Later, these skills can be refined by placing the child on more challenging surfaces, such as on a ball with a handle (answer C) or on a scooter pulled by another person (answer B) (p. 188). See Reference: Case-Smith & O'Brien. (2010). Barthel, K.A.: A frame of reference for neuro-developmental treatment.

149. (C) Lateral trunk supports. Lateral trunk supports (answer C) are correct, as they would help maintain correct alignment of the pelvis and trunk in the wheelchair. "Additional seating supports should

be used as needed to improve posture, restrict abnormal movements, and promote head control and voluntary use the limbs" (p. 492). Answer A, a reclining wheelchair, would shift the child's weight posteriorly but would not prevent lateral shifting of the trunk. An arm trough (answer B) would probably contribute to lateral shifting, although bilateral arm troughs or a lapboard could help maintain a more centered trunk position. Lateral pelvic supports (answer D) would stabilize the pelvis and prevent it from shifting sideways, but would be too low to prevent the trunk from moving laterally. See Reference: Radomski & Trombly. (2008). Dudgeon, B.J. & Dietz, J.C.: Wheelchair selection.

150. (B) Organize a game of soccer during recess with the group of children. Organizing a soccer game during recess (answer B) is correct. When occupational therapists design interventions to promote play behavior, they consider the activities, routines, and environments within the setting, recognizing that "children benefit from participating in the structured activity as contextually as possible" (p. 297). The soccer game is a naturally occurring activity during children's recess into which the OT can embed intervention strategies to promote play skills. Answers A and C do not promote interaction among the group of children. Answer D, including jigsaw puzzles in the game center, does not mean the children will use them; further, their use of the puzzles by themselves does not promote play and social skills development. See Reference: Parham & Fazio. (2007). Florey, L.L. & Greene, S.: Play in middle childhood.

151. (C) Cooperative. This individual exhibited eagerness to interact with "and agree with other members on activities,...express ideas and problem solve together, [and]...sustain interest in longer projects, across days, then weeks" (p. 53), characteristics associated with expectations in a cooperative group (answer C). Individuals participating in groups at the associative level (answer B) have less well-developed social skills, fewer problem-solving abilities, and shorter attention spans. Individuals working in parallel groups (answer A) would not be interacting with others. Individuals functioning at the mature group level would not need the level of intervention required by this individual. See Reference: Cole & Donohue. (2011). Cole, M.B.: Social participation basics.

152. (A) Perform pursed-lip breathing when doing activities. "Pursed-lip breathing (PLB) is thought to prevent tightness in the airway by providing resistance to expiration. This technique has been shown to increase use of the diaphragm and decrease accessory muscle recruitment. Persons with COPD sometimes instinctively adopt this technique, whereas others may need to be taught it" (p. 1207). The overall effect is improved endurance and tolerance for activities. Taking hot showers and avoiding air-conditioning during warm weather (answers C and D) are incorrect in that both activities are contraindicated for individuals with COPD. Using a long-handled bath sponge (answer B) may be helpful but is not the most likely tip to be included in a home program for an individual with COPD. See Reference: Pedretti. (2013). Huntley, N.: Cardiac and pulmonary diseases.

153. (C) Ulnar styloid, distal head of radius, and thumb CMC joint. "When fabricating a splint [orthosis], therapists must consider where to apply force without causing further trauma. Despite its deftness and power, the hand's lack of protective fascia means that it tolerates external pressures poorly and shearing stresses not at all. The prominent ulnar styloid, the distal radial styloid, and the thumb carpometacarpal joint are common sites for pressure" (p. 764). Answers A, B, and D also are areas that could potentially be susceptible to skin breakdown but are not primary sites of pressure when fabricating a resting hand orthosis. See Reference: Pedretti. (2013). Lashgari, D. & Yasuda, L: Orthotics.

154. (D) picking up raisins with a pair of tweezers. Answer D is correct, as this activity is the only one that targets isolated finger use. Research suggests that small-muscle development and the ability to hold utensils are among the prerequisite skills necessary for handwriting (p. 557). Drawing on sandpaper (answer A) can be used to increase kinesthetic awareness and finger strength. Copying shapes (answer B) is primarily a perceptual motor task. Rolling out clay (answer C) is an activity that promotes bilateral hand use and the development of palmar arches. See Reference: Case-Smith & O'Brien. (2010). Schneck, C. & Amundson, S.L.: Prewriting and handwriting skills.

155. (C) Providing ADL training in use of adaptive techniques for LE dressing and transfers. The primary role of the occupational therapist in working with the person with a total knee replacement is answer C, providing ADL training in use of adaptive techniques for LE dressing and transfers, as needed. Decreased knee movement may require the person to use adaptive equipment for tub transfer or special devices for lower extremity dressing (if the person cannot touch his toes), including practicing putting the knee immobilizer on and taking it off. "Helpful assistive devices or adaptive aids include a dressing stick, sock aid, long-handled shoe horn, reacher, elastic shoelaces, leg lifter, elevated toilet or commode seat, three-in-one commode, and shower chair or bench. Walker bags are helpful for people

using walkers who need to carry small items from one place to another" (p. 1083). Answer A, improving strength of the upper extremities, would not necessarily be an aspect of treatment for all individuals post-total knee replacement/arthroplasty. Answer B would be an area that the physical therapist would primarily address. A homemaking evaluation, answer D, might be performed but would not be a primary focus of intervention because the person would be expected to resume homemaking at the same level without difficulty once the period of recovery is finished. See Reference: Pedretti. (2013). Coleman Lawson, S. & Murphy, L.F.: Hip fractures and lower extremity joint replacement.

156. (A) Avoid caffeine and get into bed only when ready to go to sleep. Good sleep hygiene can help individuals with sleep disturbances. Interventions can include developing healthy routines and/or environmental adaptations. Some recommended routines include avoiding "caffeine in the afternoons and evenings" and using the bed "only for sleeping and intimacy with a partner" (answer A) (p. 750). The routine of a warm bath before bed can also be relaxing; however, exercise (answer D) "should be done earlier in the day or evening. It is alerting and should be avoided during the 2 to 3 hours just before bedtime" (pp. 750–751). A white-noise machine (answer B) can help drown out disturbing noises, and a dark room can also help to promote sleep, but these are environmental adaptations, not routines. See Reference: Brown & Stoffel. (2011). Pierce, D. & Summers, K.: Rest and sleep.

157. (D) Set clear expectations for behavior and enforce consequences. Answer D is correct. "Many children respond best when rules are clearly established and limits are defined" (p. 438). The child must clearly understand the expectations for behavior (or rules) and that there will be consistent consequences for behaviors that break the rules. Answers A and B, allowing the child to express his anger and ignoring the behaviors, would not help the child to learn new behaviors and could cause an increased loss of control. Answer C is incorrect, as a child who is out of control and responding to impulses is not able to respond to an insight-based approach such as reasoning. See Reference: Case-Smith & O'Brien. (2010). Watling, R.: Interventions and strategies for challenging behaviors.

158. (A) lying on the left side, propped up with pillows. According to American Heart Association (2013), lying on the left side, propped up with pillows, (answer A) is the correct answer. This allows the unaffected right extremities to remain free and provides weight-bearing to the affected side to assist with tone reduction. The pillows behind the individual allow support, and the individual may lean against the pillows also to provide pressure relief as needed to the affected side, because sensation may be reduced on that side along with movement. Lying on the right side (answer B) would not provide any tone reduction, which is needed during a stressful activity such as sexual intercourse. This position also would impair the movement of the unaffected extremities, which would be needed for activities involving foreplay or applying contraceptive devices. Lying in a supine (answer C) or prone (answer D) position would not provide tone reduction to an individual with spasticity and could be uncomfortable without many pillows to assist with positioning comfortably. Also, an individual lying prone has less mobility than when he or she is lying on the right side. See Reference: http://www.heart.org/HEARTORG/Conditions/More/ToolsForYourHeartHealth/Sex-After-Stroke-Our-Guide-to-Intimacy-After-Stroke_UCM_310558_Article.jsp No chapter/Pamphlet.

159. (D) Prevents stress on the extensor tendons and ligaments while decreasing edema. Burn hand orthoses prevent stress on the superficial tendons and ligaments, decreasing edema secondary to the avoidance of dependent positioning. Answer A, decreasing pain and allowing for active range of motion, is not correct because of the immobilizing nature of the static orthosis. Answers B and C, preventing scarring and skin grafting, are not primary reasons for utilizing burn hand orthoses upon admission to the intensive care unit. See Reference: Pedretti. (2013). Reeves, S.U., & Deshaies, L.: Burns and burn rehabilitation.

160. (B) Playing a simple board game. Answer B is correct because the 5-year-old child engages in cooperative play and "is able to play games with rules,...plays well with others and enjoys social interaction" (p. 127). Answer A, coloring on paper, and answer C, looking at picture books, are appropriate for younger children. Answer D, participation in a reading club, is appropriate for an older child who has developed independent reading skills. See Reference: Mulligan. (2014). Mulligan, S.: Typical child development.

161. (B) Incorporate developmental stimulation activities into family routines. Answer B is correct as "suggestions that the family can incorporate into the daily routine are the most successful" (p. 694). Separate "therapeutic activities" (answers A and D) can take up an excessive amount of time and energy and may interfere with family life. Therefore, long-term follow-through may not be as effective as will activities made to fit existing daily routines and develop into habits. Activities provided on an as-needed basis (answer C) will never become habits,

and therefore follow-through is less effective. See Reference: Case-Smith & O'Brien. (2010). Myers, C.T., Stephens, L. Tauber, S.: Early intervention.

162. (A) Provide a desirable snack for those who attend. Avolition, or decreased motivation, is one of the primary negative symptoms of schizophrenia and is clearly the issue at hand in this scenario. Individuals with schizophrenia have identified several reasons for this including "hallucinations and delusions interfered with concentration, and secondary depression lead to withdrawal. The sedating effects of medication were another cause of motivational issues. Spirit breaking by others was also associated with poor motivation" (p. 336). When individuals with schizophrenia demonstrate avoidance, rewards such as certificates and graduation ceremonies (answer A) can serve as motivational strategies. Making attendance mandatory (answer B) may improve attendance but will not address the underlying issue of motivation. Breaking the activity down into smaller steps (answer C) would be beneficial if the group members were having trouble successfully completing the tasks, resulting in a sense of failure. Providing positive feedback and avoiding criticism (answer D) are strategies that can be used to promote self efficacy. See Reference: Brown & Stoffel. (2011). Brown, C.: Motivation.

163. (B) Expected development. Answer B is correct. Rocking while supported on hands and knees is expected between the ages of 7 and 12 months. After the infant has developed the ability to maintain stable position in the shoulders, "he or she is able to bear weight (i.e., to maintain a posture). From there he or she begins to play with movement in that position.... This is referred to as 'mobility superimposed on stability'" (p. 492). This stage is essential in the development of coordinated antigravity movement. This pattern is typical of normal development and does not indicate answers A, C, or D. See Reference: Hinojosa & Kramer. (2009). Colangelo, C.A. & Shea, M.: A biomechanical frame of reference for positioning children for functioning.

164. (B) Combing the hair. An individual normally abducts and externally rotates the shoulder to comb his or her hair (answer B); therefore, the individual is more likely to have difficulty in this area than in any of the others. Shoulder abduction is not required for buttoning a shirt (answer A) or tying a shoe (answer D). Tucking in a shirt in the back (answer C) requires shoulder abduction and internal rotation. See Reference: Pedretti. (2013). Foti, D. & Koketsu, J.S.: Activities of daily living.

165. (C) Wrist orthoses to promote development of tenodesis. An orthosis to promote tenodesis is implemented in the acute phase of rehabilitation (answer C). A tenodesis grasp is developed by allowing the finger flexors to shorten. The patient is then able to achieve a functional grasp by extending the wrist. This improves the ability of an individual with a C6 or C7 spinal cord injury to grasp and hold objects. "Progressive resistive exercise and resistive activities can be applied.... Wrist extensors should be strengthened to maximize natural tenodesis function thereby maximizing the necessary prehension pattern in the hand for functional grasp and release. Strengthening wrist extensors also increases the client's ability to use the tenodesis orthosis more effectively, mechanically transferring the strength of the wrist extensors to the finger pieces of the orthosis for stronger pinch" (pp. 965–966). A volar hand orthosis (answer A) would not allow finger flexors to shorten and would interfere with the development of tenodesis. Interventions related to promoting independent performance (answer B) should begin as soon as possible, but issues related to positioning must be addressed first. An individual would not be instructed in bed mobility (answer D) until after the acute phase. See Reference: Pedretti. (2013). Adler, C: Spinal cord injury.

166. (D) Alternate tasks that require standing with those that can be performed sitting. The performance component at issue in this question is fatigue. When fatigue impedes occupational performance, energy conservation techniques should be considered. Alternating sitting and standing activities is one method that can be applied to conserve energy; others include avoiding bending and stooping, avoiding unnecessary trips, using an appropriate work height, and relaxing homemaking standards. Convincing the individual to do something she can't afford (answer A) may not be in her best interest, and it is not an example consistent with the OT concept of collaborative decision-making. Although increasing strength (answer B) may ultimately be useful, endurance is typically a more pressing issue for individuals with MS. Using the largest joints available for the task (answer C) is a joint-protection technique more appropriate for an individual with arthritis. See Reference: Pedretti. (2013). Schultz-Krohn, W., Foti, D., & Glogoski, C.: Degenerative diseases of the central nervous system.

167. (B) Provide strong color contrast at key areas to identify steps, pathways, etc. Using contrast, answer B, is a key environmental adaptation strategy for people with visual impairments. The more contrast there is, the easier it is to locate objects, steps, entrances, and pathways, thereby improving accessibility by maximizing remaining vision. "For example, clients with poor contrast sensitivity require increased contrast and lighting and have diffi-culty with curbs, stairs, and finding objects in a low light.... With the client who is having difficulty with meal preparation, consider changing the lighting, marking the controls with bright, contrasting colors, organizing the kitchen and keeping items in their assigned places, and marking containers with large print labels" (p. 731). Instructing the individual to sit during ADL (answer A) or recommending human assistance (answer C) would not directly address accessibility. Answer D, recommending training in white cane use, is a method of improving mobility for a person who is blind. See Reference: Trombly. (2008). Quintana, L.A.: Optimizing vision, visual perception, and praxis abilities.

168. (B) Tell the client that you don't mind discussing sexuality-related questions as long as his parents are comfortable with the idea. Answer B is correct; when sexuality questions arise, "if the child is under 18 years of age, therapists must obtain parental permission to discuss sexuality issues" (p. 509). Answer A, referring the client to a psychologist, would be an appropriate response if the parent(s) agreed to the idea and if the OT did not feel comfortable or knowledgeable regarding the topic. Answer C, attempting to change the subject, may encourage the child to feel inadequate, frustrated, or more confused regarding his sexuality. Answer D, answering the client's questions, would only be appropriate after seeking the permission of the child's parents to discuss the topic of sexuality. See Reference: Case-Smith & O'Brien. (2010). Shepherd, J.: Activities of daily living.

169. (D) Ask the employer to provide an isolated cubical as the work space. An isolated cubicle (answer D) is a reasonable accommodation to request for an individual who is highly distractible. The Americans With Disabilities Act (ADA) supports "the individual's right to work by prohibiting discrimination against people with disabilities.... When people with disabilities can perform the essential functions of a job with accommodations, they are allowed to apply for and maintain a job.... An employer is responsible for providing the reasonable accommodations necessary for a qualified individual to perform the job" (p. 375). A job coach (answer A) is more appropriate for an individual who needs frequent cueing or assistance to perform her job. Frequent breaks (answer B) are a reasonable accommodation suitable for individuals with anxiety who need to manage stress. Although explaining the problem of distractibility to the employer (answer C) may open the lines of communication with the employer, it does not offer a solution. See Reference: Schell, Gillen, & Scaffa. (2014). Rigby, P., Trentham, B., & Letts, L.: Modifying performance contexts.

170. (D) Dancing to a strong, fast beat. These individuals are demonstrating under-responsiveness, which is characterized by behaviors such as "difficulty paying attention...slow to respond...difficult to engage" (p. 43). Activities can be used to calm or alert. In this case, activities that help to alert would be indicated. Qualities of alerting stimuli can include "fast-paced movement of sound [answer D]...unexpectedness...novelty" (p. 106), to name a few. Activities with qualities such as slow-paced, rhythmic movement (answer A), repetition (answer B), and neutrality (answer C) are more likely to result in calming responses. See Reference: Champagne. (2011). Evaluation and dynamic systems and sensory modulation and intervention.

171. (A) "What might someone who disagrees say?" The goal of cognitive-behavioral therapy (CBT) is for the client to "identify beliefs and thoughts that interfere with desired occupational performance; to learn new beliefs and ways of thinking, feeling, and behaving; and to test and apply that learning with problems that arise in their day-to-day lives. Therapists do not tell their clients what to do; rather, they collaborate with their clients in learning how to think and talk to themselves in ways that support them doing what they want and need to do" (p. 271). Examples of responses that could help this individual revise or create new beliefs include "How could you find out whether that is true? Are there alternative explanations? What might someone who disagrees say?" (answer A) (p. 272). Assuring the individual that her family cares about her (answer B) is an example of the use of encouragement. Although the use of projective techniques, such as poetry (answer C) and mindfulness meditation (answer D), are methods used by occupational therapists for people with depression, they are not examples of CBT. See Reference: Brown & Stoffel. (2011). McCraith, D.B.: Cognitive beliefs.

172. (C) Reassess the patient's vital signs and consider modifying the activity to make it less challenging. The OT should recognize subtle signs of fatigue, such as frustration, slowing down, hurrying to finish, lessening range of motion, and use of substitution movements, which indicate the training level was too difficult and should be downgraded. Other signs include the individual's heart rate exceeding the target heart rate; increase of more than 20 bpm above resting pulse; failure to return to resting heart rate after a 5-minute rest; and systolic pressure that does not increase at all or that increases more than 20 mm Hg from baseline. Stopping the activity (answer A) is necessary if the individual experiences symptoms such as dyspnea, chest pain, lightheadedness, or diaphoresis. The activity should be upgraded (answer B) only when the individual is able to perform the activity without signs of fatigue or cardiac symptoms. Isometric exercises (answer D), which interfere with blood flow through the muscles and create a heightened demand on the cardiovascular system, should not be used in individuals with cardiac conditions. See Reference: Trombly. (2008). Huntley, N.: Cardiac and pulmonary diseases.

173. (B) Provides social interaction and support, as well as activity. Parkinson's disease frequently causes social isolation because of decreased mobility and communication; therefore, group treatment is particularly valuable for these clients (answer B). "Clients have expressed the desire to retain a sense of self and normalcy within their family, even in the face of deteriorating abilities. The focus of intervention is on developing habits and routines to foster participation in desired occupations as the disease progresses.... Involvement in community-based group may provide support needed to accommodate the changes in role and family" (p. 943). Answer A is incorrect because group treatment is not necessarily better for addressing motor problems. Presenting exercise activities (answer C) can be effective in groups, but it would not be the primary reason to select a therapeutic group for clients with Parkinson's disease. Answer D is incorrect because the therapist is responsible for leading a therapeutic group and would not leave until the group session has concluded. See Reference: Pedretti. (2013). Schultz-Krohn, W., Foti, D., & Glogoski, C.: Degenerative diseases of the central nervous system.

174. (A) Flex the child's hips. Flexing the hips breaks up the extensor pattern and, combined with knee flexion, reduces tone in the lower extremities, thus facilitating dressing (p. 503). Flexing more distal joints first (answers B, C, and D) is ineffective in reducing tone and may lead to excessive stress on the joints involved. See Reference: Case-Smith & O'Brien. (2010). Shepherd, J.: Activities of daily living.

175. (A) Standing in a standing frame with knee and hip support. A prone stander (answer A) is the best choice, as "demands on head righting are less in an upright position than in a horizontal position" (p. 546). Answer B is incorrect because, although the chest is supported by a sling, the child's shoulders, arms, and hips must be able to control the position. Answer C, prone over a wedge, is incorrect as explained above. Side-lying (answer B) allows the child to practice only lateral head rights, a component of neck stability that contributes to head control (p. 527); therefore, it is not an optimal choice. See Reference: Hinojosa & Kramer. (2009). Colangelo,

C.A. & Shea, M.: A biomechanical frame of reference for positioning children for functioning.

176. (A) Teaching wheelchair-level techniques. As the disease progresses, individuals with ALS lose the strength required for ambulation, and therefore begin to use wheelchairs, (answer A). "As the client's function declines there is a greater need for environmental support through providing durable medical equipment, modifying the home, and providing adaptive equipment" (p. 921). In phase II of ALS, the client is often prescribed "a power wheelchair if the patient wants to be independent with mobility" (p. 922). The development of meal preparation skills using a wheelchair, such as transportation of items, addressing work heights, using adaptive equipment (answer A encompasses answer B), and safety issues, is therefore the best answer. Gradually increasing standing tolerance (answer C) is not appropriate for this individual because motoric function will continue to deteriorate. Developing competence in preparing cold meals before advancing to hot meals (answer D) is more appropriate for individuals with cognitive or perceptual deficits. See Reference: Pedretti. (2013). Schultz-Krohn, W., Foti, D., & Glogoski, C.: Degenerative diseases of the central nervous system.

177. (B) A mobile arm support. An individual with C5 quadriplegia with fair shoulder flexors and abductors, and at least poor minus biceps, upper trapezius, and external rotators, will be able to operate a mobile arm support (answer B) for self-feeding and facial hygiene activities. "The mobile arm support, also called a ball-bearing feeder, is a mechanical device attached to the wheelchair. This shoulder and elbow support carries the weight of the arm and reduces friction in motion. The mobile arm support can assist the patient in driving the wheelchair, feeding, hygiene and grooming, and carrying out tabletop activities, such as writing and cooking" (p. 1189). A wrist-driven flexor hinge orthosis (answer A) would be used for a lower-level spinal cord injury (C6 to C8), in which the individual had functional use of the shoulder and arm muscles, and has fair plus or better wrist extension strength. This orthosis is indicated for individuals who lack prehension power. An electric self-feeder is indicated for individuals with a higher level of involvement (C4), and who demonstrate poor plus, or weaker, shoulder strength. Built-up utensils may be indicated for individuals with C8 or T1 injuries, because they may lack the strength to tightly grasp regular utensils. See Reference: Trombly. (2008). Atkins, M.S.: Spinal cord injury.

178. (B) Educate employees about ergonomic adaptations. Educating employees on correct positioning and equipment modification would be an ef-

fective way to introduce this population to a change in task methods related to keyboarding that may prevent CTD. Answers A, C, and D are incorrect because they represent interventions that might occur at some point following the onset of CTD. See Reference: Pedretti. (2013). Kasch, M.C. & Walsh, J.M.: Hand and upper extremity injuries.

179. (C) Suggestions for activities in which parents can engage with their child to help the child practice developing skills. Answer C is correct. "Typically, parents hope to receive recommendations for activities that help the child play, for toys that match the child's abilities, and for strategies that lead to independence in self-care" (p. 129). For most pediatric standardized tests, developmental age scores for children with multiple disabilities (answer A) highlight their limitations when compared to typically developing children. When asked, parents expressed that "service providers who focused on the negative aspects of the child's condition or compared the child to typically developing peers were viewed as not supportive" (p. 129). Answers B and D may be provided to families at some point during the intervention process, yet they are not relevant to the needs parents generally have for information to help them support their child's development. See Reference: Case-Smith & O'Brien. (2010). Jaffe, L., Humphry, R., & Case-Smith, J.: Working with families.

180. (D) randomization. Answer D, randomization, is correct, as "true-experimental design refers to the class two-group design in which subjects are randomly selected and randomly (R) assigned to either an experimental or control group condition. Before the experimental condition, all subjects are pretested or observed on a dependent measure (O). In the experimental group the independent variable or experimental condition is imposed (X). Quasi-experimental designs "are characterized by the presence of some type of comparison group and manipulation, but they do not contain random group assignment" (p. 111). See Reference: DePoy & Gitlin. (2011). Experimental-type designs.

181. (A) Referral. A referral, answer A, is a request for OT services. "The physician or other legally qualified professional requests occupational therapy services for the client. The referral may be oral, but a written record is often a necessity. Guidelines for referral vary, and in some situations occupational therapy services may require a physician's referral. The occupational therapist (OT) is responsible for responding to the referral.... State regulatory boards and licensing requirements should be reviewed prior to initiation of services to determine if a referral for service is necessary" (p. 30). Screening (answer B) is the process of observing and collecting information about the individual to determine the need for OT services. Goals (answer C) should be included in OT documentation and should be objective and measurable. Treatment planning (answer D) is the process of analyzing and determining what the individual's problems are and deciding how to solve them. See Reference: Pedretti. (2013). Schultz-Krohn, W. & McHugh Pendleton, A.: Application of the occupational therapy practice framework to physical dysfunction.

182. (C) G8988-CI. Medicare G-codes and severity modifiers must be used when submitting outpatient claims to Medicare. The G-code used for self-care, initial status, is G8987. The G-code used for goal status is G8988, and the G-code used for discharge is G8989. Modifiers indicate the level of functional limitation, and range from CH (0% impaired, limited, or restricted) to CN (100% impaired, limited, or restricted). Because the OT is setting goal status, the G-code used would be G8988. Because the individual is expected to make progress, the modifier used would be earlier in the alphabet, not later. In this case, the correct choice is G8988-CI (answer C). G8987-CI and G8987-CN (answers A and B) are both G-codes used for initial status. G8988-CN (answer D) indicates 100% impairment. See Reference: http://www.cms.gov/Regulations-and-Guidance/Guidance/Transmittals/Downloads/R165BP.pdf

183. (C) Assisting the student in developing a general understanding of client needs. According to AOTA, "The goal of Level I fieldwork is to introduce students to the fieldwork experience, to apply knowledge to practice, and to develop understanding of the needs of clients" (p. 34). Although answers A, B, and D are all significant aspects of student development, they are most representative of the expectations of a level II fieldwork experience. See Reference: AOTA ACOTE Standards. (2011).

184. (C) Program evaluation. Program evaluation (answer C) is an outcome-monitoring system that reflects the results of services on consumers by defining and reviewing the outcomes of care. Some ways of measuring outcomes include looking at "the safety and effectiveness of services rendered to clients as measured by standardized functional measures, rapidity of discharge to a lower level of care, and reduced recidivism. Another set of indicators are related to revenues and whether the program is on budget and meeting financial projections. Follow-up evaluations may include objective measures of outcome appropriate for the client population" (p. 153). Final evaluations of clients involved in the program and client satisfaction surveys (answers A and B) may both be components of the program evaluation. Utilization review (answer D) evaluates the care that is provided to ensure that services were provided in a

necessary, appropriate, and efficient manner. See Reference: Jacobs and McCormack. (2011). Giles, G.M.: Starting a new program, business, or practice.

185. (C) Interpret the results based on data collected. "An occupational therapist initiates and directs the screening, evaluation, and re-evaluation process and analyzes and interprets the data in accordance with federal and state law, other regulatory and payer requirements, and AOTA documents" (p. 4). Once the OT has assigned performance of an evaluation to a OTA, the OT is responsible for analyzing and interpreting the results (answer C). Service competency (answer A) would need to be established prior to the OTA administering the evaluation. Collecting data (answer B) is the responsibility of the OTA in this scenario. Developing the treatment plan (answer D) would follow analysis of the data. See Reference: AOTA Reference Manual of Official Documents. AOTA Guidelines for Supervision 2009.

186. (D) Use the AOTA website to obtain resources about occupational therapy. The emphasis of this question is that it is every OT practitioner's responsibility to promote the profession. Simple, daily public relations activities occur each time an OT practitioner describes the services to be provided to patients and families. More complex public relations may include developing a plan to promote community awareness regarding the profession. "As professionals, we...have the opportunity and responsibility to...work toward continually developing, shaping, and promoting the occupational therapy profession" (p. 1013) See Reference: Schell, Gillen, & Scaffa. (2014). Phipps, S.: Occupational therapy professional organizations.

187. (C) It has a standard format. Answer C is correct, as standardized tests include a "test manual,...fixed number of items,...fixed protocol for administration,...[and] a fixed guideline for scoring" (p. 221). Standardization of a test means that the test is administered in a prescribed manner and that scoring and interpretation of scores also are completed in a prescribed way. The presence of data concerning the test's "norms" and the establishment of reliability and validity (answers A, B, and D) may be, and often are, provided with standardized tests, but are not assumed to be part of the test unless this information is included. See Reference: Case-Smith & O'Brien. (2010). Richardson, P.K.: Use of standardized tests in pediatric practice.

188. (C) Needs assessment. In order to determine the need for services, needs assessment (answer C) is conducted. The needs assessment explores the needs of the targeted population from the perspective of those who work with individuals as well as the individuals themselves. The results of the needs assessment are then used "to guide the establishment of goals and objectives for programming" (p. 118). Needs assessment is the necessary first step of gathering data about a population, treatment needs, and resources available. Program planning (answer A) involves establishing goals and objectives based on the results of the needs assessment. Program implementation (answer B) occurs following program planning and involves coordination, assessment, and intervention selection. Program evaluation (answer D) occurs after implementation, and involves systematic review and analysis of the program based on achievement of program goals. See Reference: Fazio. (2008). Fazio, L.S.: Profiling the community, targeting the population, and assessing the need for services.

189. (C) Use the handout only as a resource while developing the presentation. According to the AOTA Code of Ethics, OT practitioners must "give credit and recognition when using the work of others in written, oral, or electronic media" (p. 9). The options presented in answers A, B, and D do not give the necessary credit to the author for his/her contribution. See Reference: AOTA Code of Ethics.

190. (D) Collaboratively develop an IFSP. Answer D is correct. The service plan required by federal law (IDEA 2004, Part C) and provided through early intervention programs is called an Individualized Family Service Plan. This plan is developed by the family and other team members once evaluations are complete (p. 684). Answers A and B refer to the IEP (Individualized Education Program), a service plan required for children from age 3 to 21. Answer C is incorrect because the IFSP must be developed collaboratively with other team members. See Reference: Case-Smith & O'Brien. (2010). Myers, C.T., Stephens, L., & Tauber, S.: Early intervention.

191. (D) The OT recommends the use of lumbar support and regular performance of home program. The plan section of a discharge summary contains the patient's discharge disposition (e.g., to a nursing home or to outpatient therapy), recommendations for additional therapy or actions on the part of the patient (e.g., outpatient therapy, home health, or performing a home program), equipment needs or equipment provided to the patient, and plans for discharge, answer D. Answer A is a subjective report. Answer B is an example of a statement that belongs in the objective section of a discharge summary. Answer C belongs in the assessment section. See Reference: Pedretti. (2013). Schultz-Krohn, W. & McHugh Pendleton, H.: Application of the occupational therapy practice framework to physical dysfunction.

192. (D) Cross training. "Cross training is the training of a single rehabilitation worker to provide services that would ordinarily be rendered by several different professions. Multiskilling is sometimes used synonymously with cross training but may also mean the acquisition by a single healthcare worker of many different skills. Arguments have been made for and against cross training and multiskilling. The consumer may benefit by having fewer healthcare providers and better integration of services. Involving fewer providers may reduce costs" (p. 42, answer D). Quality improvement (answer A) is a systematic approach to monitoring patient care. Peer review (answer B) is a component of quality improvement. Cost accounting (answer C) is a method of tracking the costs of specific services or costs incurred by diagnosis-specific groups. See Reference: Pedretti. (2013). Schultz-Krohn, W. & McHugh Pendleton, A.: Application of the occupational therapy practice framework to physical dysfunction.

193. (D) The OT recommends strategies that are easily embedded within the student's activities and routines in the curriculum and promote his participation. Answer D is correct. "IDEA 2004 mandates that services be provided in the least restrictive environment" (p. 668). When strategies that enable the student to participate in learning activities can be incorporated into the routine, this method is preferred as the student may continually use them throughout the day. Answers A and B represent approaches that remove the student from his peer group, and this is acceptable only when support cannot be provided in the context of the classroom activities and routines. Answer C is incorrect, as this setting does not represent the opportunities and challenges present in the student's regular classroom experiences. The OT is not able to observe the student's natural performance and promote participation in relevant learning activities. See Reference: Schell, Gillen, & Scaffa, 2014. Swinth, Y.L.: Education.

194. (D) Supportive housing. "Supported housing [answer D] is described as 'independent housing coupled with the provision of community-based mental health services'...[and] staff provide case management, support, and/or rehabilitation in a variety of different housing types, including halfway houses, group homes, and supervised apartments" (p. 476–478). This level of housing meets the criteria for both client choice and appropriate level of assistance. Custodial housing (answer C) would not provide the rehabilitation and social services this individual would require. Assisted living (answer B) is typically an option considered for older adults who require assistance with medication management, light housekeeping, meals, and activities and would provide more structure and assistance than this individual desires. Partial hospitalization (answer A) is an outpatient mental health service for individuals who still need intense daily treatment but not the level of safety provided with inpatient hospitalization. See Reference: Brown & Stoffel. (2011). Pitts, D.B.: Supported housing: Creating a sense of home.

195. (D) Order the lightweight wheelchair and hospital bed. "Generally, Medicare payments are based on the type of service provided.... Part B also covers some durable medical equipment" (p. 1059). Medicare Part B does not typically cover assistive device items such as elevated toilet seats, grab bars, or adaptive equipment because they are not considered to be medically necessary. Answers A, C, and D may all be a part of the broader statement of medical necessity not pertaining to Medicare Part B. Answers B and C are incorrect because they include items that are not considered "durable medical equipment" (e.g., reachers, a shower chair, or a handheld shower). Depending on the patient's medical condition, a bedside commode may be covered. The family may have the option of paying for nonqualifying items out of pocket (answer A) if they choose to. See Reference: Medicare Benefit Policy Manual: Covered medical and other health services, 2009, Available at: http://www.cms.gov/manuals/Downloads/bp102c15.pdf No chapter Medicare link.

196. (D) Job title, employer's expectations, productivity expectations, and how performance will be measured. "The job description describes the essential job functions of the position" (p. 211), and usually contains the title of the job, the employer's expectations, how much productivity is expected, and how the employee's performance will be measured (answer D). Items that are not required but may complement an individualized job description are personality characteristics, past experience requirements, and accomplishments. Previously established mutual goals, quality of patient care, achievement of predicted outcomes, and evidence of relationship building (answer A) are components of a performance review. Answers B and C include items such as references and accomplishments of the candidate that are not typically found in a job description but are more appropriately located on a résumé. See Reference: Jacobs & McCormack. (2011). Fisher, T.F.: Personnel management.

197. (C) Confidentiality, time, and money. Answer C, "concerns about confidentiality and security of medical information...[and] investment in time

and money" (p. 472), contains legitimate concerns related to the implementation of an electronic documentation system (as opposed to the traditional paper and pen form of documentation). Answers A, B, and D are all potential advantages, versus disadvantages, to using an electronic documentation system within a clinical setting. See Reference: Schell, Gillen, & Scaffa. (2014). Sames, K.M.: Documentation in practice.

198. (C) Internal validity. Internal validity is the "ability of the research design to answer the research question accurately.... If a design has internal validity, the investigator can state with a degree of confidence that the reported outcomes are the consequence of the relationship between the independent variable and dependent variable and not the result of extraneous factors" (pp. 90–91). Some of these factors relate to internal validity: history, testing, instrumentation, maturation, regression, mortality, interactive effects. Answers A, B, and D are not representative of internal validity. See Reference: DePoy & Gitlin. (2011). Language and thinking processes.

199. (B) Child's writing, dressing, and self-feeding performance. Answer B is correct. As the therapist prepares a summary report for the school, information should focus on important occupations that are relevant for roles and performance this student will use in the school setting. Education personnel rely on the OT to provide information that helps them include the student in curricular and extracurricular activities (p. 658). Answers A and D describe information that is relevant in overall discharge planning but is not specifically relevant to the information the school district needs from the OT. Answer C is not something the OT could evaluate. See Reference: Schell, Gillen, & Scaffa. (2014). Swinth, Y.L.: Education.

200. (C) Ask whether the company can delay the start date until her license arrives. All OT practitioners must hold a current, updated state license if residing in a licensed state (answer C). According to the AOTA Code of Ethics, Principle 5 (procedural justice) states, "Occupational therapy personnel shall comply with institutional rules, local, state, federal, and international laws and AOTA documents applicable to the profession of occupational therapy" (p. 7). Students completing fieldwork II placements should apply for a temporary license prior to beginning their job search. Answers A, B, and D would all be both unethical and illegal. See Reference: AOTA Code of Ethics. (2010).

Simulation Examination 2

Directions: Circle the correct answer to the following questions. When you have completed this examination, check your answers against the answer key that follows. As you will see, an explanation is given for each answer along with a reference for further study. The book author is listed as well as the chapter author. See the bibliography for complete references. Study the areas in which your comprehension was low, then test yourself again by taking Simulation Examination 3.

EVALUATION

1. An OT measures an individual's elbow PROM three times and gets three different measurements, varying by up to 10 degrees. The BEST action for the therapist to take is to:
- A. check the alignment of the goniometer.
- B. use a larger goniometer.
- C. use a smaller goniometer.
- D. attempt to force the individual's arm further into flexion.

2. An OT practitioner is evaluating assistive technology needs for an adult with severe motor limitations. The OT will MOST likely:
- A. make recommendations for ways of operating the technology.
- B. assist with vocational goals.
- C. seek job placement for the client.
- D. solve mechanical or software problems.

3. A child with autism spectrum disorder craves tactile stimulation, rubbing objects on his arms and legs; however, he avoids being touched by others. This behavior MOST likely indicates a sensory integration problem related to what area?
- A. Sensory modulation.
- B. Sensory registration.
- C. Sensory seeking.
- D. Overresponsiveness.

4. The OT staff in an outpatient facility are developing goals for a new, multidisciplinary work-hardening program. Which of the following goals is MOST appropriate for this program?
- A. ADL retraining to increase the ability to perform household skills independently.
- B. Progressive resistive exercise to increase endurance for self-care skills.
- C. Work simulation and conditioning to increase strength and endurance for work-related skills.
- D. Vocational retraining to increase the ability to reenter the job market.

5. During a perceptual evaluation, an OT practitioner determines that an individual exhibits constructional apraxia, body scheme disturbances, and unilateral neglect. During the functional part of the evaluation, these deficits are MOST likely to be exhibited as self-care difficulties related to:
- A. spatial relations.
- B. dressing apraxia.
- C. anosognosia.
- D. figure-ground discrimination.

6. During an initial session with an individual diagnosed with major depression, the OT observes that the individual is unwashed and dressed in dirty clothing, suggesting obvious ADL performance deficits. What is the BEST evaluation tool to use with this individual?
- A. Functional Independence Measure (FIM).
- B. Skilled observation and closed-ended questions.
- C. Canadian Occupational Performance Measure (COPM).
- D. Family member interview regarding the individual's ADL performance.

7. An individual with an intellectual disability has a job assembling packets that include a plastic knife, fork, and spoon and a napkin. He uses a visual sample for guidance. The OT notes that when he runs out of knives, he continues to assemble the packets anyway, even though they are incomplete. At which of Allen's Cognitive Levels is this individual functioning?

    A. Level 2.
    B. Level 3.
    C. Level 4.
    D. Level 5.

8. The OT is assessing an individual who demonstrates normal range of motion when flexing the elbow, but hyperextends by 15 degrees when the elbow is extended. The practitioner will MOST LIKELY record the measurement as:

    A. −15 to 0 to 140 degrees.
    B. 0 to 140 degrees.
    C. 15 to 140 degrees.
    D. −15 to 120 degrees.

9. During evaluation, an individual who had a severe myocardial infarction 2 weeks ago displays good memory of information processed before the MI, poor recall of the first week after the MI, but good recall of information from the past week. What would be the best way for the OT to document this deficit?

    A. Disorientation.
    B. Impaired long-term memory
    C. Anterograde amnesia.
    D. Retrograde amnesia.

10. An OT is evaluating a school-age child with cerebral palsy. Which procedure should DEFINITELY be included in the process?

    A. Screening of gross and fine motor performance.
    B. The Canadian Occupational Performance Measure.
    C. Interview with child's parent.
    D. Bruininks-Oseretsky Test of Motor Proficiency-2.

11. A child with autism engages in limited and repetitive acts during an occupational therapy evaluation. How would the OT MOST likely document the child's behavior?

    A. The child rocks and bangs his head against the wall throughout the evaluation.
    B. The child frequently cries, without an obvious reason that creates the tearfulness.
    C. The child does not verbally respond to the questions initiated by the OT.
    D. The child does not make eye contact with the OT throughout the evaluation.

12. An OT is determining the level of cognitive function in an individual with an intellectual disability, using the Allen's Cognitive Disability Model. In which way will this be the MOST helpful to the therapist?

    A. Identifying difficult behaviors that might interfere with intervention.
    B. Planning a training program to improve prevocational skills.
    C. Identifying the type of environmental supports that can maximize the client's level of function.
    D. Developing an educational plan to improve social skills.

13. An individual with schizophrenia has worked as a janitor for about a year. The case manager requested an OT consultation when the individual was transferred to an area with carpets and began having difficulty with job performance, specifically vacuuming, reporting that the vacuuming triggered auditory hallucinations. What is the MOST appropriate area for the OT to assess?

    A. Sensory processing.
    B. Cognitive level.
    C. Social participation.
    D. Balance.

14. When completing a screening following the teacher's concern over a third grader's handwriting skill, what is the PRIMARY goal of the OT?

    A. Provide strategies to promote student's fine motor development.
    B. Document the appropriateness of the teacher's referral.
    C. Establish the student's hand skill and penmanship baselines.
    D. Determine the need for further formal evaluation.

15. An individual presents with a visual impairment and complains of cloudiness in the lens of the eye, dulling of colors, and overall blurry vision when performing all tasks. Which of the following is the individual most likely experiencing?

    A. Age-related macular degeneration.
    B. Glaucoma.
    C. Diabetic retinopathy.
    D. Cataracts.

16. A child running in the playground trips and falls forward, landing on outstretched arms. How is this reaction BEST described?

A. Attitudinal reflex.
B. Righting reaction.
C. Equilibrium reaction.
D. Protective extension response.

17. The OT asks an individual with schizophrenia to describe what brought her to the hospital for admission. The individual responds by saying, "I took a cab." How would the OT MOST likely identify this response?

A. Delusional thinking.
B. A distractible response.
C. A concrete response.
D. An insightful response.

18. The director of an assisted living facility has asked an OT to help them develop a falls prevention program. The OT should FIRST:

A. evaluate residents of the facility who have fallen in the past 6 to 12 months.
B. interview facility administration and staff to determine goals for the program.
C. determine how frequently falls occur, how many individuals are affected, and how the problem is currently being addressed.
D. provide the director with a menu of recommendations that will address the problem of falls in the facility and determine a starting point.

19. A newly referred patient complains of frequently dropping lightweight items and reports a numb feeling in both hands. Which of the following instruments is MOST important to use in evaluating this individual?

A. Goniometer.
B. Dynamometer.
C. Pinch gauge.
D. Aesthesiometer.

20. The teacher reports to the OT that a 5-year-old child with Down syndrome and low muscle tone sits only in a "W" sitting position for any floor activity. What does this observation MOST likely indicate?

A. Increased muscle tone in the lower extremities.
B. Need for this position to achieve stability.
C. Lack of control over lower extremity movement.
D. A posture that is typically seen in early motor development.

21. A 3-year-old child demonstrates the ability to use the toilet independently except for wiping and readjusting clothing afterward. This behavior indicates the child is performing at which level?

A. Significantly below age level.
B. Slightly below age level.
C. At age level.
D. Above age level.

22. An OT has been hired to work with clients with mental health conditions in an organization whose philosophy of care is based on the recovery model. What is the MOST appropriate evaluation tool for this population?

A. Making Decisions Empowerment Scale.
B. Comprehensive Occupational Therapy Evaluation.
C. Bay Area Functional Performance Evaluation.
D. Worker Role Interview.

23. An individual confides to the OT practitioner that he is concerned that lower extremity flaccidity may cause problems during sexual activity. After evaluating the client's tone, the BEST strategy to recommend is to:

A. use a side-lying position.
B. use pillows to prop up body parts into the desired position.
C. incorporate slow rocking into movements.
D. avoid movements that elicit a quick stretch.

24. An OT is assessing a 3-year-old child born with fetal alcohol syndrome. In addition to the parent interview, which is the NEXT strategy to gather assessment data?

A. Complete an activities and interests survey with the child.
B. Record the child's developmental milestones on a standardized chart for comparison.
C. Refer to the child's medical records and reports from early intervention services.
D. Watch the child engage in play, eating, and bathing activities.

25. An OT documents that an individual exhibits elbow flexion strength of grade 1. According to the manual muscle test system of letters and numbers, the word that would be the equivalent to grade 1 would be:

A. absent.
B. trace.
C. good.
D. normal.

26. Which of the following questions is most appropriate for evaluating self-awareness in an individual recovering from a brain injury?
   A. "How often do you find yourself forgetting appointments?"
   B. "What would you do if you smelled smoke coming from the kitchen?"
   C. "Are you any different now compared to what you were like before your injury?"
   D. "How would you find out which bus to take in order to get to work by 9 a.m.?"

27. During a mealtime feeding evaluation of an individual who has sustained a brain injury, the OT observes that the client picks up his fork but does not attempt to eat, though the food is accessible and he has expressed that he is hungry. In what area is the individual MOST likely exhibiting problems?
   A. Attention.
   B. Concentration.
   C. Initiation.
   D. Apraxia.

28. An OT observes a child climb into a high chair and jump up and down on the floor. However, when presented with a new rocking horse, the child is unable to mount the horse and ride. This MOST likely indicates a problem in which area?
   A. Muscle strength.
   B. Motor control.
   C. Reflex integration.
   D. Praxis.

29. An individual with a TBI is able to pick up a toothbrush and apply toothpaste independently, but takes 15 minutes to brush his teeth. This behavior most likely indicates difficulty in which of the following areas?
   A. Sequencing.
   B. Following directions.
   C. Problem-solving.
   D. Terminating an activity.

30. An OT practitioner is working with an individual who has tested positive for HIV. The individual accidentally cuts his finger with a knife while helping with a meal preparation activity. Which of the following are the MOST appropriate precautions to follow?
   A. Suicide.
   B. Universal.
   C. Escape from unit.
   D. Medical.

31. At a team meeting, a teacher reports that a child is having difficulty copying letters, completing paper mazes, and using scissors. This behavior MOST likely indicates a problem in which area?
   A. Visual-motor integration.
   B. Visual acuity.
   C. Visual tracking.
   D. Visual discrimination.

32. While completing tasks on a standardized test, the child suddenly becomes uncooperative and complains that the test is "too hard." What is the MOST appropriate response?
   A. Change pace of test activities according to test manual specification.
   B. Terminate the session and score the remaining items at zero points.
   C. Follow administration instructions without deviation.
   D. Adapt the remaining test items to ensure the child's success.

33. In planning the evaluation for an adolescent with psychosocial problems, which is the school-based OT MOST likely to include?
   A. Prevocational and career skills.
   B. Observation in the cafeteria and during classroom free-play period.
   C. Standardized measures of visual-motor performance related to school tasks.
   D. Community mobility checklist.

34. An OT is conducting an interview with a patient upon admission to an inpatient psychiatric unit. The individual answers the questions in an unfocused, tangential manner. In order to get as much information as possible before the session is over, what type of question should the OT incorporate?
   A. Open-ended.
   B. Closed-ended.
   C. Directed.
   D. Double.

35. A child is lacing a series of geometric beads by copying from a stimulus card and is unable to identify a moon-shaped bead when it is turned sideways on the table. What area of visual perception is MOST difficult for the child?
   A. Figure-ground.
   B. Form constancy.
   C. Position in space.
   D. Visual sequencing.

TREATMENT PLANNING

36. An OT practitioner is planning a program to address the needs of persons with Alzheimer's disease, and their families, as part of a hospital outreach program. What area of intervention would be MOST beneficial to maintaining safety and supporting function at home for people in the moderate to severe stages of Alzheimer's disease?

    A. Strength and endurance activities.
    B. Cognitive rehabilitation techniques.
    C. Environmental modification.
    D. Assertiveness skills.

37. When developing play activities for a child with acute juvenile rheumatoid arthritis, what types of activities should the OT avoid?

    A. Light touch.
    B. Vestibular.
    C. Resistive.
    D. Elevated temperatures.

38. An OT is planning intervention for an 11-month-old child who was born 3 months prematurely and spent 2 months in the NICU. When thinking about expectations, how does the therapist need to consider the baby's development?

    A. As an infant who is 8 months old.
    B. As an infant who is 9 months old.
    C. As an infant who is 11 months old.
    D. According to norms for premature infants.

39. An individual in a partial hospitalization program who is interested in obtaining employment is observed grabbing tools from others, acting out of turn, and rejecting feedback. Which of the following occupation-based interventions is MOST appropriate for addressing this individual's skills deficits and preparing him for a work environment?

    A. Operating the photocopy machine in a clerical group.
    B. Handing out trays and utensils to people in a food service group.
    C. Placing books back on the shelves in a library group.
    D. Reconciling income and expenses at the end of the day in a thrift store group.

40. What is a priority in the OT intervention plan for a new student who travels to elementary school using a wheelchair?

    A. Opportunities to practice maneuvering the wheelchair through an obstacle course made of cones.
    B. Plans for routine wheelchair maintenance and subsequent needed repairs.
    C. Training for the school bus driver to ensure that that student travels to school safely and comfortably.
    D. Plans to design and create a writing surface that can be attached to the wheelchair for student's use during seat work.

41. A short-term goal of the treatment plan of a child with cerebral palsy is to improve the ability to manipulate objects during play, and increased flexor tone interferes with the child's ability to grasp objects. What activity would be MOST appropriate to meet this objective?

    A. Building a block tower.
    B. Active release of blocks into a container.
    C. Traction on the finger flexors.
    D. Weight-bearing over a small bolster in prone position.

42. A parent of three young children complains of severe low back pain. What is the BEST way to get a toddler up from the floor onto the changing table for a diaper change?

    A. Carry the child as close to her body as possible.
    B. Lift the child from the floor using a wide base of support, one foot slightly in front of the other.
    C. Lift the child from the floor by bending the knees, not the back.
    D. Have the child climb up onto her lap.

43. A family and their young child are ready to transition from Part C early intervention to a preschool program. Which option will MOST likely support the family in the process?

    A. Home-based OT advises family that services and paperwork differ in preschool so they are prepared to expect changes.
    B. Home-based OT contacts OT at preschool agency and offers to answer any questions after the toddler begins in the preschool.
    C. Preschool staff invite the parent and child to come and visit the preschool before they end their current services.
    D. IFSP team ensures that all paperwork is complete and in the child's file before the anticipated transition date.

44. Which of the following reflects a primary goal area appropriate for wellness programs with the older adult population?
- A. Augmenting strength following strokes.
- B. Increasing overall physical activity levels and fitness.
- C. Enhancing social interactions for depressed elders.
- D. Increasing independent performance of ADL and mobility.

45. An OT is preparing an individual who recently sustained a partial thickness burn injury to perform a home program of positioning and use of orthosis. The MOST appropriate recommendation to prevent deformity would be to:
- A. discontinue the positioning and use of orthosis program upon returning home.
- B. continue the same positioning and use of orthosis program that was indicated at discharge.
- C. continue with the positioning and use of orthosis program only during the day.
- D. continuing with the positioning and use of orthosis program only at night.

46. A 1-year-old boy with delayed motor development recently mastered independent sitting. What is the next significant motor performance his family should expect to see him develop?
- A. Creeping.
- B. Rolling from back to stomach.
- C. Cruising.
- D. Moving from supine to sitting.

47. An OT practitioner is planning a program for an individual who needs to increase shoulder strength, range of motion, and endurance. Which of the following activities is MOST suitable for periodic upgrading?
- A. Blowing up and tying balloons of various sizes.
- B. Shooting a game of balloon darts.
- C. Painting faces on balloons.
- D. Playing balloon volleyball.

48. An OT is teaching several older adult individuals with COPD energy conservation techniques in home-management skills. Following learning principles for older adults, the MOST effective way to present the information would be to:
- A. present all the important principles to be covered together in a single presentation.
- B. keep the presentation loosely structured, rather than highly organized.
- C. attempt to persuade individuals about the importance of those points on which they do not seem to agree.
- D. present important principles in small units that are spaced at a slower than normal pace.

49. The goal for an elderly individual with lower extremity weakness is to be independent with bathing, but this requires the tub to be more accessible to the individual, who uses a walker. Which environmental adaptation(s) would the OT practitioner MOST likely recommend to achieve this?
- A. Tear out the tub and install a walk-in shower.
- B. Install shower doors for privacy and for support getting in and out of the tub.
- C. Provide a transfer tub bench and install grab bars.
- D. Place nonskid decals in the tub and mats on the floor to prevent slipping on the wet floor.

50. An individual who is hospitalized with schizophrenia is attending occupational therapy in order to learn how to manage stress. The OT has decided to use a behavioral approach. Which of the following interventions is the best example of a behavioral approach?
- A. Journaling about situations that produce anxiety.
- B. Reducing auditory stimuli and dimming the lights.
- C. Participating in a deep breathing and muscle relaxation group.
- D. Providing tokens for attendance at an exercise group.

51. In planning a therapeutic dressing intervention for a first-grade child who has Down syndrome, what should the OT consider FIRST?
- A. Adaptive equipment.
- B. Adaptive clothing.
- C. Proper positioning.
- D. Adapted teaching techniques.

52. When planning an intervention, what is an important consideration to help the OT establish a positive, therapeutic relationship with a group of middle school youth in an inner-city afterschool program?

    A. Contracts to establish expectations, written in age-appropriate language.

    B. Verbal and nonverbal language and physical contact with the students.

    C. Culturally sensitive rewards and reinforcements for students who attend groups.

    D. Inclusion of older students in the group to serve as role models for the middle schoolers.

53. A long-term goal for an individual with back pain is to be able to return to work as an illustrator, which requires long periods of sitting. Which of the following is the BEST example of a short-term goal for this individual?

    A. Client will draw sitting at a worktable.

    B. Client will draw for 1 hour, taking stretch breaks every 20 minutes.

    C. Instruct client in stretching techniques to be performed every 20 minutes.

    D. Instruct client in the use of proper body mechanics that apply to prolonged sitting.

54. An OT has recommended strategies for use throughout the school day to support a young child with autism to participate in learning activities. When designing the plan to collect data regarding the effectiveness of the intervention, what must the OT include?

    A. Confirmation that the teacher approves the plan.

    B. A time line to readminister standardized tests.

    C. Documentation that the intervention was implemented as planned.

    D. Criteria for modifying the intervention.

55. The OT's intervention plan is focused on developing executive function to help a 17-year-old student with autism spectrum disorder increase his organization and work habits for greater success in the high school curriculum. What type of activities would the OT program MOST likely include?

    A. Visual attention, memory skills, and problem-solving.

    B. Tactile and proprioceptive input while the student makes a goal-directed, adaptive response.

    C. Leisure and high interest activities into which problem-solving tasks are embedded.

    D. Identification of own strengths, anticipating challenges and strategies that support performance.

56. An OT is working with a group of 3-year-old children in a preschool setting. The OT has decided to initiate a group that facilitates symbolic play. Which would be the MOST appropriate activity to introduce first?

    A. Scissors and cutting activities with construction paper.

    B. Jump-rope games with complex footwork.

    C. Make-believe group with stuffed animals and imaginary friends.

    D. Building towers with blocks that resemble pictures in books.

57. An outpatient OT has administered, scored, and interpreted data from interview, observation, and assessments. What is the FIRST step in developing recommendations for the child?

    A. Describe and prioritize the child's problem and needs.

    B. Document evaluation findings in a language and manner that are useful for team members, including the child's parents.

    C. Consider the roles and occupations required for this child and develop recommendations that increase the child's competence in these areas.

    D. Analyze the effects of the child's difficulty on developmental tasks and performance.

58. An OT has received an order to evaluate an individual who is 2 days post-total hip arthroplasty and expected to be discharged to home in 2 days. What areas are MOST important to address prior to discharge?

    A. Cognitive and perceptual functioning.

    B. Work, self-care, and leisure performance.

    C. Upper and lower extremity strength, ROM, and coordination.

    D. Adaptive equipment needs and assistance from others.

59. A homeless individual with mental illness has recently begun coming to a shelter. Which type of group is MOST likely to engage this individual?

    A. Highly structured craft group.

    B. Volunteer activity group.

    C. Simple meal preparation group.

    D. Social skills group.

60. An OT is leading a group for individuals who have difficulty coping with chronic pain. Based on a cognitive-behavioral frame of reference, with which of the following steps would the therapist BEGIN?

A. Providing the individuals with information on activity pacing to minimize pain.

B. Developing awareness about how thoughts and behaviors affect one's perceptions of and ability to cope with pain.

C. Practicing relaxation techniques to be used when the individual is experiencing stress.

D. Setting up a method to monitor and report on how successful the individual's use of recommended techniques was at home.

61. An OT working on laundry skills with an adult with cognitive disabilities has determined that the individual is unable to recognize or judge when clothing is dirty. What is the NEXT step that should be taken to maximize the individual's independence in doing laundry?

A. Instruct the individual to wear clothes for 2 days and then to launder those items.

B. Assess the individual's ability to recognize dirty clothing.

C. Recommend that the individual take clothes to the dry cleaner rather than wash them at home.

D. Recommend to the staff that they do the individual's laundry from now on.

62. A client presents with post-cerebrovascular accident edema in her dominant hand. The OT has introduced a manual edema mobilization (MEM) method in attempts to activate the lymphatic system. Which of the following is most representative of what the OT would perform via the MEM program?

A. Retrograde massage, use of orthosis, and positioning.

B. Massage, compression bandaging, exercise, and external compression.

C. Ultrasound, fluidotherapy, and AROM.

D. Elevation, use of orthosis, PROM, and desensitization.

63. An OT consulting with a community center is developing a club for youth at risk for violence, with the primary goal of engaging the children in meaningful occupations designed to build their participation in community enhancement. Which activity is MOST consistent with this goal?

A. Develop a community-based chess competition.

B. Plant flower seeds in small pots to be taken home once they sprout.

C. Provide a psychoeducational intervention on anger management.

D. Convert an empty lot filled with trash into a community garden.

64. An individual with Alzheimer's disease has limitations in shoulder range of motion. The OT goal for this individual is to improve active shoulder motion in order to resume self-care activities. Which strategy would be MOST effective in actively engaging the individual?

A. Telling the individual to perform repetitions of active UE range-of-motion exercises independently.

B. Training the individual to use long-handled adaptive devices to compensate for decreased shoulder motion.

C. Incorporating simple, familiar activities such as hanging up clothing or catching a ball.

D. Instructing the caregivers to perform PROM exercises on the individual.

65. A construction worker reports experiencing severe anxiety when climbing ladders. The OT has only received authorization for one session to work on a self-management strategy that the individual can use to reduce anxiety while on the job. What is the MOST appropriate strategy to teach this client?

A. Autogenic training.

B. Meditation.

C. Deep breathing.

D. Progressive muscle relaxation.

66. An OT practitioner is instructing an individual with a total hip replacement (posterior lateral approach) how to perform a passenger-side car transfer. Which of the following is the BEST method for entering the car?

A. Stand the body parallel to the car, hold on to a stable section of the car, lift and place the involved leg into the car, and slowly sit and follow with opposite leg.

B. Back up the body to the passenger seat, hold on to a stable section of the car, extend the involved leg, and slowly sit in the car.

C. Back up the body to the passenger seat, hold on to a stable section of the car, flex both legs simultaneously, and slowly sit in the car.

D. Back up the body to the passenger seat, hold on to a stable section of the car, flex the involved leg, and slowly sit in the car.

67. The school-based OT meets with the classroom teacher to gain information to help plan services for a student with learning disabilities in the middle school general education curriculum. The IEP includes occupational therapy to support the student's participation in the language arts curriculum. Which question is MOST likely to elicit useful information that will also promote collaboration for the student's benefit?

A. What are you most concerned about with this student's performance in the language arts curriculum?

B. Does the student perform better on spelling tests when answers are typed rather than written?

C. Are the student's parents in favor of moving to computer use for assignments that require a good deal of written expression?

D. What is the student's approach when writing an outline that will guide a short research report?

68. An OT is working with a medically stable child who sustained bilateral upper extremity, partial-thickness burns 3 days ago while playing with a lighter. Which ADL intervention should the OT introduce FIRST?

A. Instruct the child to use adapted equipment for all ADLs.

B. Encourage independent compression garment application.

C. Perform bilateral upper extremity PROM exercises twice a day.

D. Encourage independent ADLs with minimal reliance on adapted utensils and tools.

69. The OT is working with an individual who is in recovery and about to be discharged from an inpatient substance abuse program. The patient's goals are to find a place to live and abstain completely from alcohol use. What is the MOST appropriate information for the OT to provide as part of the discharge planning process?

A. How to manage medication and a schedule.

B. The elements of the recovery model and its importance.

C. Healthy leisure participation and Alcoholics Anonymous.

D. Group homes that use a harm reduction model and availability.

70. An OT has been asked to perform an ergonomic evaluation and provide ergonomic interventions to a job site where the rate of cumulative trauma disorders is unusually high. Which of the following actions BEST addresses this request?

A. Introduce relaxation seminars for employees to decrease stress while on the job.

B. Treat corporate clients for cumulative trauma disorders.

C. Provide work-simulation activities.

D. Suggest furniture and accessories that promote better positioning at work.

71. A child with autism spectrum disorder presents as clumsy and has difficulty with moving through space and executing efficient gross motor control. The OT can BEST support this child through which approach?

A. Look at pictures of children playing on an obstacle course and talk about what they are doing with this child just prior to beginning the activity.

B. Include ample opportunities for practice and repetition in parts of an obstacle course before trying multiple segments together.

C. Prior to beginning, remind the child about what an obstacle course is and demonstrate various ways of moving through its segments.

D. Limit tactile sensory experiences in the obstacle course segments, preferring primarily vestibular experiences.

72. An orthotic for an individual with carpal tunnel syndrome should position the wrist in:

A. no more than 20 degrees of extension.

B. 10 degrees of flexion.

C. 5 to 10 degrees of extension.

D. 10 to 15 degrees of extension.

73. An individual is participating in an assertiveness training group within a psychiatric rehabilitation program. In what area is the individual MOST likely to improve?

    A. Engaging in relevant conversations with coworkers.

    B. Using appropriate facial expressions when disagreeing with coworkers.

    C. Expressing disagreement with coworkers in a productive manner.

    D. Using courteous behavior when disagreeing with coworkers.

74. During intervention planning, before the OT develops goals and objectives for a 6-year-old child with autism spectrum disorder, what other steps need to be completed?

    A. Identify a practice model and frame of reference and select intervention activities.

    B. Engage in the clinical reasoning process to identify priorities for this student.

    C. Collaborate with other team members to develop long-term goals and project duration of services.

    D. Review school's requirements to understand the preferred format and style for goal writing.

75. What principles are MOST important to include when training an individual in joint protection?

    A. Using the strongest joint and avoiding positions of deformity.

    B. Preparing muscles and joints with massage before exercise.

    C. Practicing vivid imagery and relaxation exercises during difficult functional activities.

    D. Applying heat before treatment and cold after range-of-motion treatment.

76. Specific recommendations have been made for electronic assistive technology for an adult with muscular dystrophy. After the devices are ordered and modified as necessary, the NEXT step in the process of implementation is for the OT practitioner to:

    A. assess how well the whole system works.

    B. evaluate whether the assistive technology devices match the needs of the client.

    C. train the client in the operation of the assistive technology system and in strategies for its use.

    D. determine whether funding is available for the recommended assistive technology.

77. An OT is working with an individual who has dysphagia. What should the OT anticipate that the individual will have difficulty doing?

    A. Coordinating the two sides of the body.

    B. Expressing him- or herself orally.

    C. Swallowing crushed ice.

    D. Speaking clearly.

78. An OT is working with a family and their 1-month-old infant who have just enrolled in early intervention. Which is MOST likely a first step in her initial home visit?

    A. Update the developmental assessment completed 2 weeks ago by the evaluation team to establish current baseline.

    B. Ask the parents to describe the infant's daily schedule and identify routines that are going well and those that are challenging.

    C. Confirm the parents' schedule and review the dates of planned visits for months before the next Quarterly Review.

    D. Handle the infant to assess muscle tone and provide visual, touch, and movement stimuli to observe sensory responses.

79. A toddler with feeding difficulties due to limited oral motor control and oral defensiveness now demonstrates the ability to eat dry cereals with milk. How would the OT progress the child's diet?

    A. Applesauce and mashed bananas.

    B. Cut-up meats and sandwiches.

    C. Strained fruits and vegetables.

    D. Scrambled eggs and pureed bacon.

80. Based on evaluation data, the IEP team has developed goals for a new student with autism spectrum disorder and is now developing a service plan. Which represents the MOST likely next step?

    A. Team leader identifies the classrooms in the school district that are available for students with autism.

    B. IEP team leader describes the services the school typically provides to students with similar needs.

    C. Family and other team members discuss the service options to identify those that match established priorities and support student's achievement.

    D. IEP team approves services that are available in the school and refers the family to community resources for those they cannot provide.

81. Which of the following community activities provides an appropriate level of challenge for a client BEGINNING assertiveness training?

- A. Asking a store salesperson for information about an item before buying it.
- B. In a restaurant, requesting that food be sent back to be rewarmed.
- C. Returning an item to a department store for cash with the receipt.
- D. Questioning a waitress about whether a restaurant bill is accurate.

82. Which type of play is the OT MOST likely encouraging during a play period with blocks in the preschool?

- A. Construction play.
- B. Symbolic play.
- C. Social play.
- D. Recreational play.

83. An OT practitioner is starting an inpatient group for individuals with schizophrenia whose psychosis has been controlled through medication, but who continue to display negative symptoms, including difficulty sustaining attention, limited ability to express feelings and ideas, depressed affect, and low interest and energy levels. Which type of activities would the OT be MOST likely to plan for the members of the group at this beginning stage?

- A. Skill-building activities with concrete goals, such as time management training.
- B. Self-management activities, such as relaxation training.
- C. Expressive/projective activities such as journal writing.
- D. Verbal activities such as discussing movies or current events.

84. An OT in a residential community mental health setting is planning activities for clients within a psychodynamic frame of reference. Which of the following types of activities would the practitioner would be MOST likely to use?

- A. Activities designed to explore and express feelings.
- B. Activities matched to the specific cognitive level of group members.
- C. Activities that can serve as reinforcers for desired behaviors.
- D. Activities that can teach the use of problem-solving strategies.

85. A 3-year-old child with Down syndrome is dependent in all areas of dressing. When using a developmental approach with this child, which skill should FIRST be addressed?

- A. Pulling shoes off feet.
- B. Putting on a T-shirt.
- C. Removing sweat pants.
- D. Putting on hat.

86. An OT is working on keyboarding activities with an individual with asymmetrical muscle tone who keeps falling to the side while sitting in a wheelchair. Which adaptation would MOST effectively stabilize the upper body in a midline position?

- A. Change to a reclining wheelchair.
- B. Use an arm trough.
- C. Provide lateral trunk support.
- D. Attach lateral pelvic support.

87. Following a brain injury, an individual complains she is unable to concentrate on balancing her checkbook for more than a few minutes. What is the most appropriate intervention using a strategy training approach?

- A. Make sure the desk is free of clutter before balancing the checkbook.
- B. Ask questions such as "What am I currently doing?" and "What am I supposed to do next?"
- C. Turn off television, music, and phone alerts.
- D. First calculate all additions to the account, then calculate all subtractions from the account.

INTERVENTION

88. A first-grade student has difficulty completing seated tabletop activities in the classroom because of limited sitting balance. Which should the OT provide to promote postural adjustments in sitting?

- A. Sturdy chair without armrests while the child completes seat work.
- B. Corner floor seat with built-in desk surface while the child eats lunch.
- C. Bolster for back support while the child colors.
- D. Air-filled cushion on the child's seat during seat work periods.

89. An OT is working with a client with a C4 spinal cord injury to determine the best way for him to operate a power wheelchair. What is the MOST effective recommendation for the OT to make?

    A. No assistive device would be suitable for a C4 spinal cord injury.

    B. Head, chin, or breath-control device.

    C. Generator/battery backup device.

    D. Mouth stick.

90. An OT is working with a group of children in a preschool program. All of the children in the group are able to sit independently on the floor except for one child with cerebral palsy. The child has told the OT that he wants to sit on the floor with his peers and not in his wheelchair during morning circle time. What would the OT MOST likely recommend for the child to use?

    A. Hammock seat.

    B. Floor sitter.

    C. Wheelchair insert.

    D. Prone stander.

91. An OT practitioner is instructing an individual with left hemiplegia how to remove a pullover shirt. The correct sequence is:

    A. (1) remove shirt from unaffected arm; (2) remove shirt from affected arm; (3) gather shirt up at the back of the neck; and (4) pull gathered-back fabric off over head.

    B. (1) remove shirt from affected arm; (2) remove shirt from unaffected arm; (3) gather shirt up at the back of the neck; and (4) pull gathered-back fabric off over head.

    C. (1) gather shirt up at the back of the neck; (2) pull gathered-back fabric off over head; (3) remove shirt from affected arm; and (4) remove shirt from unaffected arm.

    D. (1) gather shirt up at the back of the neck; (2) pull gathered-back fabric off over head; (3) remove shirt from unaffected arm; and (4) remove shirt from affected arm.

92. The OT is teaching the parents of a child with spastic quadriplegia how to effectively position the child sitting in a wheelchair so that participation in family tabletop games is facilitated. What is the OT MOST likely to recommend?

    A. Keep the head upright.

    B. Place arms on the armrests.

    C. Ensure the back is straight.

    D. Secure the pelvis in the seat.

93. An OT is using leather stamping as part of a group activity for individuals with neurological deficits and needs to increase the degree of problem-solving demand within the group. What is the BEST approach for encouraging problem-solving in a craft media group?

    A. Teach them to break the activity down into smaller, more manageable steps.

    B. Begin with gross motor activities and progress to fine motor activities.

    C. Structure the number and kinds of choices available.

    D. Gradually increase the time used in the activity by 15-minute increments.

94. An individual with chronic regional pain syndrome (CRPS) has been referred to occupational therapy in order to return to work as an administrative assistant in an educational environment. The client has expressed that returning to work is the primary goal, but has concerns about being able to perform all of the required tasks due to pain. Using a Model of Human Occupation approach, on what should OT intervention focus?

    A. Job retraining for a more appropriate position.

    B. Strategies to promote resumption of the worker role.

    C. Voice-activated software and environmental adaptations.

    D. Communication and assertiveness training.

95. An OT is working with a client who recently had a myocardial infarction and fatigues easily. The long-term goal is to be able to dress independently while applying energy conservation techniques. Which statement is the BEST example of a short-term goal?

    A. The patient will demonstrate energy conservation techniques during performance of all ADLs 100% of the time.

    B. The patient will perform lower extremity dressing with assistance for shoes and socks.

    C. The patient will perform lower extremity dressing with verbal cuing for energy conservation techniques 50% of the time.

    D. Instruct patient in the use of energy conservation techniques that apply to dressing.

96. An OT is working with an individual who is preparing for discharge from a psychiatric facility. The patient has been repeatedly readmitted to the hospital when acute symptoms emerged after forgetting to take prescribed medication on a regular basis. Which one of the following approaches to medication adherence would be most appropriate?

  A. A psychodynamic approach to help her address the stigma related to taking her meds.
  B. A psychoeducational approach to teach her about the medications she needs to take.
  C. An environmental approach that provides an auditory cue when it is time to take her medications.
  D. A cognitive-behavioral approach that addresses the patient's attitudes about taking medications with negative side effects.

97. An OT is planning to begin work on self-care activities with an individual who recently had a traumatic brain injury and who has cognitive and visual-perceptual impairments. What is the MOST effective way for the OT to present directions during the activity?

  A. Tell the patient about the activity he will be working on and ask him to begin.
  B. Rely on facial expressions and body gestures, rather than words, to get the patient started.
  C. State simple, concrete directions allowing time for delayed responses.
  D. Provide a written list of steps with pictures for the patient to follow.

98. Which one of the following is the BEST bathing technique for an individual with chronic obstructive pulmonary disease and low endurance?

  A. Tub bathing with hot water.
  B. Standing for a quick shower.
  C. Using a bath chair with the door open.
  D. Tub bathing using lukewarm water.

99. An individual diagnosed with borderline personality disorder tells an OT that she is the only one she can trust. The next day, she accuses the therapist of lying to her. What is the BEST way for the OT to respond?

  A. Tell the individual her feelings have been hurt.
  B. Remain matter of fact and consistent in approach.
  C. Ask the individual how she felt when lied to in the past.
  D. Apologize and try to determine how the misunderstanding occurred.

100. A child with ataxic CP exhibits tremors in the upper extremities. When she feeds herself, tremors cause most of the food to fall off the swivel spoon before it reaches her mouth. Which adaptations should the OT recommend?

  A. Replace the spoon with a blunt-ended fork.
  B. Build up the handle of the swivel spoon.
  C. Provide hand-over-hand assistance.
  D. Bend the spoon handle at a 45-degree angle.

101. When structuring intervention to promote sensory modulation for a child with tactile defensiveness, what is the BEST initial approach?

  A. Apply intense light touch stimulation, such as tickling on the abdomen, for desensitization.
  B. Avoid all forms of tactile stimulation to accommodate the child's preferences.
  C. Allow the child to self-apply tactile stimuli to maximize the child's tolerance.
  D. Eliminate all deep-pressure tactile stimuli to decrease defensiveness.

102. An OT is working with a group of individuals who present with decreased strength due to a variety of issues related to deconditioning. The OT plans to invite them to participate in aquatic therapy one day a week as the environment of a pool has the potential to decrease:

  A. hypersensitivity.
  B. proprioception.
  C. edema.
  D. gravitational force.

103. An OT is explaining to a teacher about high-technology that can be used to help a student with multiple disabilities to communicate in the classroom. Which intervention would the OT MOST likely recommend for this child?

  A. Environmental control unit.
  B. Wanchik writer.
  C. Head pointer.
  D. Augmentative communication device.

104. A local business has hired an OT to assist with needs related to the Americans with Disabilities Act to determine reasonable accommodations and whether an employee is considered as a Qualified Individual with a Disability (IWD). Which of the following BEST represents an individual who would qualify as IWD?

 A. The individual has a broken leg from a car accident.
 B. The individual has a physical or mental impairment that substantially limits major life activities and has a history of having had such an impairment.
 C. The individual has a history of knee or hip replacement.
 D. The individual has reported to be a user of illegal drugs and alcohol, which interfere with the ability to perform worker roles.

105. An OT practitioner is performing a home management evaluation of an ambulatory individual with cerebral palsy who is cognitively intact but exhibits an ataxic gait pattern. The PRIMARY focus of the evaluation should be:

 A. safety and stability.
 B. the individual's ability to reach and bend.
 C. whether the individual has adequate strength to perform homemaking tasks.
 D. fatigue and endurance levels.

106. An OT is working with a 4-year-old child who has significant hearing loss. The child also demonstrates decreased fine motor coordination when compared with typically developing children her age. Which activity would the OT MOST likely implement to address these needs?

 A. Parachute activities to provide vestibular input, alert the child, and encourage gross motor practice.
 B. Dressing practice with child's right and left shoes color coded to compensate for decreased reception of verbal cues.
 C. Introduce the child to other children via socialization groups to increase social interaction and game playing.
 D. Play hide-and-seek with clay balls in which the child "digs" for various coins and then places them in a piggy bank.

107. An OT places a 6-month-old-infant in the supine position and arranges attractive toys overhead to provide an opportunity to work against gravity. This position will MOST likely encourage antigravity movement of:

 A. shoulder flexion and protraction.
 B. shoulder extension and retraction.
 C. head control.
 D. trunk control.

108. An OT is providing instruction to caregivers in a long-term care facility about how to assist a resident whose severe attention span deficits impair the ability to participate in self-feeding. The therapist is MOST likely to recommend which method?

 A. Demonstrating the feeding process.
 B. Providing verbal feedback.
 C. Providing hand-over-hand assistance.
 D. Using backward chaining.

109. An individual with a low back injury lives alone and must be able to do laundry independently. To prevent reinjury, what should the OT instruct the individual to do?

 A. Place the clean laundry basket on the floor next to a chair and sit for folding.
 B. Stop the activity when pain becomes severe.
 C. Divide the laundry into several small loads for carrying.
 D. Carry the laundry in one or two large loads.

110. An OT is educating a client who presents with weakness in the left hand due to a CVA about the possibility of using a dynamic orthosis, such as the SaeboFlex™, during feeding and grooming tasks. The SaeboFlex™ would assist the client to do which of the following?

 A. Grasp and release objects such as a fork or toothbrush.
 B. Lift heavy cookware without pain.
 C. Reach above (over 90 degrees of shoulder flexion) to place dishes and cups into overhead cabinets.
 D. Flex and extend the elbow in order to brush hair.

111. What are the PRIMARY functions of an OT leading a therapeutic group in the beginning stages of group development?

    A. Set the atmosphere, model appropriate behavior, and develop the rules.

    B. Facilitate expression of feelings and conflict resolution.

    C. Provide balance between support and confrontation, and encourage new skills.

    D. Reinforce change and how it can apply to everyday life.

112. An OT is conducting an ongoing assertiveness training group. Which of the following strategies would be MOST helpful in facilitating group cohesion and exchange of feedback among group members?

    A. Define assertiveness, passivity, and aggression for the group members.

    B. Encourage all group members to release their aggressive feelings physically and verbally toward inanimate objects.

    C. Demonstrate commonly used assertiveness techniques to the group members.

    D. Encourage group members to share similar experiences and reactions with each other.

113. A child with limited sitting balance is unable to put on and remove lower extremity clothing. Which approach BEST addresses this functional issue?

    A. Teach the child to dress in a side-lying position.

    B. Add loops to the waistbands of pants and skirts.

    C. Use hook and loop fasteners in place of zippers.

    D. Teach the child to dress in a standing position.

114. A child is on a pureed diet because of an inability to chew food. What would be the MOST effective method to facilitate the child's ability to chew?

    A. Encourage removal of food from spoon with teeth.

    B. Stimulate texture management with vegetable soup.

    C. Use infant mesh feeder bag.

    D. Place a raisin between child's teeth.

115. An OT practitioner is initiating training with a worker with an intellectual disability. The game packaging task involves first putting a pencil in a box, followed by putting a score pad in the box. Which of the following reinforcement schedules would be used initially to achieve the goal of learning this task sequence?

    A. Intermittent reinforcement with correct responses.

    B. Reinforcement every 10 minutes.

    C. Reinforcement for every fourth correct response.

    D. Continuous reinforcement of correct responses.

116. An OT is working with a 17-year-old girl with impaired mobility, dexterity, and communication skills. The teenager has low average cognitive abilities. Which would the OT MOST likely recommend to the family regarding emergency alert systems in the event of a fire?

    A. Position a wireless cell phone within the girl's reach.

    B. Establish an exit routine in order to get out of the house quickly in the event of a fire.

    C. Review "fire prevention within the home" literature.

    D. Recommend that the girl wear an emergency alert system pendant around her neck.

117. An OT is working with an individual who has COPD and has become severely deconditioned. During the OT evaluation, the patient identified a goal to be able to prepare meals for the family, along with a strong interest in woodworking. How can the OT incorporate this interest into a plan to increase strength and endurance for meal preparation?

    A. Assemble presanded pieces of a wooden ship while standing at a worktable for increasingly longer periods of time.

    B. Sand, assemble, and stain parts of a wooden birdhouse, starting out with 2-pound wrist weights.

    C. Select a small wooden kit activity that can be sanded and painted in one session, alternating between sitting and standing.

    D. Sand pieces for a three-piece stool using an incline board, gradually raising the angle of the incline.

118. The OT is working with an individual who experiences panic attacks when near dogs, and it has begun to interfere with socialization. Using a cognitive-behavioral approach, what is the BEST way for the OT to help this individual handle this challenge?

A. Select a picture of a calm, gentle dog, then practice mentally shifting from the image of a scary dog to the image of the gentle dog.

B. Help to identify strategies that will allow avoidance of dogs in everyday life.

C. Provide instruction of how to use mindfulness when she is in the presence of dogs.

D. Start by touching a therapy dog for just one second, then gradually transition to petting the dog for increasingly longer periods of time.

119. A child has difficulty controlling food in her mouth when swallowing. In helping the parents plan snacks, what would the OT MOST likely recommend?

A. Tapioca pudding.

B. Peanut butter.

C. Carrot sticks.

D. Pudding.

120. During the clean-up portion of a cooking activity, an elderly woman with a diagnosis of depression and dementia begins to dry the plates and utensils she has already dried. What should the OT do NEXT?

A. Tell the client that the same dishes and utensils are being redried.

B. Put the dried dishes away and begin to hand her wet dishes.

C. Suggest the client stop the activity because it seems too difficult.

D. Ask the client to describe what she is doing.

121. An infant born 12 weeks prematurely has a history of multiple medical issues, including retinopathy of prematurity, mechanical ventilation for 5 weeks, and poor feeding skills. The infant is now chronologically 4 months old (1-month adjusted age). She is a medically stable and engaging infant, with a G-tube and oxygen supplement of 2 liters by nasal cannula. What is the MOST appropriate intervention to provide at this time?

A. Teach parent positioning and handling to promote motor development.

B. Instruct parent how to perform PROM of all extremities.

C. Include family's concerns into recommended caregiving practices.

D. Provide interventions that incorporate multi-sensory stimulation.

122. An individual with chronic mental illness is moving into a group home and would like to learn to take a bus to a friend's home three stops away. In the first training session, the OT accompanies the client to the bus stop and onto the bus, demonstrates how to pay, points out when they have arrived at their destination and walks with the client from the bus stop to the friend's home. Using the scaffolding approach, which one of the following should the OT do differently during the next training session?

A. Stand back while the client pays for the ride.

B. Encourage the client to walk from the point of disembarkation to his friend's home independently.

C. Teach the client to recognize the first, last, and intervening bus stops on the map inside the bus.

D. Instruct the friend to watch from the window until the client is able to get to the house independently.

123. Which activity is MOST appropriate to recommend for vocational skills training of high school students with severe learning disabilities who are developing skills for community-based employment?

A. Stocking the shelves at a local grocery.

B. Packaging items in a local sheltered workshop.

C. Cleaning the school cafeteria after lunch.

D. Role-playing interviews with a mentor.

124. An OT is working with an elderly patient with mild to moderate severity of Alzheimer disease who was admitted to the hospital after accidentally setting a kitchen fire. What is the MOST appropriate information to provide caregivers with after discharge regarding cooking?

A. Recommend outpatient OT services to teach kitchen safety.

B. Seek volunteer companion services for home supervision.

C. Identify transportation services to bring the person to a community meal site.

D. Refer to home-delivered meal services.

125. A high-functioning 10-year-old child with a behavior disorder has an innately difficult temperament. Which treatment approach is MOST appropriate for the OT to initiate?

A. Utilize time-out consistently in response to maladaptive behavior in the classroom.

B. Help the child develop cognitive strategies for anxiety-producing activities.

C. Help care providers develop an unpredictable routine to promote problem-solving strategies.

D. Provide a play environment in which the parent and child can act out conflicts.

126. The OT is working on lower body dressing with an individual who is s/p CVA and has some residual cognitive deficits. When using a forward chaining approach to dressing with pajama bottoms, how should the OT begin?

A. Using hand over hand, allow the client to complete as much of the activity as possible.

B. Guide the client to position the pajama bottoms in front and insert one leg.

C. Assist the client with all but the very last step of the activity.

D. Review all the steps of the activity prior to beginning.

127. Which one of the following individuals would MOST likely need a transfer board?

A. An individual who is unable to follow commands.

B. An individual who cannot bear weight on the lower extremities.

C. An individual who has good lower extremity strength but is fearful of fatigue.

D. An individual who is able to perform a stand-pivot transfer.

128. An OT is working with a 12-year-old whose upper extremity physical disabilities limit the ability to independently read books while lying in bed. What would be the BEST adaptation for this child who enjoys book reading before sleep?

A. Teach the child how to use a book holder and mouth stick.

B. Fabricate an adapted book holder for use in his bed.

C. Purchase talking books related to the student's areas of interest.

D. Have the child's parent read a book the child selects each night.

129. A 4-year-old child with ADHD exhibits visual inattention and perceptual deficits that interfere with completing classroom worksheets. What activity would the OT MOST likely recommend for this child to train visual attention?

A. Playing a game in which images are matched by memory.

B. Assembling a 200-piece puzzle.

C. Finding "Waldo" against a complex visual background.

D. Blowing cotton balls into a target.

130. A preteen with a history of TBI is relearning how to prepare simple foods but has been having difficulties with sequencing. The OT has provided her with a chart of steps to follow and she has just learned to prepare her favorite sandwich without "losing her place" in the process. She continues to require occasional verbal cues to look at the chart and to ensure safety. At this point, how would her level of independence be documented?

A. Independent.

B. Independent with setup.

C. Supervision.

D. Minimal assist.

131. An individual with severe and persistent mental illness and no work experience has indicated a strong interest in paid employment. Following evaluation, the OT determines the client is not ready for mainstream employment. What is the NEXT step in progressing the client toward the goal of mainstream employment?

A. Transitional employment.

B. Sheltered employment.

C. Income requirements determination.

D. Job coach identification.

132. The IEP team is developing long-range planning for a student with moderate intellectual disabilities. Given the student's learning capacities, what will MOST likely be learned?

A. Perform school skills at a middle school level.

B. Understand basic concepts related to money.

C. Perform mathematic operations that use simple division.

D. Write an accurate short story about his summer vacation.

133. A child with attention deficit-hyperactivity disorder (ADHD), hyperactivity type, is receiving occupational therapy to increase his attention span. Keeping this in mind, the OT introduces a construction activity. When a puzzle with many pieces is placed in front of the child, the child sweeps many of them to the floor and starts throwing the remaining ones around the room. How can the OT MOST effectively restructure the activity to facilitate a successful experience for this child?

A. Use soft foam puzzle pieces.

B. Provide puzzle pieces of one color only.

C. Use larger interlocking puzzle pieces.

D. Present only a few puzzle pieces at a time.

134. **An OT is planning to review kitchen activities with an individual who underwent a total hip replacement and is to return home tomorrow. Because the chart says that this person is toe-touch weight-bearing (TTWB), how will the weight-bearing restriction impact participation in kitchen-related activities?**

    A. The person should perform all kitchen activities from a sitting position.

    B. Standing kitchen activities can be performed by placing about 50% of the person's body weight on the affected leg.

    C. Standing kitchen activities can be performed by placing the majority of weight through both arms, using toes for balance (about 10% of weight).

    D. The person will be able to perform all standing activities without weight-bearing restriction.

135. **To practice transfers using a transfer board, the OT practitioner must have the individual use a wheelchair that has:**

    A. detachable footrests.

    B. detachable armrests.

    C. antitip bars.

    D. brake-handle extensions.

136. **An OT practitioner is working with an older adult who has diabetes and subsequent issues related to vision, specifically contrast sensitivity. Owing to this, he is having difficulties discriminating between medications each morning. The BEST adaptation for the therapist to provide is:**

    A. braille labels.

    B. labels with white print on a black background.

    C. a pill-organizer box.

    D. brightly colored pills with each type of medication a different color.

137. **An OT is working with an individual who has had a brain injury and is unable to remember what day it is and frequently tries to put on pajamas after the midday meal. What is the MOST appropriate compensatory intervention to facilitate awareness of person, place, and time?**

    A. Provide verbal cues, external aids, and opportunities to practice using the aids.

    B. Reduce the number of distractions by moving the individual to a quiet room when reviewing information.

    C. Present information about the environment in short units, spaced with time between each segment.

    D. Connect new orientation information to previously learned knowledge.

138. **The OT is administering the Allen's Cognitive Level Screen to an elderly individual diagnosed with dementia. The OT determines that the individual is functioning at Allen's Cognitive Level 4.8. (goal-directed activity—personalizing). The family reports that the individual has been in multiple car accidents within the past few months and they are concerned about his driving safety. When taking the client-centered approach, what is the MOST appropriate intervention for the OT to recommend?**

    A. Instruct the family to hide the car keys.

    B. Explain to the client the danger that is presented when driving.

    C. Initiate OT intervention that focuses on memory and problem-solving skills.

    D. Recommend that a family member ride in the car when the client is driving.

139. **An OT is formulating a home program of play activities for the parents of a 4-year-old child with developmental delay. What type of activities would be BEST for development of symbolic play skills?**

    A. Building blocks.

    B. Board games.

    C. Paint-by-number kits.

    D. Dollhouse and dress-up clothes.

140. **A client recently underwent bilateral below-knee amputations (BKAs). The client presents with good UE strength and sitting balance. In which of the following transfer techniques would the OT most likely instruct the client FIRST?**

    A. Stand pivot.

    B. Slide or transfer board.

    C. Dependent.

    D. Sit to stand.

141. **When evaluating an individual for phantom limb pain, the OT would expect the individual to report:**

    A. feelings that the entire limb is still intact postamputation.

    B. a perception that the amputated extremity is painful, crampy, hot, or achy.

    C. feelings of sharp pain at the residual limb site.

    D. a perception that the distal amputated limb is actually intact.

142. An OT is working with a group to develop grocery shopping skills. In addition to classroom teaching and homework exercises, what is the MOST important component to include?

    A. Participating in simulated grocery shopping activities.

    B. Finding the lowest-priced items.

    C. Practicing in an actual grocery store.

    D. Knowing where and how to find items.

143. Which of the following is MOST important to include at the onset or, acute inflammatory stage for an individual with complete upper and lower extremity paralysis as a result of Guillain-Barré syndrome?

    A. ADL training.

    B. Balance and stabilization activities.

    C. Developing communication tools, as needed, and proper positioning of trunk/head and upper extremities.

    D. Resistive activities for the intrinsic hand muscles.

144. The OT is working on handwriting skills with a school-age child with decreased proprioception in the hand and wrist. Which adaptation would the OT recommend for writing?

    A. Wide pen.

    B. Attach a rubber band to the eraser and the child's wrist.

    C. Soft triangle grip.

    D. Weighted utensil holder.

145. Which of the following would the OT MOST likely recommend an individual use at home after discharge following a total hip arthroplasty (posterior lateral approach) for BADL completion?

    A. A wire basket attached to a walker.

    B. A padded foam toilet seat 1 inch in height.

    C. A short-handled shoehorn.

    D. A long-handled reacher.

146. An OT is ordering a mobility device for a child with cerebral palsy. The child has some arm control and hand grasp function and frequently expresses the desire to be independent in mobility, especially within the school setting. What type of device will the OT will MOST likely recommend that the family order?

    A. Power wheelchair.

    B. Standard wheelchair.

    C. Caster cart.

    D. Powered scooter.

147. Upon discharge, an individual will be performing sliding board transfers with assistance from family members. When ordering a wheelchair, which features will be MOST important to include?

    A. One-arm drive and low backrest.

    B. Reclining backrest and elevating footrests.

    C. Swing-away footrests and removable armrests.

    D. Elevating footrests and removable armrests.

148. An individual with right unilateral neglect is able to track from the left side to the midline of the body on paper-and-pencil tasks. What is the BEST treatment activity to promote crossing the midline to improve writing skills?

    A. Practice wheeling a wheelchair following a taped line on the floor.

    B. Place commonly used self-care items on the left side.

    C. Trace lines across the page with the right index finger from the left to the right side.

    D. Place playing cards in a horizontal row from right to left in sequence.

149. To avoid overstimulation when handling a stable, 12-week premature infant in the neonatal intensive care unit setting, the OT FIRST:

    A. teaches parents to use firm, steady touch without rocking to help infant during feeding and diapering.

    B. helps the infant establish a calm state by playing a musical mobile.

    C. encourages auditory stimulation through singing and playing music around the infant.

    D. establishes a bond through visual orientation to the therapist's face.

150. An OT working in acute care sees several patients bedside each hour. When moving from one patient's room to the next, what is the MOST important action to take to prevent the spread of infection?

    A. Place all lines and equipment in the correct location.

    B. Wear protective clothing.

    C. Wash hands between patient contacts.

    D. Dispose of any waste in proper containers.

151. While participating in activities to improve strength, an individual with multiple sclerosis who was recently admitted to the hospital complains of fatigue. Which of the following actions is the MOST appropriate for the OT to take?

A. Instruct the individual to work through the fatigue to complete the session.
B. Instruct the individual to work through the fatigue for another 5 to 10 minutes.
C. Discontinue strengthening activities.
D. Give the individual a rest break.

152. While evaluating an individual's ADL status on the first day of treatment following open heart surgery, it is MOST important for the OT practitioner to:

A. keep the MET level below 3.0.
B. observe for shortness of breath.
C. listen for complaints of chest pain.
D. monitor heart rate, blood pressure, and symptoms.

153. An individual with Alzheimer disease becomes confused with multistep instructions during self-care activities. Which is the MOST effective method that the OT practitioner can recommend to the caregiver for giving directions to the individual at home?

A. Give simple, step-by-step instructions and physical guidance.
B. Provide three-step instructions with gestures for demonstration.
C. Offer written instructions for the individual for any tasks that contain more than three steps.
D. Have the individual verbally repeat instructions after the caregiver gives them.

154. An OT is preparing the discharge summary for a preadolescent child with limited upper extremity strength and endurance. Which home adaptation is MOST important to recommend?

A. Mount lever handles on doors and faucets.
B. Remove all throw rugs.
C. Install nonskid pads on steps.
D. Use a tabletop easel for written homework.

155. The OT is working with a client who sustained a polytrauma, secondary blast injury. Which of the following might the OT expect to see?

A. Brain injury and injuries as a result of fragments impacting the body.
B. Trauma similar to what one might see in a car accident.
C. Pulmonary and gastrointestinal issues.
D. Multiple fractures of upper and lower extremities.

156. An OT working with a young child with autism learns from the parent that falling asleep at night is difficult for the child. Which is the FIRST strategy the OT would try to assist the child to fall asleep?

A. A mini-trampoline to tire the child out before going to bed.
B. Positive bedtime routines that are predictable.
C. Let child pull a prebedtime activity from a bag containing favorite items.
D. Play with multisensory tactile media before bedtime.

157. After a radial nerve injury, an individual initially had trace muscle strength in elbow extension. One week later, strength is noted to have increased to poor minus. The individual is ready for which activity?

A. Passively self-ranging the injured arm through a full arc of motion.
B. Actively extending the elbow in midrange 30 to 40 degrees with the forearm resting on the table.
C. Pushing a cup filled with pennies with the back of the hand, with arm resting on the table to full extension.
D. Lifting a book placed on the back of the hand up off the table.

158. The OT has been asked to identify strategies to reduce agitation in residents of an SNF with mid- to late-stage Alzheimer's disease. What are the MOST appropriate environmental modifications?

A. Provide rocking chairs, music, dimmed light, and reduced clutter.
B. Train caregivers in use of validation and reinforcement.
C. Install monitoring devices such as door alarms, pressure gates, and video monitors.
D. Institute mealtime positioning and adaptive feeding strategies.

159. An OT is making a home visit to an elderly individual who lives alone and has severe hand weakness resulting from arthritis. When planning to address safety in the home, the MOST important area to consider is the individual's ability to:

A. work locks and latches on doors and windows.
B. use built-up utensils while eating.
C. demonstrate energy conservation techniques.
D. manipulate fasteners on clothing.

160. After attending several OT group sessions, a client with a history of low self-esteem is showing more self-confidence and asks for the OT's phone number. What is the MOST appropriate response for the OT to make?

A. Give him the phone number and instruct him to call when he is feeling depressed.
B. Ignore the request, but reinforce what progress he is making.
C. Explain that the OT has someone special in her life.
D. In private, explain the nature of the client-therapist relationship.

161. An OT is demonstrating bathing techniques for a 2-year-old child with seizure disorder and hypertonic muscle tone. Which suggestion is MOST appropriate for the OT to recommend to the child's parents?

A. Place child on back in tub filled with only several inches of water.
B. Bathe the child quickly to avoid an increase in tone.
C. Handle the child slowly and gently in warm water.
D. Stand and lean over the tub to support and wash the child.

162. An OT working with a community mental health agency has a caseload of individuals planning on moving into supportive housing apartments. The role of the OT with these individuals is to work on skills related to budgeting, interpersonal relationships, domestic routine, and leisure/social practices. Which is the BEST time and place for the OT to work on the skills?

A. In the apartments after they have moved in.
B. In the partial hospitalization program before they move into the apartments.
C. In the adult day program after they have moved into the apartments.
D. In a clubhouse model environment after moving into the apartments.

163. An OT working with an individual following a UE amputation is determining whether a hook terminal device or a functional prosthetic hand would be most appropriate. The individual's primary concern is his ability to return to work and function as a carpenter. What is the MOST important factor in the therapist's recommendation?

A. Cosmetic appearance.
B. Prehensile function.
C. Weight of the terminal device.
D. Ease of cleaning.

164. An OT is working with a client with an intellectual disability in an alternative work environment. When a new member joins the work line the OT observes a sudden change in behavior—the client's eyes get wide, his voice gets high, and he repeatedly asks if he is doing the job correctly. How should the OT respond to the client in this situation?

A. Use a directive approach, increase structure and repetition, and provide guidance to the client.
B. Reassure the client that you can see his worry about the new worker.
C. Remove the client immediately from the work environment.
D. Change the background music to something more soothing.

165. A young child exhibits tactile defensiveness with all dressing tasks. What is the MOST effective technique to facilitate the task?

A. Tickle the child prior to dressing and undressing.
B. Play loud music when undressing the child.
C. Lightly stroke the child's arms and legs during dressing tasks.
D. Use deep firm pressure when holding and moving child during dressing.

166. An individual is participating in a work-hardening program after an accident resulting in physical limitations. The individual's goal is to return to his job as an auto mechanic. Which of the following BEST represents a work-simulation activity?

A. Lifting weights.
B. Working on a mock car engine.
C. Visiting the work site garage.
D. Preparing lunch for work, in a standing position.

167. An individual who sustained a mild brain injury continues to have difficulty with remembering appointments and activities. Which compensatory strategies would be appropriate for the OT to recommend to assist this person with memory following discharge to home?

  A. Visual imagery.
  B. Calendars.
  C. Mnemonics.
  D. Repetition.

168. In the middle of a wheelchair-to-bed transfer, a morbidly obese patient begins to slip from the grasp of an average-size OT practitioner. The BEST action for the OT to take is to:

  A. ease the patient onto the floor.
  B. reverse the transfer, getting the patient back into the wheelchair.
  C. continue the transfer, getting the patient to the bed.
  D. call next door for assistance.

169. An individual with cognitive limitations has been participating in a social skills training group to improve the ability to make conversation. Residential home staff report to the OT that they are seeing minimal progress. In order to promote development of conversation skills what should the OT do NEXT?

  A. Have the client watch movies that include simple conversations.
  B. Encourage staff to practice conversation skills with the client in a local market with local people.
  C. Have staff provide only positive feedback.
  D. Instruct staff to discourage the individual from conversing with others until the skill has been mastered.

170. An individual with serious and persistent mental illness demonstrates the ability to participate in an inpatient task-oriented group. She is able to stay within her own space and use her own materials, with minimal verbal exchange. She prefers to focus on the activity rather than on the other group members. Which level of group should the OT provide to enable this individual to participate as fully as possible?

  A. Parallel.
  B. Associative.
  C. Basic cooperative.
  D. Mature.

171. An OT group is planning an outing to a local horse show. Because many of the group participants take antipsychotic (dopamine-blocking) medications to reduce symptoms of schizophrenia, what is the MOST important precaution for the OT to take?

  A. Avoid prolonged sun exposure.
  B. Limit access to sharp objects.
  C. Plan for frequent bathroom stops.
  D. Avoid flashing lights.

172. Which adapted technique would the OT MOST likely select in order to teach independent dressing to an 8-year-old girl with hemiparesis?

  A. Encourage the child to do most of her dressing while lying in her bed.
  B. Teach the child to dress her hemiparetic extremities first.
  C. Educate the child's mother regarding how to assist with dressing skills.
  D. Instruct the child to dress her nonhemiparetic extremities first.

173. An OT is evaluating the sensation of an individual who recently sustained a cerebrovascular accident (CVA) and has adapted the method of response to include nodding and pointing to a card with a picture of the correct answer. This method of response would be MOST appropriate for an individual who has:

  A. expressive aphasia.
  B. receptive aphasia.
  C. agnosia.
  D. ataxia.

174. The MOST effective method of compensation for both unilateral neglect and absence of sensation in an upper extremity with good motor control is to:

  A. avoid the use of sharp tools or scissors and to avoid extreme water temperatures.
  B. provide a warning tone, such as noisy bracelets on the wrist, or as a reminder to visually scan toward the affected side.
  C. use an electric shaver.
  D. wear elbow pads on the affected side.

175. The rehab team in a skilled nursing facility is preparing to discharge an individual following rehabilitation for a hip replacement. Although the individual lived independently prior to admission, at the time of discharge he is demonstrating mild confusion. The patient is able to walk safely indoors with a walker but needs meals prepared and housekeeping done for him. Which housing option is MOST appropriate for this individual?

A. Assisted living.
B. Memory-care facility.
C. Long-term care facility.
D. Senior housing.

176. A 16-year-old boy who had a traumatic brain injury 5 years ago is ready to begin shaving, but has difficulty as a result of limited range of motion in his shoulders and elbows. Which is the BEST adaptation for him to use?

A. Electric razor attached to universal cuff.
B. Safety razor with built-up handle.
C. Safety razor with extended handle.
D. Safety razor attached to universal cuff.

177. An OT practitioner is working with an individual who is at risk for aspiration during swallowing. The BEST way for the OT to assist the client during feeding activities is for the OT to:

A. place the client in slight neck extension.
B. recline the client in bed.
C. position the client by using a side or front hold.
D. facilitate the client to move into full neck flexion.

SERVICE MANAGEMENT AND PROFESSIONAL PRACTICE

178. An OT is working with individual with a visual-field deficit who neglects the left side of the plate when eating. Based on the client's interests, the OT has the client working on a mosaic activity to address this deficit. When documenting the client's performance in the objective part of the SOAP note, which example is most likely to justify reimbursement to a third-party payer?

A. "Patient has progressed from moderate assist level to occasional verbal cues for left-side neglect while eating."
B. "Patient would benefit from continued skilled occupational therapy in order to achieve preadmission level of independence."
C. "Patient required occasional tactile cues to look to the left to compensate for visual field deficit, and was able to acquire and correctly position all 50 tiles from the container placed on the left side."
D. "Patient demonstrates ability to pick up half-inch tiles using pincer grasp, and accurately follow a simple repeating pattern for 10 minutes with occasional verbal cuing."

179. The OT investigator is exploring the lived experiences of individuals diagnosed with terminal cancer in order to prioritize end-of-life OT interventions. Which of the following forms of naturalistic or qualitative injury would be most appropriate?

A. Phenomenological.
B. Ethnographic.
C. Participatory action research.
D. Grounded theory.

180. The lead OT investigator gave a group of patients who were diagnosed with C5 to C6 tetraplegia a test prior to a scar management intervention and another test after the intervention. What kind of test design was the investigator MOST likely using?

A. Pretest-posttest.
B. Survey.
C. Nonexperimental.
D. Ex post facto.

181. An OT arrives for a home health visit, but the individual is not feeling well so the visit is rescheduled for the following day. The charges for the week are due that afternoon. Anticipating a follow-up visit with the individual the next day (1/15/15) and reluctant to wait another 2 weeks to submit for payment, the practitioner bills for treatment using the 1/14/15 date. How would the OT's actions be described?

    A. Acceptable because treatment has been scheduled for the next day.

    B. Acceptable if the agency she works for allows it.

    C. Unacceptable because it violates the AOTA Code of Ethics.

    D. Unacceptable because if the individual is still ill and unable to participate in therapy on 1/15/15, a delay of more than 1 day is unacceptable for billing purposes.

182. Upon completion of the initial interview and chart review, what is the NEXT step to be taken in the OT process?

    A. Analyze the data.

    B. Develop a treatment plan.

    C. Perform selected assessments.

    D. Select appropriate assessment tools or screening procedures.

183. The administrator of an assisted living facility has asked an OT practitioner to help implement programming that will decrease the number of residents needing to move from the assisted living facility to nursing homes. The MOST important area for the practitioner to address is:

    A. adaptive equipment needs.

    B. falls prevention.

    C. meaningful use of leisure time.

    D. balancing work, leisure, and rest.

184. A participant in a study requires an MRI of the brain four times a month in a study that strives to combat the symptoms of depression. The lead investigator of the study informs the participant of the potential risks and anticipated high level of involvement required by the study. This interaction, in which the lead investigator of the study comprehensively informs the participant about her involvement in the study, is commonly referred to as a:

    A. review of remediation of risks.

    B. confidentiality of study participant.

    C. full disclosure.

    D. withdrawal of rights for participation.

185. The OT has provided services to an individual with Medicare benefits on an outpatient basis 10 times. The individual has achieved his initial self-care goals, and the OT expects him to progress further in the area of self-care performance. The claim for the initial session included a self-care G-code and modifier, but no claims have included any G-code and modifier since then. According to Medicare guidelines, what does the OT now need to do?

    A. Submit a claim with final status G-code/modifier and discharge the patient.

    B. Submit a claim including new G-code/modifier for current status and G-code/modifier for new goals.

    C. Identify a new, different G-code set, such as mobility or carrying/moving/handling, and establish related goals.

    D. Request an extension or exemption to continue to provide services.

186. The OT researcher wishes to strengthen a study. What does employment of "random assignment" assume?

    A. There is no need for inclusion criteria.

    B. Research subjects always receive the experimental treatment.

    C. The sample is not representative of the larger population.

    D. There is equivalency between the study group and the control group.

187. An OT qualitative researcher has more than 80 hours of narrative interviews related to a sequence of life events that were shaped by sociopolitical events in a client diagnosed with polio. This type of research is commonly referred to as:

    A. ethnographic.

    B. life history.

    C. phenomenological.

    D. participatory action.

188. When working within a school system to help include child with spina bifida within a general education first grade, the OT consults with the classroom teacher. What is the OT's priority outcome of this consultation?

A. The OT learns about the first-grade curriculum and daily schedule of first-grade students.
B. The teacher understands more about how occupational therapy can support students in the classroom.
C. The OT evaluates the student and writes a complete summary report for the school record.
D. The OT and the teacher identify new strategies to help the student access and participate in classroom learning centers.

189. An OT/OTA team needs to report discharge information and document the information in the patient's chart. At what level can the OTA participate in the discharge planning process?

A. An entry-level OTA may perform the task independently.
B. An intermediate-level OTA may perform the task independently.
C. An OTA may contribute to the process, but not complete the task independently.
D. An OTA cannot perform the task owing to regulatory statutes.

190. An OT has been hired to develop social skills training programs for persons with serious, persistent mental illness in a community mental health setting and needs to select a behavior to assess as an outcome measure. Improvement in which area would BEST indicate that the program was successful in achieving goals for this population?

A. Attain a balance of rest, work, play, and leisure.
B. Achieve verbal and nonverbal communication skills.
C. Identify areas for vocational exploration.
D. Perform daily self-care and home management activities.

191. An OT learns that a nursing home resident fell during the night and may have sustained a new fracture. The individual still wishes to engage in therapy. What is the BEST course of action for the OT to take?

A. Provide treatment as originally planned based on the wishes of the individual but stop if increased pain is elicited.
B. Withhold treatment, but gather information on the course of events for documentation and consultation with the treatment team.
C. Provide treatment by observing self-feeding, an area not listed as an OT treatment goal.
D. Withhold treatment and wait for the OT director to return from vacation to gather information and plan treatment.

192. An OT manager is preparing the outpatient OT staff for a visit from an accrediting agency. The accrediting agency that surveys inpatient and comprehensive outpatient rehabilitation programs is BEST represented by which of the following?

A. AOTA.
B. JCAHO.
C. CARF.
D. NBCOT.

193. An OT and OTA share and coordinate therapy for a caseload. Which of the following tasks would be MOST appropriate for the OTA to perform:

A. Reviewing charts for pertinent information.
B. Completing the nonstandardized portions of the evaluation.
C. Interpreting the results of the nonstandardized portion of the evaluation.
D. Independently designing a treatment plan for the individual.

194. The OT is developing a survey to ask about child-care patterns, health, and wellness. The researcher should attempt to avoid the use of double-barreled questions. Which of the following is MOST representative of a double-barreled question?

A. How many times do you bathe your child each day?
B. How many times a month to you seek outside assistance for emotional support?
C. How many times a day do you feel frustrated and/or discouraged by your encounters with your child?
D. How many times a week do you complete a.m. care (hygiene and dressing) and transportation to school for your child?

195. The OT manager is training colleagues about the use of electronic health records as the outpatient rehabilitation department transitions from a handwritten documentation system. Some important considerations must be taken to assure the client health record, such as:

A. legibility of entries.

B. creating updated care plans.

C. completing a discontinuation summary.

D. logging in and out each time an electronic entry is made.

196. An individual with intellectual disability is living in a supervised community environment. Upon evaluation, the OT determines that the individual can perform work tasks involving repetitive processes and demonstrates good social interaction skills. The family and client are most interested in an integrated work environment. What is the MOST appropriate service delivery model for the OT to recommend?

A. An adult activity center.

B. Supported employment.

C. Volunteer work.

D. A sheltered workshop.

197. A OTA working in outpatient rehabilitation teaches herself how to use paraffin by reading books on physical agent modalities (PAMs), carefully reading the instructions that came with the paraffin bath unit, and practicing on herself for several weeks. Is it now acceptable for this OTA to provide paraffin treatments?

A. No, OTAs may not administer PAMs.

B. No, it violates the AOTA's Position Paper on modalities.

C. Yes, she has demonstrated service competency.

D. She must have an OT on duty when she uses the PAM.

198. As a fieldwork assignment, a level II student introduces a new assessment tool for evaluating work skills of individuals with intellectual disabilities to the fieldwork educator. The fieldwork educator wants to test the reliability of the instrument. What is the BEST way to do this is?

A. Ask several experts within the department for their opinion and document them.

B. Ascertain that a new therapist is able to obtain the same results as those of an experienced therapist.

C. Demonstrate that a patient will perform in a consistent manner when being evaluated twice over the course of 2 weeks.

D. Determine an area to evaluate, assess the need for an evaluation tool, and determine an evaluation format.

199. An OT manager in a large department is trying to determine which of the four staff therapists will be able to supervise level II fieldwork students in the upcoming months. Which therapist CANNOT be assigned a level II fieldwork student?

A. The therapist who graduated 9 months ago, has taken the Fieldwork Educator Certificate Program course, and has supervised two level I students.

B. The therapist with 2 years of practice experience, has taken the Fieldwork Educator Certificate Program course, but has no experience supervising level I fieldwork students.

C. The therapist who graduated 3 years ago, has supervised two level I OTA students, but has not taken the Fieldwork Educator Certificate Program course.

D. The OT with 5 years of experience who trained at a foreign university.

200. An OT practitioner documenting the progress of a client using the SOAP note format would include which of the following in the "subjective information" section?

A. The OT practitioner will establish a daily self-feeding routine using verbal and physical cues to encourage the client to open containers on the lunch tray.

B. The client has been able to identify closed liquid beverage containers on the meal tray for four of six presentations.

C. The client is able to identify and drink liquids presented in cups without lids but leaves beverages in closed containers untouched.

D. The client asks for more beverages during meals and appears surprised when the OT practitioner indicates beverages in closed containers are on the meal tray.

Answers for Simulation Examination 2

1. (A) check the alignment of the goniometer. If the goniometer is not aligned correctly, any joint measurements will demonstrate a discrepancy, so rechecking (answer A) would be correct. "When reading the goniometer, always state your results as a range using two numbers.... The most common method of determining ROM is the Neutral Zero Method recommended by the Committee on Joint Motion of the American Academy of Orthopedic Surgeons.... For measurements of ROM to be considered to reflect actual change, the amount of change must exceed measurement error, which was found to be 5 degrees for both the upper and lower extremities. For example, if in a reevaluation the patient has shown an increase of 10 degrees in shoulder flexion, it is considered a minimal improvement, as 5 degrees may be accounted for by measurement error" (p. 124). Changing the size of the goniometer to larger (answer B) or smaller (answer C) during measurements could make the discrepancy greater, because it could make aligning the arms of the goniometer with the landmarks more difficult. It is much faster to check the alignment of the goniometer first when using one of the proper length for the job. Forcing the individual's arm further into flexion (answer D) would be painful to the individual because measurements are taken at the end of the individual's full range of motion and the joint would be unable to go further. See Reference: Trombly. (2008). Flinn, N.A., Trombly Latham, C.A., & Podolski, C.R.: Assessing abilities and capacities: Range of motion, strength and endurance.

2. (A) make recommendations for ways of operating the technology. The OT practitioner on the assistive technology team typically determines which part of the body has sufficient motor control for operating the technology and then recommends the type of input access device (switch, keyword, software, etc.) that will best meet the client's needs. Answer B, assisting with vocational goals, is most often the job of the vocational rehabilitation counselor. A vocational rehabilitation agency typically assists in job placement (answer C). Answer D, solving mechanical and software problems, is usually the role of the rehabilitation engineer. See Reference: Trombly. (2008). Buning, M.E.: High-technology adaptations to compensate for disability.

3. (A) Sensory modulation. Answer A is correct. Studies indicate that "many children frequently demonstrate behavioral characteristics of both underresponding and overresponding, often within the same sensory system. This may be particularly the case for children with autism" (p. 344). Answer B is incorrect, as sensory registration refers to the central nervous system knowing "when to "pay attention" to a stimulus and when to "ignore" it (p. 344). Answer C is incorrect as children who seek sensation engage in intense stimulation, "showing signs of pleasure from the sensations, but the input does not affect the nervous system to the extent that it does for most other children" (p. 345). Answer D, overresponsiveness, describes only part of this child's behavior. See Reference: Case-Smith & O'Brien. (2010). Parham, D. & Mailloux, Z.: Sensory integration.

4. (C) Work simulation and conditioning to increase strength and endurance for work-related skills. Work simulation is considered to be a goal of work hardening, in addition to increasing productivity and feasibility through work-simulated activities, as, "actual equipment from the job is preferred during the work simulation to maximize cooperation of the worker and more closely replicate the actual demands of the job...work conditioning is more often defined as physical conditioning alone, which covers strength, aerobic fitness, flexibility, coordination, and endurance" (p.348). Answers A and B, ADL retraining and progressive resistive exercises, are not typical goals associated with the description of a work hardening program. Answer D, vocational retraining, is incorrect. It is vital that a work hardening program be viewed as an adjunct to vocational retraining, not as a vocational training program in and of itself. OT practitioners typically measure and assess a client's overall physical ability to perform the requirements of a particular job. See Reference: Pedretti. (2013). Haruko Ha, D., Page, J.J., & Wietlisbach, C.M.: Work evaluation and work programs.

5. (B) dressing apraxia. Answer B, is correct, as "dressing apraxia contributes to the inability to plan effective motor actions required during the complex perceptual task of dressing one's upper and lower body" (p. 641). Difficulty with spatial relations (answer A) is a problem with awareness of the relationship of one's self to another object. A person with anosognosia (answer C) is unaware of any deficits. Figure-ground discrimination (answer D) is the ability to distinguish an object from its background. See Reference: Pedretti. (2013). Phipps, S.C.: Assessment and intervention for perceptual dysfunction.

6. (C) Canadian Occupational Performance Measure (COPM). "In depression, typically the barrier is not lack of knowledge or ability to perform the

ADL but a lack of volition, interest, or drive for engagement in self-care" (p. 660). Therefore, the COPM (answer C), which is the most client-centered and occupation-based option provided, is the best choice, because it "is self-directed and person centered and assists the individual in determining what life areas are important to focus on" (p. 551). The FIM (answer A) assesses ADL performance from a physical perspective. Skilled observation (answer B) is an effective way of assessing ADL performance; however, open-ended questions would elicit more meaningful information about volition and interests. Interviewing a reliable informant, such as a family member (answer D), may be useful but may be "limited by the amount of knowledge the rater has about the individual and the demands created by the physical and social environment (p. 663). See Reference: Brown & Stoffel. (2011). Brown, C.: Activities of daily living and instrumental activities of daily living.

7. (C) Level 4. Clients functioning at Level 4 "perform goal directed actions in response to visual cues.... These clients are able to complete short tasks.... Attention is up to one hour, and steps toward a goal can be imitated in short sequences.... Visual stimuli are the focus, but nonvisible properties in the environment, like heat and electricity, may pose a danger. Directions for getting places or doing tasks must be demonstrated visually because verbal and written directions are not followed" (p. 200). See Reference: Cole. (2012). Allen's cognitive disabilities group.

8. (A) −15 to 0 to 140 degrees. Negative range-of-motion documentation may vary from one setting to another. However, this range may be written as a negative (minus) sign preceding the degree (−15 degrees) or as a positive number preceding the neutral position (15 degrees to 0 degrees to 140 degrees) (p. 503). Therefore, answers B, C, and D are incorrect. See Reference: Pedretti. (2013). Philips Killingsworth, A., Pedretti, L.W., & McHugh Pendleton, H.: Joint range of motion.

9. (C) Anterograde amnesia. Anterograde amnesia is the inability to recall events after a trauma. Retrograde amnesia (answer D) is the inability to recall events prior to trauma. Long-term memory (answer B) is the storage of information for recall at a later time. Disorientation (answer A) is a problem in the awareness of person, place, and time (pp. 262–263). See Reference: Trombly. (2008). Radomski, M.V.: Assessing abilities and capacities: Cognition.

10. (C) Interview with child's parent. Interviewing the parent (answer C) is the correct response. Interviews with parents are an essential part of every evaluation, regardless of the setting. They enable the OT to "gather vital information about...client's expectation related to [OT's] involvement, and about his or her priorities, and...begin to understand how...client sees his or her situation" (p. 224). Answer A is inappropriate as the child's diagnosis already suggests that assessment of gross and fine motor performance is likely, and further, information from parent and teacher will help the OT address this concern. Answers B and D suggest specific evaluation tools that a therapist may use with some children with cerebral palsy, yet they are not essential for all students with cerebral palsy. See Reference: Mulligan. (2014). Mulligan, S.: Conducting interviews and observations.

11. (A) The child rocks and bangs his head against the wall throughout the evaluation. Answer A is most representative of restrictive-repetitive acts such as rocking, hand flapping, biting, dumping, throwing, and self-talk, which are a "core feature of the ASDs" (p. 102). Answers B, C, and D are most representative of behaviors related to socialization deficits frequently seen in children with autistic spectrum disorders (p. 88). See Reference: Kuhanek & Watling. (2010). Audet, L.R.: Core features of autism spectrum disorders: Impairment in communication and socialization, and restrictive acts.

12. (C) Identifying the type of environmental supports that can maximize the client's level of function. OTs use tools such as the Allen Cognitive levels screening assessment to "determine what kind of structure and environmental cues are needed to engage the client in task completion (answer C)" (p. 33). A cognitive level assessment will not give information on difficult behaviors specifically (answer A), though it may provide insight into how the person reacts to cognitive challenges. Answers B and D are incorrect because the cognitive level assessment evaluates how a person processes information cognitively within the framework of functional activity, rather than evaluating specific prevocational skills or level of social interaction skills. See Reference: Cara & MacRae. (2013). MacRae, A. & Boggis, T.D.: Environmental and cultural considerations.

13. (A) Sensory processing. Individuals with schizophrenia often find sensory stimuli "unpleasant and engage in behaviors to avoid the sensation" (p. 289). Sensory processing assessments (answer A) can identify sensory processing issues and preferences. Because the individual has been performing his job successfully for about a year, and only the environment has changed, a cognitive evaluation (answer B) would not be indicated, nor is there anything to suggest that the individual's social skills (answer C) are of concern. Vacuuming may challenge balance (answer D), but if other activities such as mopping are not problematic, there is nothing to suggest balance would be an issue. See Reference: Brown & Stoffel. (2011). Brown, C. & Nicholson, R.: Sensory skills.

14. (D) Determine the need for further formal evaluation. Answer D is correct; a screening includes observation of skills to determine "what standardized test and further analysis should be pursued" (p. 295). Answers A, B, and C are incorrect as a screening does not include the measurement and analysis needed to define baseline, develop recommended strategies for skill development, or determine the appropriateness of the referral. See Reference: Case-Smith & O'Brien. (2010). Exner, C.: Evaluation and intervention to develop hand skills.

15. (D) Cataracts. Individuals who present with "clouding of the lens in the eye, causing blurred vision; generally related to aging; dull colors and blurs visual details throughout the visual field" (p. 1187), typically present with cataracts (answer D). Age-related macular degeneration (answer A) is "a disease associated with aging that affects...sharp, central vision," whereas answer B, glaucoma, "causes gradual failing of peripheral vision," and answer C, diabetic retinopathy, "results in blurred vision or spotty areas, called scotomas" (p. 1187). See Reference: Schell, Gillen, & Scaffa. (2014). Meibeyer, E.: Visual impairments.

16. (D) Protective extension response. Answer D, protective extension response, is correct. This is a postural reaction used to stop a fall or to prevent injury when equilibrium reactions fail to do so (p. 255). Equilibrium reactions (answer C) maintain the center of gravity over the base of support. Righting reactions (answer B) "bring the head and trunk back into an upright position" (p. 74). Answer A, attitudinal (primitive) reflexes, are automatic movements that "appear within the first year and are designed to align the head with the body (limbs) and the upper body with the lower body. Most attitudinal reflexes are suppressed early in infancy" (p. 255). See Reference: Case-Smith & O'Brien. 2010). O'Brien, J. & Williams, H.: Application of motor control/motor learning in practice.

17. (C) A concrete response. Literal responses to general inquiries reflect the type of concrete thinking (answer C) that persons with schizophrenia may exhibit. Concrete thinking is characterized by "extremely literal verbal responses due to concrete thinking patterns. The speaker does not recognize the nuances of language, including abstractions or metaphors" (p. 177). Difficulty in understanding questions with several possible meanings also suggests disorganized thought processes seen in persons with schizophrenia. Delusional responses (answer A) would most likely be completely off topic. A distractible re-

sponse (answer B) would change the topic or stop in the middle of responding. An insightful response (answer D) would include reasons that led up to being hospitalized. See Reference: Cara & MacRae. (2013). MacRae, A.: Diagnosis and psychopathology.

18. (C) determine how frequently falls occur, how many individuals are affected, and how the problem is currently being addressed. The first step in program development is to profile the community, answer C. This includes collecting demographic information about the target population and information about the characteristics of the problem (frequency of occurrence, number of individuals involved, factors contributing to the problem, etc.). "The process by which this occurs mirrors individual evaluation and intervention but requires focus on the needs and interests of groups of individuals as well as epidemiological data that suggest what kinds of problems are most common" (p. 955). Next, the consultant should perform a needs assessment by collecting data from individuals with a variety of viewpoints, including staff, administration (answer B), and the population. Goals are established and recommendations (answer D) are made once the needs assessment is complete and goals have been established, and may include evaluation of individual residents (answer A). See Reference: Schell, Gillen, & Scaffa. (2014). Bonder, B.R.: Providing occupational therapy for older adults with changing needs.

19. (D) Aesthesiometer. An aesthesiometer is an "instrument designed for sensory testing. The term usually indicates a tool consisting of a ruler type of scale and two prongs that can be moved progressively closer or farther apart that is used for assessing two-point discrimination" (p. 213). People with sensory loss in the hand often drop things because they are not receiving adequate sensory input. An aesthesiometer (answer D) measures two-point discrimination with a moveable point attached to a ruler that has a stationary point at one end. The dynamometer (answer B) and pinch gauge (answer C) are both used to measure strength. An individual with a loss of strength would drop heavy, not lightweight, items. A goniometer (answer A) is a tool with two arms used to measure movement at a joint. One arm is held stationary while the other arm moves around an axis of 360 degrees. See Reference: Pedretti. (2013). Bentzel, K.: Assessing abilities and capacities: Sensation.

20. (B) Need for this position to achieve stability. Answer B is correct because "W" sitting is a posture that "children use to maintain stable sitting but is not recommended because it may dislocate hips and limit trunk strengthening" (p. 248). The child is likely compensating for postural control limitations that affect dynamic balance. Answer A is incorrect because the child has already been identified as having low muscle tone, a frequent characteristic in children with Down syndrome. Exclusive "W" sitting would not be considered either typical or age-appropriate for a 5-year-old child with Down syndrome. Answer C is incorrect as "W" sitting is not a functional strategy to control lower body movement. Answer D is incorrect as this is not an expected pattern in typically developing 5-year-old children. See Reference: Case-Smith & O'Brien. (2010). O'Brien, J. & Williams, H.: Application of motor control/motor learning in practice.

21. (C) At age level. Answer C is correct. At 3 years of age, a child is expected to know when he or she has to use the toilet and be able to get on and off the toilet. Three-year-old children may need assistance to cleanse themselves effectively and to manage fasteners or difficult clothing. Complete independence in using the toilet (answer D) is usually achieved by the age of 4 to 5 years. By the age of 2 years (answer B), most children have daytime control over elimination, with occasional accidents, so they still need to be reminded to go to the toilet. One-year-old infants (answer A) typically indicate discomfort when wet or soiled (p. 496). See Reference: Case-Smith & O'Brien. (2010). Shepherd, J.: Activities of daily living.

22. (A) Making Decisions Empowerment Scale. All answers include assessments that can be used with individuals with mental health conditions. However, the recovery model specifically addresses the areas of hope, empowerment, and self-determination. "Hope is an essential ingredient in initiating one's recovery, which is further fostered by a sense of empowerment, being connected with others, having access to resources, practicing self-determination, and having a clear sense of one's values and life goals.... Researchers and practitioners have generated evidence and tools to measure recovery and aspects of recovery, such as hope, empowerment, and self-determination" (p. 11). The Making Decisions Empowerment Scale (answer A) is one of the standardized assessment tools designed to measure empowerment, a key element in the recovery model. The Comprehensive Occupational Therapy Evaluation (answer B) and the Bay Area Functional Performance Evaluation (answer C) both measure occupational/functional performance. The Worker Role Interview (answer D) addresses psychosocial factors that impact work performance. See Reference: Brown & Stoffel. (2011). Stoffel, V.: Recovery.

23. (B) use pillows to prop up body parts into the desired position. An individual with low tone may benefit from supportive positioning devices such as pillows, towels, or bolsters that can help to prevent overstretching and fatigue. Slow rocking (answer C) and avoidance of quick stretch (answer D) are both methods for reducing tone and would not be beneficial to an individual having a problem with low tone. A side-lying position (answer A) would be a very difficult position for an individual with lower extremity flaccidity to maintain during sexual activity, but may be preferable for someone requiring energy conservation. See Reference: Pedretti. (2013). Tipton-Burton, M. & Umphred Burton, G.: Sexuality and physical dysfunction.

24. (D) Watch the child engage in play, eating, and bathing activities. Answer D is correct. Watching the child engage in play, eating, and bathing tasks is the only choice that reflects the components of skilled observation. "Skilled observations provide a window into many aspects of the child's function.... Observations can inform the therapist in matching other assessment methods to the ability level of the client" (p. 291). Answer A, performing a questionnaire, is most representative of interviewing, not observing. Although answer B, obtaining performance information, is considered a comparative measurement assessment method, the question is asking for the next strategy that the OT would use. Finally, answer C, referring to medical records and early intervention program reports, reflects those items most closely linked to record review, not skilled observation. See Reference: Kuhanek & Watling. (2010). Watling, R.: Occupational therapy evaluation for individuals with an autism spectrum disorder.

25. (B) trace. Trace muscle strength equals a 1 on the numerical scale of muscle testing. A grade of trace or "T" is defined as "contraction [that] can be observed or felt, but there is no motion" (p. 536). The other answers would be incorrect because answer A, absent strength, would equal 0, answer C, good strength, would equal a 4, and answer D, normal strength, would equal a 5. See Reference: Pedretti. (2013). Phillips Killingsworth, A., Williams Pedretti, L., & McHugh Pendleton, H.: Evaluation of muscle strength.

26. (C) "Are you any different now compared to what you were like before your injury?" Many of the tools developed to measure self-awareness are questionnaires. Most authors agree on the importance of determining "an individual's knowledge or understanding of strengths and deficits" (answer C) along with an understanding of the consequences of limited self-awareness and the ability to set realistic goals (pp. 76–79). An individual would need to have self-awareness in order to know how often he or she is missing appointments (answer A). Asking what to do in case of emergency (answer

B) would be used to assess safety skills. Asking someone to use a bus schedule (answer D) addresses problem-solving and planning skills. See Reference: Gillen. (2009). Self-Awareness and insight: Foundations for intervention.

27. (C) Initiation. "Survivors of brain injury tend to have difficulty initiating and terminating functional activities throughout their days. Initiation [answer C] refers to the ability to begin an activity at an appropriate time in the day to accomplish a specific goal" (p. 559). An individual with initiation problems may be able to plan or carry out activities, but may be unable to begin until prompted by another person. Problems with attention (answer A), concentration (answer B), or apraxia (answer D) would be evidenced if the eating activity were performed incorrectly or incompletely. See Reference: Cara & MacRae. (2013). Phipps, S.: The cognitive, behavioral, and psychosocial sequela of brain injury.

28. (D) Praxis. Answer D is correct. "Praxis is the ability to conceive of, plan, and organize a sequence of goal-directed motor actions...to adapt and quickly react to novel environmental demands in a meaningful and efficient manner" (p. 115). Muscle strength (answer A) is incorrect, as the child's ability to climb into the high chair and jump reflect sufficient force and strength to move and control his body in space. Motor control (answer B) is incorrect as this refers to the "ability to regulate or direct the mechanisms essential to movement" (p. 391), and the child demonstrates this capacity when climbing into the high chair and jumping. To express the functional mobility required to get into the high chair and jump (answer C), the child must have integrated primitive reflexes, so answer C is incorrect. See Reference: Hinojosa & Kramer. (2009). Schaaf, R.C., Schoen, S.A., Smith Roley, S., Lane, S.J., Koomar, J., & May-Benson, T.A.: A frame of reference for sensory integration; Kaplan, M.: A frame of reference for motor skill acquisition.

29. (D) Terminating an activity. This individual demonstrated difficulty ending the task of brushing his teeth (answer D), as evidenced by perseveration (p. 893). Trying to put toothpaste on the toothbrush before taking off the cap would have been an example of a deficit in sequencing (answer A). Difficulty following directions (answer B) could be evident if the individual attempted to brush his hair or shave rather than brush his teeth. An example of impaired problem-solving ability (answer C) is that of an individual trying to squeeze the tube of toothpaste too softly so that nothing comes out, and then giving up on the task. See Reference: Pedretti. (2013). Tipton-Burton, M., McLaughlin, R., & Englander, J.: Traumatic brain injury.

30. (B) Universal. Health-care personnel should follow universal precautions (answer B) when blood or body fluids are present regardless of diagnosis. Suicide, escape, and medical precautions (answers A, C, and D) are guidelines developed for individuals identified with risks that are not noted in this question. See Reference: Pedretti. (2013). George, A.H.: Infection control and safety issues in the clinic.

31. (A) Visual-motor integration. Answer A is correct. Visual motor integration is the "discrete motor skill that enables the coordination of the visual stimulus with the corresponding motor action" (p. 361) and each of the problem areas requires the child's use of eyes and hands together to complete the task. Visual acuity (answer B) refers to the "ability to discriminate fine details of objects in the visual field" (p. 357). A child with limited visual acuity would be observed bringing objects and papers close to his eyes in order to see them better. Visual tracking (answer C) is the "continued fixation on a moving object" (p. 357). Children with tracking difficulties lose focus while following a moving object. Visual discrimination (answer D) refers to the "ability to detect distinctive features of a visual stimulus and to distinguish whether the stimulus is different from or same as others" (p. 359). Limitations in this area may result in difficulty recognizing objects or matching and sorting objects. See Reference: Hinojosa & Kramer. (2009). Schneck, C.: A frame of reference for visual perception.

32. (A) Change pace of test activities according to test manual specification. Answer A is correct. "Most standardized tests have some flexibility about the order and arrangement of items.... Tests provide guidelines for administering the test in two sessions, and examiners should be familiar with these guidelines before starting the test" (p. 237). In addition, changes in the child's behavior represent important test data and should be recorded. Although a test session may need to end before the child completes all items (answer B), scoring incomplete items at zero points does not reflect the child's performance on those items. Again, the child's behavior should be documented and the test administration reported as incomplete. The responses described in answers C and D may make the test results invalid, unless they are specified in the test manual. See Reference: Case-Smith & O'Brien. (2010). Richardson, P.K.: Use of standardized tests in pediatric practice.

33. (B) Observation in the cafeteria and during classroom free-play period. Observation in selected classroom activities (answer B) is correct. This provides an opportunity for the OT to observe how the child structures time and interacts with peers. "One of the most valuable assessment methods with children and adolescents who have social participation problems is to observe them interacting with peers or family members during motivating activities such as crafts, board games, or preparing and enjoying food" (p. 424). Data from this observation help the therapist identify the student's strengths along with areas that warrant in-depth evaluation. There is no evidence to support a specific focus on prevocational and career skills (answer A) or tests to measure visual-motor performance (answer C). Answer D, community mobility checklist, is appropriate for a student who has, or is at risk for, movement limitations. See Reference: Case-Smith & O'Brien. (2010). Davidson, D.A.: Psychosocial issues affecting social participation.

34. (B) Closed-ended. "Closed questions [answer B], which can be answered with a 'yes' or 'no' are most appropriate when seeking specific information and tend to discourage communication." Open-ended questions require "a longer, more detailed answer"..." and are used to encourage self-disclosure with clients" (p. 52). It may be necessary to use closed questions to help an individual focus on the topic or when time is running out. Leading questions (answer C) suggest the desired response. A double question (answer D) asks two questions at once or forces a choice. See Reference: Cole & Donohue. (2011). Cole, M.B.: Social participation basics.

35. (B) Form constancy. Answer B is correct. Form constancy is the "recognition that forms and objects remain the same in various environments, positions, and sizes. It is the ability to see a form and being able to find it, even though the form may be smaller, larger, rotated, reversed, or hidden" (p. 359). Answer A is incorrect as figure-ground is the "ability to perceive a form visually, and to find this form hidden in a conglomerated ground or model" (p. 359). Position in space (answer C) is the "determination of the spatial relationship of figures and objects to oneself or other forms and objects" (p. 359). Visual sequencing (answer D) is an activity that requires the ability to copy the same sequence of beads. Although these abilities are all required for this bead-stringing task, the error described in the question refers to a form constancy error. See Reference: Hinojosa & Kramer. (2009). Schneck, C.: A frame of reference for visual perception.

36. (C) Environmental modification. Environmental modification (answer C) is the area of intervention that can best assist in maintaining safety and supporting function at home by providing the physical and sensory environments to compensate for deficits. At this stage of the disease process, intervention should focus on "ensuring safety in the home and other environments by making adaptations suited to the level of client functioning (alarms, restricted use of heating devices and sharp instruments, cabinet latches, identification bracelet, visual cues for locating items, and visual camouflaging" (p. 928). Strength and endurance activities (answer A) will have no direct effect on safety in the home. Cognitive rehabilitation techniques (answer B) are not indicated for conditions with progressive cognitive deterioration. Use of assertiveness skills (answer D) would be inappropriate for dealing with the kinds of communication problems encountered with persons who have Alzheimer disease. See Reference: Pedretti. (2013). Schultz-Khron, W., Foti, D., & Glogoski, C.: Degenerative diseases of the central nervous system.

37. (C) Resistive. Answer C is correct. Activities requiring the manipulation of highly resistive materials, such as clay, leather, and copper sheets, should be avoided. Joint inflammation, stiffness, and weakness around the involved joints are common features of juvenile rheumatoid arthritis (JRA) (p. 153). Pressure applied to the joints could exacerbate the condition; therefore, reducing fatigue and stress on joints is indicated (p. 154). The OT should always use techniques for joint protection and energy conservation with a child with acute juvenile rheumatoid arthritis. Light touch (answer A) is likely to be disturbing to a child with tactile defensiveness (p. 346). Rapid vestibular stimulation (answer B) is contraindicated for a child who is prone to seizures. The need to avoid above-normal body temperature (answer D) is more relevant to a client with multiple sclerosis, because high temperatures exacerbate the symptoms. See Reference: Case-Smith & O'Brien. (2010). Rogers, S.L.: Common conditions that influence children's participation; Parham, D. & Mailloux, Z.: Sensory integration.

38. (A) As an infant who is 8 months old. Answer A is correct, because 3 months (number of months premature) are subtracted from the child's chronological age to adjust for prematurity (p. 222). This child is then given the benefit of time lost because of a shorter gestation period. Answers A, B, and D do not reflect appropriately calculated adjusted age to account for prematurity. See Reference: Case-Smith & O'Brien. (2010). Richardson, P.K.: Use of standardized tests in pediatric practice.

39. (B) Handing out trays and utensils to people in a food service group. This individual demonstrates limitations in the area of interpersonal skills. Adequate interpersonal and social skills are necessary for successful employment. In order to develop these skills, the individual should be provided with opportunities to practice them in a structured environment. Handing out trays and utensils (answer B) requires minimal interaction, and would provide an opportunity for this individual to practice interacting with others at a limited level in a natural environment. "Occupational therapy practitioners may find that they can aid generalization of skills by following group skills training with coaching and reinforcement in the actual occupational environments" (p. 308). None of the other options provides the opportunity to develop interpersonal skills. See Reference: Brown & Stoffel. (2011). Stoffel, V.C. & Tomlinson, J.: Communication and social skills.

40. (C) Training for the school bus driver to ensure that that student travels to school safely and comfortably. Answer C, related to safe travel on the school bus, is the correct answer. The OT should ensure the driver follows specific positioning and strapping procedure for the student's safety in the wheelchair, and the wheelchair's safety in the bus (p. 643). Without any evidence that this student needs to practice efficiently maneuvering the wheelchair within a busy environment, there is no rationale for answer A, practice negotiating an obstacle course. Plans for routine wheelchair maintenance (answer B) are an ongoing concern for the family and not an immediate concern relative to school-based services. Creating a lap tray for the student to use to complete seat work in her wheelchair (answer D) is not a preferred option, as this does not support her inclusion with peers in the classroom desk/table and chair arrangement used by other peers in the classroom. The OT should ensure that needed adaptations are in place so the student has a safe and comfortable seating option that includes her in learning activities with her peers. See Reference: Case-Smith & O'Brien. (2010). Wright-Ott, C.: Mobility.

41. (D) Weight-bearing over a small bolster in prone position. Answer D is correct. Research has shown that "children with cerebral palsy demonstrated increased use of wrist extension and finger extension after upper extremity weight bearing" (p. 300). Weight-bearing on the arms can help with overall inhibition of tone before participating in hand skill activities. Answers A and B are incorrect because they require voluntary control of the release of objects without inhibition. Answer C is incorrect because traction on the finger flexors may increase spasticity in the flexor muscles, and make opening of the hand more difficult. See Reference: Case-Smith & O'Brien. (2010). Exner, C.: Evaluation and intervention to develop hand skills.

42. (D) Have the child climb up onto her lap. All answers describe the use of good body mechanics. Answer D, having the child climb onto her lap, is preferable, though, because it minimizes the amount of bending and lifting required. See Reference: Trom-

bly. (2008). Maher, C. & Bear-Lehman, J.: Orthopaedic conditions.

43. (C) Preschool staff invite the parent and child to come and visit the preschool before they end their current services. Preschool staff extending an invitation to the family to visit the program (answer C) is correct. "Communication is powerful and can make or break our relationships with children and families" (p. 86). When staff in the preschool reach out to families and invite their participation, they facilitate relationship building. At best, change is often difficult and strategies that facilitate the process are optimal. Answer A is not constructive and highlights differences in the upcoming change. Answer B is incorrect, as the OT should not work in isolation from other team members. Answer D is incorrect, as filing reports is a procedural task and by itself, does not support collaborative relationships/program planning. See Reference: Dunn. (2011). Dunn, W.: Structure of best practice programs.

44. (B) Increasing overall physical activity levels and fitness. Wellness programs focus on developing personal control of behaviors through educational approaches and active participation in activities that promote health, such as increasing levels of physical activity to improve physical fitness, answer B. "Smoking, poor diet, and physical inactivity are the root causes of a third of deaths in the United States. Such information would be useful in framing goals of senior center activities, educational programs, and health screenings" (p. 955). Answers A, C, and D reflect traditional occupational therapy therapeutic interventions to improve performance in specific deficit areas, rather than promoting general good health. See Reference: Schell, Gillen, & Scaffa. (2014). Bonder, B.R.: Providing occupational therapy for older adults with changing needs.

45. (B) continue the same positioning and use of orthosis program that was indicated at discharge. It is necessary to continue positioning and use of orthosis after discharge because active scar development continues for many weeks, depending on the severity of the burn. The same positioning and use of orthosis devices used at the hospital are used at home, with changes made as needed during follow-up visits. Individuals stay in the hospital until their conditions can be managed at home, with outpatient visits to maintain status. Individuals are not kept in the hospital until they are completely healed, which would be the only situation in which a home program would not be necessary (answer A). If an individual follows the home program only as he or she deems appropriate during the day or night (answers C and D), instead of as scheduled by the therapist, the position time may not be sufficient to prevent deformity from occurring. See Reference: Pedretti. (2013). Reeves, S. & Deshaies, L.: Burns and burn rehabilitation.

46. (A) Creeping. Creeping on hands and knees (answer A) is correct and typically emerges after 7 months. "Most 10-12 month old infants crawl rapidly across the room, over various surfaces, and even up and down inclines" (p. 68). Answer B, rolling from back to stomach, is typically accomplished by 6 months (p. 67), before the infant is able to sit independently. Cruising, supported stand, and sideward stepping (answer C) occurs just before the child walks. "By 12 months, the infant can rise to sitting from a supine position" (p. 68). See Reference: Case-Smith & O'Brien. (2010). Case-Smith, J.: Development of childhood occupations.

47. (D) Playing balloon volleyball. An activity such as balloon volleyball (answer D) may be graded for improving strength by adding resistance to the arm in the form of weights. Endurance may be improved by adding more repetitions of the movement. "Activities should allow for one or more kinds of grading, such as for resistance, range, coordination, endurance, or complexity.... If an activity is selected in which the client has an interest, the client is more likely to experience sufficient satisfaction to sustain performance. The therapist's job is to guide the client to suitable therapeutic activities at just the right level of challenge so that the client will achieve satisfaction by engaging in the activity" (p. 738). Raising the height of the net can increase the range of motion required. Blowing up and tying balloons (answer A) and painting faces on balloons (answer B) are primarily fine motor activities. An individual who throws darts at balloons (answer C) would be able to increase the resistance needed for shoulder strengthening by adding weight to the arms or using balloons with thicker rubber. However, this activity is less suitable to increase the number of repetitions, because the repeated loud noise associated with bursting the balloons would be annoying. See Reference: Pedretti. (2013). Breines, E.B.: Therapeutic occupations and modalities.

48. (D) present important principles in small units that are spaced at a slower than normal pace. According to learning principles for older adults, learning will be more effective if the information is presented in small units at a slower pace. Answer A is incorrect because learning will be impeded if information is presented too quickly and in large chunks. Answer B is incorrect because presentations that are highly organized will enhance retention of information more than loosely structured presentations. Attempts to persuade individuals on points that may not be in agreement with their preconceived

ideas, values, or habits also may impede learning (answer C), whereas a more collaborative approach may result in better learning of concepts. See Reference: Trombly. (2008). Goodman, G. & Bonder, B.R.: Preventing occupational dysfunction secondary to aging.

49. (C) Provide a transfer tub bench and install grab bars. The best adaptation to achieve access to the tub would be providing the individual with a transfer tub bench, which is recommended for individuals who cannot step over the edge of the tub. Bathroom grab bars also should be installed to provide stability during the move into the tub. Tearing out the original tub and installing a walk-in shower (answer A) would be an unreasonable expense when answer C is an option. Shower doors (answer B) would make it very difficult to transfer into the tub using a transfer bench, which is the safest option. Nonskid decals and mats are primarily safety measures to prevent slipping and falling (answer D). See Reference: Pedretti. (2013). Foti, D. & Koketsu: Activities of daily living.

50. (D) Providing tokens for attendance at an exercise group. "The use of behavioral approaches are often helpful with clients who need structure and an external locus of control.... In token economies (answer D), clients may be given direct reinforcement following positive behavior or tangible symbol that counts toward the purchase of some larger reinforcement (p. 321). In addition, exercise has been shown to be effective in managing stress (p. 323) Journaling (answer A) is an example of a psychodynamic-object relations approach, where "therapists can use expressive techniques in collaboration with the client to develop insights and understanding, and facilitate adaptive behaviors to meet goals" (p. 321). Reducing auditory stimuli and dimming the lights (answer B) may help to reduce visual and auditory stimuli that overwhelm the individual, and are examples of a sensory and environmental adaptation approaches. Deep breathing and muscle relaxation (answer C) "can decrease the stress response and facilitate adaptive coping" (p. 323), and are examples of cognitive-behavioral approaches. See Reference: Brown & Stoffel. (2011). Haertl, K. & Christiansen, C: Coping skills.

51. (D) Adapted teaching techniques. Answer D is correct because a child with intellectual disability characteristically has difficulty with processing and performance, applying concepts, and organizing and sequencing tasks (p. 502). Teaching methods such as "chaining" or behavior modification are used. Video modeling (VM) and video self-modeling (VSM) are researched techniques used with children. "For children with intellectual limitations, dressing was learned more quickly when the speed of the VSM was slower" (p. 502). Answers A, B, and C are of secondary importance because physical coordination may be impaired, or there may be other physical challenges, such as abnormal muscle tone or problems with balance. These additional concerns may require adaptive equipment, clothing, or techniques. However, all aspects of dressing depend on the child's ability to learn procedures of dressing; therefore, it is initially necessary to consider task analysis and the optimal teaching approach. See Reference: Case-Smith & O'Brien. (2010). Shepherd, J.: Activities of daily living.

52. (B) Verbal and nonverbal language and physical contact with the students. The correct answer is B, as this focuses on the therapist's behavior and this question concerns the therapist's presence to help facilitate change among the students. OTs need to be "mindful of their actions, reactions and nonreactions.... Included in the conscious use of self are preplanned (not spontaneous) verbal and nonverbal responses to a person or the environment.... A therapist cannot change a child's behavior or skills; rather, he or she can only become part of an environment in which the child can change" (p. 171). Answers A, C, and D are all potential considerations in the intervention plan. However, they are incorrect as they do not present options that directly influence or develop the interaction between the OT and group members. See Reference: Lane & Bundy. (2012). Hinojosa, J. & Segal, R.: Building intervention from theory.

53. (B) Client will draw for 1 hour, taking stretch breaks every 20 minutes. Goals refer to what the therapist anticipates the individual will accomplish and should be functional, measurable, and objective; thus, answer B meets those criteria. Answer A is not measurable. Answers C and D describe what the OT practitioner will do and would be included in the plan section of a note. See Reference: Pedretti. (2013). Smith, J.: Documentation of occupational therapy services.

54. (C) Documentation that the intervention was implemented as planned. Answer C is correct. "In addition to carrying out the intervention, data about the treatment integrity of the intervention should be collected,...which means that the treatment program is being followed the way it was intended and with the frequency and duration that was established" (p. 749). Although teacher agreement with the implementation plan (answer A) is part of the collaboration between OT and teacher, this documentation does not contribute to the measurement plan. Readministering standardized tests (answer B) is not a necessary element in progress monitoring, as many standardized tests do not reflect changes in

function, nor are standardized tests appropriate for all students. The OT considers plan modification (answer D) when progress-monitoring data indicate that desired change in function has not occurred. See Reference: Kuhanek & Watling. (2010). Frolek-Clark, G: Using data to guide your decisions.

55. (D) Identification of own strengths, anticipating challenges and strategies that support performance. Enhancing metacognitive skills to increase task performance is among the approaches recommended for students with ASD and executive function difficulties; therefore, answer A is correct. Studies describe the process to include "assisting students in developing awareness of the strategies that they automatically use to cope with task challenges.... Youths learn how to anticipate their needs for strategies and how to go about applying cognitive strategies to improve occupational performance" (p. 687). Answers A, B, and C are incorrect, as they do not directly relate to the executive function challenges that are the focus of this question. See Reference: Kuhanek & Watling. (2010). Orentlicher, M.L. & Wilson, L.J.: Transition from school to adult life for students with an autism spectrum disorder.

56. (C) Make-believe group with stuffed animals and imaginary friends. Answer C is correct. Symbolic play is typically imaginative in nature, thus making any activity that involves pretending that dolls and stuffed animals are real is appropriate. Symbolic play that "involves the use of objects as symbols...becomes more elaborate with the involvement of more children, detailed roles to play out, and decreasing reliance on objects. Both drama and imitation are features of symbolic play" (p. 354). Answer A, scissors and cutting tasks, would most likely be used to facilitate fine motor and in-hand manipulation skills, whereas answer B, jumping rope, would involve gross motor skills typically seen in older children. Answer D, building towers to resemble an actual picture, is an activity that would be more representative of constructive play and/or manipulation skills. See Reference: Parham & Fazio. (2007). Spitzer, S.L.: Play in children with autism: Structure and experience.

57. (C) Consider the roles and occupations required for this child and develop recommendations that increase the child's competence in these areas. Answer C is correct, as this first step helps the therapist ensure that recommendations are "functional" for this child. "Functionality refers to the relevance of the recommendation to the child's life" (p. 202). Answers A and D are part of the evaluation and planning processes and the therapist considers these factors in relation to the child's roles and occupations in which the child is expected to engage. Answer B is a final step in the evaluation results and recommendations process (p. 205). See Reference: Case-Smith & O'Brien. (2010). Stewart, K.B.: Purposes, processes, and methods of evaluation.

58. (D) Adaptive equipment needs and assistance from others. "For at least 6 weeks, and for some patients longer, movement is restricted. As these restrictions preclude bending over or bringing the foot closer to the hands, adaptations are required to resolve problems in bathing, dressing, functional mobility, and home management" (p. 1118). In light of the reality that the hospital stay following total hip arthroplasty is usually less than a week, the OT practitioner must prioritize what can reasonably be accomplished in that time. Determining an individual's need for adaptive equipment and determining how much assistance is required for ADLs (answer D) are the highest priority for occupational therapy evaluation and are reasonable goals for such a short length of stay. Although work and leisure performance (answer B) are important aspects of occupational performance, they may need to be addressed later by the OT practitioner working with the individual in home health, as an outpatient, or in an extended care facility. Addressing deficits in strength, ROM, or coordination (answer C) also may be necessary to enhance occupational performance, but the need for intervention would likely extend beyond acute care as well. Although cognitive/perceptual functioning (answer A) is critical to safe ADL and IADL performance, these areas are more thoroughly assessed prior to surgery to determine the client's ability to adhere to the prescribed precautions postsurgery. See Reference: Trombly. (2008). Maher, C. & Bear-Lehman, J.: Orthopaedic conditions.

59. (C) Simple meal preparation group. Obtaining food is a basic survival need and is often the focus of a homeless individual's day. "Homeless individuals identify occupational performance problems related to finances, housing, personal care, difficulties satisfying basic needs, and health concerns" (p. 610). Therefore, although all the above groups may meet a need, activities related to food are likely to be more highly valued by this individual. Craft groups (answer A) may be useful in developing healthy leisure interests. Volunteer activities (answer B) can help develop necessary work habits. Social skills groups (answer D) address interpersonal skills necessary for living in society. See Reference: Brown & Stoffel. (2011). Helfrich, C.A.: Homeless and women's shelters.

60. (B) Developing awareness about how thoughts and behaviors affect one's perceptions of and ability to cope with pain. All of the answers are aspects of the cognitive-behavioral process

in addressing chronic pain. However, treatment begins with an educational approach that teaches clients how their thoughts and behaviors impact their perception of being and their ability to manage it (answer B). When using the CBT approach, the client will need to "express concerns related to occupational performance strengths and limitations; to identify beliefs and thoughts that interfere with desired occupational performance; to learn new beliefs and ways of thinking, feeling, and behaving; and to test and apply that learning with problems that arise in their day-to-day lives" (p. 271). Therapy should then move to learning alternative ways of responding to pain (answer A), followed by rehearsal of techniques (answer C), and finally implementation of techniques and coping strategies to decrease pain and stress during daily occupations (answer D). See Reference: Brown & Stoffel. (2011). McCraith, D.B.: Cognitive beliefs.

61. (A) Instruct the individual to wear clothes for 2 days and then to launder those items. "By understanding the components of a task, it is often possible to modify a task to compensate for cognitive impairments" (p. 253). In answer A, the patient is told to rely on a schedule rather than judgment. Teaching the individual to recognize and judge when clothing needs to be laundered has been unsuccessful, indicating that the individual may not have the capacity to learn this skill. If the OT practitioner determines that the individual can usually wear clothes for 2 days before they need to be laundered, then providing a rigid schedule based on this average removes the need for judgment, and provides an environmental compensation—a schedule that will result in the individual wearing clean clothes most of the time, if not always. Assessment of the individual's clothing management capabilities (answer B) would have been performed before the implementation of the initial intervention. Taking the clothes to the dry cleaner (answer C) would be cost prohibitive and would still require judgment to determine when they needed to be cleaned. Turning the responsibility over to the staff (answer D) would not promote independence in clothing management. See Reference: Brown & Stoffel. (2011). Brown, C.: Cognitive skills.

62. (B) Massage, compression bandaging, exercise, and external compression. Answer B is most representative of a MEM edema reduction method. "These methods include the principles of manual lymph-edema treatment (MLT) massage, medical compression bandaging, exercise, and external compression adapted to meet the specific needs of subacute and chronic postsurgical and poststroke UE edema. The goals are to stimulate the initial lymphatics to absorb excessive fluid and large molecules from the interstitium and to move this lymph centrally....

MEM is used to prevent or reduce subacute or chronic edema. MEM is used to prevent or reduce subacute or chronic high-protein edema as seen in postsurgical, trauma, or post-cerebrovascular accident (CVA) hand edema" (p. 1059). Answers A, C, and D are not representative of a manual edema mobilization method of edema reduction. See Reference: Pedretti. (2013). Kasch, M.C., & Walsh, J.M.: Hand and upper extremity injuries.

63. (D) Convert an empty lot filled with trash into a community garden. Answer D, converting an empty lot into a garden, is correct. "Each environment and/or context provides unique barriers and supports to occupational performance. Therefore, modification of the environment and/or context can impact the occupational performance and participation of all members of an organization, community, or population" (p. 345). Further, this activity is based on the concepts of building and creating and results in one shared outcome. Answer A promotes competition and answer B promotes individual reward, rather than team building. Anger management skills are important for children at risk for violent behavior; however, a psychoeducational format (answer C) will not directly contribute to community building. See Reference: Schell, Gillen, & Scaffa. (2014). Scaffa, M.: Occupational therapy interventions for organizations, communities, and populations.

64. (C) Incorporating simple, familiar activities such as hanging up clothing or catching a ball. "The primary goal of OT intervention for clients with AD (Alzheimer's Disease) is to maximize the quality of life and engagement in occupation and to promote safety;...task simplification: diminish demands ADL and other tasks through establishing daily routines or increasing visual, verbal, or tactile cues and support from caregivers; [and] use of assistive technology or adaptive devices (e.g., pill boxes)" (p. 1099), meaning that simple activities would be most effective for gaining active cooperation and participation from a person with Alzheimer disease (answer C). Telling the person to perform repetitions of active exercises (answer A) might not be effective because she or he may not be able to remember to perform repetitions of exercises or may not understand the purpose and become confused. Training in the use of adaptive devices (answer B) would not increase active shoulder motion and could be confusing if cognitive deficits were present. PROM exercises performed by the caregivers (answer D) would not lead to improvement of active range of motion. See Reference: Schell, Gillen, & Scaffa. (2014). Meibeyer, E.: Alzheimer's disease.

65. (C) Deep breathing. All four answers are examples of self-management techniques utilizing re-

laxation training. Deep breathing (answer C) is most appropriate for this situation because it can be taught quickly and used in a relatively short amount of time (p. 285). Progressive muscle relaxation (answer D) usually takes about 30 min. Autogenic training (answer A) and meditation (answer B) require more extensive periods of training. See Reference: Cara & MacRae. (2013). Cara, E.: Anxiety disorders.

66. (B) Back up the body to the passenger seat, hold on to a stable section of the car, extend the involved leg, and slowly sit in the car. Answer B is the safest way to perform a car transfer after surgery for a total hip replacement. The posterolateral approach is the most frequently performed technique. The surgeon typically recommends that the individual avoid positions of hip adduction, internal rotation, and flexion. Answers A, C, and D are contraindicated owing to their lack of adherence to total hip replacement precautions. See Reference: Pedretti. (2013). Lawson, S.C. & Murphy, L.F.: Hip fractures and lower extremity joint replacement.

67. (A) What are you most concerned about with this student's performance in the language arts curriculum? Answer A, representing an open-ended question, is correct. This wording doesn't assume any particular difficulties and asks the teacher to speak about specific, current concerns. OTs formulate questions in particular ways to elicit different types of information. Open-ended questions "promote interaction...[and the OT] allow[s] for some silence now and again without being too quick to jump in with a comment or another question" (p. 227). Answers B and C are closed-ended questions that lead the teacher to speak about specific areas the OT identifies. The way these questions are worded evokes a specific short answer and does no promote interaction or discussion without further questioning. Although answer D is an open-ended prompt designed to elicit the teacher's perspectives and begin discussion, limited information is gathered as the OT has targeted only a specific focus that may or may not be of concern to the teacher. See Reference: Mulligan. (2014). Mulligan, S.: Conducting interviews and observations.

68. (D) Encourage independent ADLs with minimal reliance on adapted utensils and tools. Encouraging independence in ADLs with minimal use of adapted utensils and tools (answer D) is the most appropriate ADL intervention. Intervention goals for a child with burns concern "optimizing active ROM,...ensuring good use of the hands, and optimizing skills for self-care and for home and school activities" (p. 184). It is important to avoid an overreliance on adapted equipment so the child can experience full active range of motion when engaged in

ADL. Answer A, instruct the child to use adapted equipment for all ADLs, may interfere with the achievement of full AROM. Answer B, encourage independent compression garment application, is typically contraindicated with open wounds and is implemented once wounds close. Answer C, perform bilateral upper extremity PROM exercises twice a day, is not considered an ADL intervention. See Reference: Case-Smith & O'Brien. (2010). Rogers, S.L.: Common conditions that influence children's participation.

69. (C) Healthy leisure participation and Alcoholics Anonymous. Studies have shown the "effectiveness of CBT, 12-step programs, and mixed 12-step/CBT programs...were equally effective in reducing patients' substance use, psychological symptoms, and increasing the proportion of patients who avoided legal problems and are not incarcerated or homeless to be comparable" (p. 848). Providing information about healthy leisure pursuits and Alcoholics Anonymous (answer C) is an example of a combination of a cognitive-behavioral therapy (CBT) approach and a 12-step program approach. A nurse would most likely be the individual involved with instructions on medication management (answer A). Information about the recovery model (answer B) would have been introduced earlier in the individual's hospitalization. Although information about group home options could be important, the harm reduction model (answer D), which does not subscribe to complete abstinence, is not in alignment with this individual's goals. See Reference: Cara & MacRae. (2013). Hoppes, S. et al: Substance abuse and occupational therapy.

70. (D) Suggest furniture and accessories that promote better positioning at work. The best recommendation is for ergonomically correct furniture and accessories (answer D). Additional adaptations may include tool modification and the training of workers in appropriate positioning. Answers A and C, setting up stress management and work simulation activities, are not considered to be ergonomic interventions. Answer B is not an example of an ergonomic intervention, but is instead a treatment intervention. See Reference: Meriano & Latella. (2008).

71. (A) Look at pictures of children playing on an obstacle course and talk about what they are doing with this child just prior to beginning the activity. Answer A is correct. Children with autism spectrum disorders have difficulty planning and sequencing new and unfamiliar movements to complete a task and visual cues provide helpful support. "Visual cues can aid the process of ideation, which is often difficult for children with an ASD. Forming an initial idea of what to do is often the first step in fa-

cilitating praxis" (p. 498). Answer B is incorrect because "motor skills that are executed in isolation or out of context are less likely to be meaningful" (p. 497) for children with ASDs. Answer C is incorrect, as the directions do not help the child with ideation to move through the obstacle course. Answer D is incorrect, as the "sensory environment used in therapy is structured in a way that enhances the child's possibilities to achieve praxis and organization of behavior through proprioceptive, vestibular, and tactile sensations" (p. 489). See Reference: Kuhanek & Watling. (2010). Mailloux, Z. & Smith Roley, S.: Sensory integration.

72. (A) no more than 20 degrees of extension. Carpal tunnel syndrome is a condition that results from compression of the median nerve at the wrist. Wrist orthotics should position the wrist in neutral. "Conservative intervention is usually attempted first and includes splinting [use of orthosis] of the wrist in no more than 20 degrees of extension" (p. 1065), to minimize intratunnel pressure and alleviate symptoms. "A semiflexible or neoprene splint [orthosis] rather than a completely rigid splint [orthotic device] may be used to provide support while allowing a small amount of flexion and extension for greater functional use in carpal tunnel syndrome" (p. 1065). See Reference: Pedretti. (2013). Kasch, M.C. & Walsh, J.M.: Hand and upper extremity injuries.

73. (C) Expressing disagreement with coworkers in a productive manner. "Assertiveness as a social characteristic empowers people to stand up for themselves.... Using assertiveness, people act on their own behalf to satisfy their needs, accomplish their intentions, and achieve their goals while remaining respectful of the needs, rights, and opinions of others" (p. 56). Assertiveness training focuses on developing the ability to articulate one's needs while respecting the rights of others and express feelings in an appropriate and productive manner (answer C). Answers A, B, and D are examples of additional social interaction skills; however, they do not address an assertiveness component. Answers A and B are examples of actions taken when engaging in conversation, and answer D is an example of proper social conduct. See Reference: Cole & Donohue. (2011). Cole, MB : Social participation basics.

74. (C) Collaborate with other team members to develop long-term goals and project duration of services. Answer C is correct. "Intervention planning, first and foremost, should be a collaborative effort" (p. 256) as this ensures a comprehensive program representing multiple perspectives toward metal priorities. "[L]ong-term goals are what you hope your client will achieve and what you anticipate the child's functional status to be at the time therapy is discontinued" (p. 257). The OT uses this expectation to develop the incremental steps (short-term objectives) that lead to long-term goal achievement. An OT practice model and frame of reference "determine[s]...[the] approach to intervention, and that will guide...actions throughout the intervention process" (p. 262). Answer A is incorrect as a practice model and specific activities are not selected before intervention goals are established. Answer B, engage in clinical reasoning, is incorrect as the OT uses clinical reasoning through the OT process and not to identify student priorities. Further, priorities are best developed through collaboration with other members of the school team and not by the OT in isolation. The OT needs to understand the systems documentation requirements (answer D); however, this is not a next step in view of the other options. See Reference: Mulligan. (2014). Mulligan, S.: Intervention planning and documentation.

75. (A) Using the strongest joint and avoiding positions of deformity. The significance of using these principles, using the strongest joint and avoiding positions of deformity (answer A) for individuals with preexisting joint conditions and adverse musculoskeletal changes, may help to restore function as well as prevent further impairments. "Use of stronger, larger joints can handle greater forces. Examples of this include lifting objects from the floor by using the hips and knees instead of bending at the spine; pushing and pulling objects rather than carrying them; and using a belted waist pack rather than holding the purse with a hook grasp" (p. 1223). Answers B, C, and D involve common muscle relaxation and stress management techniques not always associated with joint protection techniques. See Reference: Trombly. (2008). Yasuda, Y.L.: Rheumatoid arthritis, osteoarthritis and fibromyalgia.

76. (C) train the client in the operation of the assistive technology system and in strategies for its use. Assistive technologies "are expected to be used over prolonged periods by individuals with limited training and possibly with limited cognitive skills. The technology, therefore, must be designed so that it will not inflict harm on the user through casual misuse. The controls of the device must be readily understood such that although some training may be required to use the device, constant retraining will not be. The device should not require deep understanding of its principles and functions to be useful" (p. 429). That being said, training activities in the use of the assistive devices/technology are the next critical step after setup of the system (answer C) and are essential because the complex nature of assistive technologies can require many hours of practice to master. Evaluating how well the whole system works

(answer A) usually occurs after training is completed during the follow-up phase. Evaluating the match between the client and the technology (answer B) is done earlier in the process to ensure maximum success and because expensive technological devices may be ordered only once. Funding sources (answer D) also are determined before ordering equipment. See Reference: Pedretti. (2013). Anson, D.: Assistive technology.

77. (C) Swallowing crushed ice. Dysphagia is the "difficulty with any stage of swallowing, interferes with functional independence for many recipients of occupational therapy services" (p. 1322), so answer C is correct. Answer A is representative of bilateral integration or the ability to coordinate both sides of the body. Aphasia, answer B, is the inability to express oneself orally, and answer D, the inability to speak clearly, or dysarthria, is best described as slurred speech secondary to cerebral lesions. See Reference: Schell, Gillen, & Scaffa. (2014). Avery, W.: Dysphagia.

78. (B) Ask the parents to describe the infant's daily schedule and identify routines that are going well and those that are challenging. Learning about the family's routines and how they are going (answer B) is correct. Research suggests that "children learned best when opportunities to practice new skills were woven into daily life" (p. 53); therefore, learning about infants' routines is an essential first step when meeting new families. "Families not only provide context in which children live but also are a constant presence over a child's life span, and they spend more time with their child than do any of the professionals in the child's life" (p. 49). Answers A, C, and D are incorrect as they conflict with family-centered, family-strengths and relationship-based concepts that are central in early intervention programs. (pp. 49–51) See Reference: Lane & Bundy. (2012). Morrison, C.D.: Early intervention.

79. (B) Cut-up meats and sandwiches. Answer B is correct. To increase oral tolerance and control of food, textures are gradually modified from smooth and consistent (answer C), to smooth and slightly varied (answers A and D), to increasingly resistive foods and a combination of contrasts, for example, hard and crunchy mixed with soft or liquid. After the child has mastered this level of control and tolerance, he or she can safely proceed to an even greater variety of textures, tastes, and temperatures, such as cut-up meats and sandwiches, answer B (p. 463). See Reference: Case-Smith & O'Brien. (2010). Schuberth, L.M., Amirault, L.M., & Case-Smith, J.: Feeding intervention.

80. (C) Family and other team members discuss the service options to identify those that match

established priorities and support student's achievement. Answer C is correct. "The Individuals with Disabilities Education Act...outline(s) a clear process of clarifying the ways that people obtain access to their environments for daily life" (p. 3). Using federal regulations and best practice approaches (p. 4), the family is an integral part of the IEP team. Professionals are responsible for providing information and discussing options with parents to agree on a plan of services that matches the student's unique needs and enables participation in the education curriculum for all students. Answers A and B are incorrect as they do not address the student's individual needs and they do not include parents in the decision making. Answer D is incorrect as it does not include parent participation and also refers parents to secure services that the school should provide, yet is unable to do so at the time. See Reference: Dunn. (2011). Dunn, W.: Best practice philosophy for community services for children and family.

81. (A) Asking a store salesperson for information about an item before buying it. Intervention to develop assertive behavior is a process of gradually empowering clients to make their own decisions, request assistance, avoid being taken advantage of, and provide constructive criticism when it is warranted in a variety of situations. Activities to assist in this process need to be graded for success by starting with situations that are less threatening to the client. "When grading, the OT practitioner increases the demands of the task at hand to potentially reduce an underlying impairment performance skill deficit" (p. 323). Asking for information about an item without buying it (answer A) is the least challenging of the options, requiring a request for information that is well within the expectations of a department salesperson, making it a suitable exercise for beginning assertiveness training. Answers B, C, and D each require the client to make a special request, and question or criticize a service, which requires more skill and confidence. See Reference: Schell, Gillen, & Scaffa. (2014). Gillen, G.: Occupational therapy interventions for individuals.

82. (A) Construction play. Construction play (answer A) is correct. A child engaging in this type of play "makes products, specific designs [are] evident, [and] builds complex structures" (p. 60). An unstructured period with blocks and building toys is an example of construction play. Symbolic play (answer B) is associated with the development of language and concepts (e.g., use of "dress-up" materials). Creative play (answer C) and interests are characterized by refinement of skills in activities that allow construction, social relationships, and dramatic play (e.g., finger painting). Recreational play (answer D) is leisure ex-

periences that allow the exploration of interests and roles such as arts and crafts or sports. See Reference: Parham & Fazio. (2007). Knox, S.: Development and current use of the revised Knox Preschool Play Scale.

83. (A) Skill-building activities with concrete goals, such as time management training. "Individuals who display negative symptoms often need highly structured activities with concrete expectations and goals [answer A]. Specific skill training and psychoeducation are very beneficial to people with negative symptoms, but many individuals need ongoing support to utilize their skills" (p. 214). Answers B, C, and D are all treatment formats that could be used with clients who have schizophrenia, but may present too high a level of challenge at this stage. See Reference: Cara & MacRae. (2013). MacRae, E. & Andoinian, L.: Schizophrenia.

84. (A) Activities designed to explore and express feelings. Psychodynamic theory (answer A) "provides a framework by which therapists can use expressive techniques in collaboration with the client to develop insights and understanding and facilitate adaptive behaviors to meet goals" (p. 320). Activities that encourage the exploration and expression of feelings (answer A) are most reflective of psychodynamic theory. Activities matched to the specific cognitive level of group members (answer B) reflect a cognitive disabilities approach. Activities that can serve as reinforcers for desired behaviors (answer C) would be used with a behavioral frame of reference. Activities that can teach the use of problem-solving strategies (answer D) would be used within a cognitive-behavioral context. See Reference: Brown & Stoffel. (2011). Haertl, K. & Christiansen, C.: Coping skills.

85. (A) Pulling shoes off feet. Answer A is correct because, according to most developmental scales, children first learn to remove garments, especially socks and shoes (p. 501—Typical Development Sequence for Dressing). Answers B (putting on T-shirt) and D (putting on hat) are incorrect, because children are typically able to remove garments before they are able to put them on. Answer C, removing sweatpants, is a skill that follows shoe and sock removal (p. 501). See Reference: Case-Smith & O'Brien. (2010). Shepherd, J.: Activities of daily living.

86. (C) Provide lateral trunk support. A lateral trunk support (answer C) in the frontal plane stabilizes the side, helping to maintain correct alignment of the pelvis and trunk in the chair by counteracting the twisting effect of asymmetrical muscle tone. By providing upper extremity support, the lateral trunk support also would prevent improper loading on to an unstable shoulder joint. "Lateral trunk supports can be used to reduce scoliosis and lateral trunk flexion caused by imbalanced tone of the intrinsic muscles of the back" (p. 900). Using a reclining wheelchair (answer A) is incorrect because doing so would shift the individual's weight to the posterior, but would not prevent the lateral shift of the trunk. An arm trough (answer B) may help maintain a more centered position of the trunk, but the weight of the affected extremity would result in instability and improper alignment of the shoulder, which could lead to shoulder pain. A lateral pelvic support (answer D) would provide stabilization of the pelvis to prevent it from shifting sideways, but this support would be too low to prevent the trunk from moving laterally. See Reference: Pedretti. (2013). Tipton-Burton, M., McLaughlin, R., & Englander, J.: Traumatic brain injury.

87. (B) Ask questions such as "What am I currently doing?" and "What am I supposed to do next?" Strategy training for attention "involves helping a person learn to control, monitor, or prevent the emergence of attentional symptoms" using techniques such as "self protection, self questioning (answer B), specific goal setting, and self evaluation" (p. 794). Answers A, C, and D are also appropriate strategies but are environmental or task adaptations, not training strategies. See Reference: Schell, Gillen, & Scaffa. (2014). Toglia, J.P., Golisz, K.M., & Goverover, Y.: Cognition, perception, and occupational performance.

88. (D) Air-filled cushion on the child's seat during seat work periods. Answer D is correct, as OTs "modify the position in which the child balances to challenge stability and improve balance control whether the child is stationary or moving through space" (p. 257). Use of the seat cushion requires that the student continually adjust to the subtle movements of an unstable surface. Once this intervention is trialed, the OT needs to collect data about the child's performance to assess the benefit of its continued use. Answers A, B, and C provide additional external support (i.e., they provide adaptations using a compensatory approach, rather than facilitating the development of new skills). See Reference: Case-Smith & O'Brien. (2010). O'Brien, J. & Williams, H.: Application of motor control/motor learning in practice.

89. (B) Head, chin, or breath-control device. "Level C4...Wheelchair propulsion...power recline and/or tilt wheelchair with head, chin, or breath control" (p. 971). Answer A, no device, would be likely for an individual who sustained a C1 to C3 spinal cord injury, as this level of injury presents with, "total paralysis of trunk, upper extremities, lower ex-

tremities; dependent on ventilator" (p. 969), and answer C, a generator or battery back-up is also indicated with a C1 to C3 spinal cord injury due to ventilator dependent status. Answer D, mouth sticks, are usually used for direct access on keyboards or on environmental control unit (ECU) control panels. See Reference: Pedretti. (2013). Adler, C.: Spinal cord injury.

90. (B) Floor sitter. Answer B, a floor sitter, is correct. An OT "can make an important contribution to the overall functioning of children through the recommendation and provision of appropriate adaptive equipment" (p. 707). The floor sitter may enable the child to play on the floor near his peers. A hammock (answer A) would not allow the child to feel as if he "fits in" in view of his desire to sit on the floor with his peers, perhaps making him feel even more different than he does when he sits in his wheelchair. Introducing an adapted wheelchair insert or a prone stander (answers C and D) ignores the child's desire to sit on the floor with his peers. Wheelchair inserts are often used for positioning a child in a wheelchair to permit increased trunk support and stability, thus allowing for more independent use of the upper extremities. A prone stander allows the child to assume a standing or weight-bearing position, but would not assist with positioning him with his classmates who are sitting on the floor. See Reference: Case-Smith & O'Brien. (2010). Teeters Meyers, C., Stephens, L., & Tauber, S.: Early intervention.

91. (D) (1) gather shirt up at the back of the neck; (2) pull gathered-back fabric off over head; (3) remove shirt from unaffected arm; and (4) remove shirt from affected arm. Answers A, B, and C are examples of incorrect sequences that would most likely result in failure to remove the shirt successfully. See Reference: Pedretti. (2013). Foti, D. & Koketsu, J.S.: Activities of daily living.

92. (D) Secure the pelvis in the seat. Positioning the pelvis securely (answer D) is correct. "The key points in achieving functional seating are the position and stability of the pelvis" (p. 641). Positioning the pelvis against the back of the seat with a seat belt enables a stable pelvis and facilitates the positioning of the other body parts (answers A, B, and C) so that the child can participate in family games. See Reference: Case-Smith & O'Brien. (2010). Wright-Ott, C.: Mobility.

93. (A) Teach them to break the activity down into smaller more manageable steps. "Training in problem-solving strategies involves teaching the person to break down complex activities into smaller, more manageable steps" (p. 805). Gross and fine motor activities (answer B) can heighten awareness of self and develop coordination. Increasing the time spent on the activity (answer D) helps development of attention span. Structuring the number and kinds of choices (answer C) is a method for developing decision-making skills. See Reference: Schell, Gillen, & Scaffa. (2014). Toglia, J.P. et al: Cognition, perception, and occupational performance.

94. (B) Strategies to promote resumption of the worker role. The Model of Human Occupation recognizes how the relationship between an individual's performance abilities, habits, motivation, interests, values, and personal causation impact his or her occupational and role performance. Therefore, the overarching concept this answer needs to address is role performance (answer B). Adapted software (answer C) and communication and assertiveness training (answer D) are both strategies that could be used to support resumption of role performance. Job retraining (answer A) could be necessary, but is not indicated based on the information available. See Reference: Brown & Stoffel. (2011). Brown, C.: Motivation.

95. (C) The patient will perform lower extremity dressing with verbal cuing for energy conservation techniques 50% of the time. Goals should be functional, measurable, and objective. Answer C meets those criteria. Answer B does not provide measurable criteria. Answer D describes what the practitioner will do. Short-term goals must relate to the long-term goal being addressed. Because the long-term goal being addressed is independence in dressing, the short-term goal must relate to dressing, not all activities of daily living (answer A). See Reference: Pedretti. (2013). Smith, J.: Documentation of occupational therapy services.

96. (C) An environmental approach that provides an auditory cue when it is time to take her medications. Medication noncompliance is a primary factor related to frequent readmissions for individuals with psychiatric conditions. Cognitive limitations, such as poor memory, can be a major barrier to successful medication management. An environmental approach (answer C), such as "pillboxes that...beep when it is time to take a medication" (p. 663), is most appropriate for this client because the reason she is noncompliant is poor memory. Other major barriers to medication compliance include the stigma associated with taking psychiatric medications, for which a psychodynamic approach could be used (answer A); lack of knowledge about medications, for which a psychoeducational approach (answer B) could be used; and negative attitudes about medications and their side effects, for which a cognitive-behavioral (answer D) approach could be

used. See Reference: Brown & Stoffel. (2011). Brown, C: Activities of daily living and instrumental activities of daily living.

97. (C) State simple, concrete directions allowing time for delayed responses. Answer C is correct, because "most people with TBI experience some degree of difficulty processing external information from the environment. A delay in response time is often noted and can range from a few seconds to several minutes.... Many individuals with TBI exhibit concrete thinking, in which they are able to interpret information only at the most literal level. For example, individuals with impaired executive and abstract function may be able to complete a meal preparation activity accurately and safely only if step-by-step directions are provided" (p. 894). Because processing of information is also an area of difficulty, allowing time for delayed responses is frequently necessary. Answer A, telling the person what is expected and asking him to begin, would require abstract thinking and initiation of activities—both areas that are likely to be impaired. Answers B and C, relying on gestures and providing written directions with pictures, may not be effective if visual perception is impaired. See Reference: Pedretti. (2013). Tipton-Burton, M., McLaughlin, R., & Englander, J.: Traumatic brain injury.

98. (C) Using a bath chair with the door open. The best bathing method for a person with COPD considers the energy demands of the task, as well as the effect of water temperature, in light of the individual's functional status. People with COPD have difficulty breathing when the environment is hot or humid, or when there is a high degree of steam. Answer A is incorrect because the energy demand of transferring into a tub and the use of hot water may cause difficulty breathing. Answer B, standing for a quick shower, also is incorrect because even if brief, standing would be more energy demanding than sitting, and an overhead shower can increase humidity. A lukewarm tub bath (answer D) would provide lower humidity by using the coolest water temperature, but the need to transfer in and out of the tub may make the task very energy demanding. See Reference: Trombly. (2008). Huntley, N.: Cardiac and pulmonary diseases.

99. (B) Remain matter of fact and consistent in approach. Individuals with borderline personality disorder demonstrate inconsistent behavior, have difficulty maintaining stable relationships, and have poor self-image. "Maintaining trust and addressing pervasive nature of personality disorders requires intervention that is predictable" (p. 151). It is important in this case that the OT recognizes this behavior as part of the pathology and not take it personally. Because the accusation is a result of pathology, the

OT has nothing to apologize for, and is unlikely to uncover any reasonable explanation for a misunderstanding (answer D). In addition, the practitioner should not complain of hurt feelings to a client (answer A). Delving into exploration of the individual's past (answer C) is not a recommended approach for occupational therapy. See Reference: Brown & Stoffel. (2011). Urish, C.: Personality disorders.

100. (A) Replace the spoon with a blunt-ended fork. Answer A is correct. For a child with incoordination and tremors, stabbing food with a blunt-ended fork is often more effective for feeding than using a spoon. The food will not fall off the fork, and the blunt tines will prevent any injury to the child. Building up the spoon handle (answer B) is more appropriate for a child with a weak grasp. A swivel spoon (answer C), and bending the handle 45 degrees (answer D) are more appropriate for a child with limited forearm and wrist motion (p. 461). See Reference: Case-Smith & O'Brien. (2010). Shepherd, J.: Activities of daily living.

101. (C) Allow the child to self-apply tactile stimuli to maximize the child's tolerance. Answer C is correct because "allowing the child to self-initiate and self-administer the input may make the activity less aversive" (p. 159). Answer A is incorrect because light touch sensations are particularly disturbing for children with tactile defensiveness, and may create overwhelming feelings of anxiety. Answer B is incorrect because avoiding all forms of tactile sensation is virtually impossible, and such complete avoidance would not help the child to develop coping skills. Answer D also is incorrect because "when treating a child with tactile over-responsivity or defensiveness, the therapist would use increased pressure touch...and increased proprioceptive aspects of the activity to help the child manage and adapt to tactile stimuli during activities" (p. 159). See Reference: Hinojosa & Kramer. (2009). Schaaf, R.C., Schoen, S.A., Smith Roley, S., Lane, S.J., Koomar, J., & May-Benson, T.A.: A frame of reference for sensory integration.

102. (D) gravitational force. "Aquatic rehabilitation approaches may be employed for the remediation of strength. Though aquatic rehabilitation does not currently require specific conditions, continuing education is recommended prior to implementing intervention within a water environment. Water inherently provides an environment that is free of gravitational force.... The simple elimination of this force, often taken for granted by individuals without strength limitations, presents an ideal opportunity to foster strength while also engaging in a leisure activity. Strength is fostered directly by the viscous properties of water, or the tendency of water molecules to

adhere to one another" (p. 61), answer D. Answers A, B, and a C do not relate to the overall goal of increasing strength, owing to deconditioning. See Reference: Meriano & Latella. (2008). Proulx-Sepelak, D.: Foundational skills for functional activities.

103. (D) Augmentative communication device. Answer D is correct. An augmentative communication keyboard is a high-technology aid that can compensate for expressive deficits and assist a student with communication (p. 526). Answer A is incorrect because an environmental control unit is a device that allows a person with severe disabilities to operate appliances or devices. It may be used to turn on a tape recorder for note taking, but it would not be used as the primary method for conversation and graphics in the classroom. Answers B and C are incorrect because both the Wanchik writer and a head pointer are low-technology aids for communication, rather than high-technology devices. See Reference: Radomski & Trombly. (2008). Buning, M.E.: High-technology adaptations to compensate for disability.

104. (B) The individual has a physical or mental impairment that substantially limits major life activities and has a history of having had such an impairment. In order for reasonable accommodations decision progression to take effect, the individual must meet one or more of the following criteria: "a physical or mental impairment that substantially limits one or more major life activities, a history of having had such an impairment and/or regarded as having such an impairment.... If the worker is not an IWD, the employer does not have to accommodate" (answer B, p. 387). Answers A, C, and D disqualify an individual from ADA coverage. "The ADA provides its protection against disability discrimination only for those who meet the criteria.... This means that individuals with temporary impairments, such as a broken leg or after a knee replacement that is likely or expected to heal normally, will not find that the ADA protects them. Individuals who have impairments that are not substantially limiting, such as a visual limitation correctable with eyeglasses, will not find benefits under the ADA.... The ADA further excludes from its protection illegal drug users, compulsive gamblers, kleptomaniacs, pyromaniacs, and alcoholics whose alcohol use prevents them from performing their jobs" (p. 386). See Reference: Pedretti. (2013). Kornblau, B.L.: Americans with Disabilities Act and related laws that promote participation in work, leisure, and activities of daily living.

105. (A) safety and stability. Incoordination, tremors, ataxia, and athetoid movements may result from conditions that affect the central nervous system, such as Parkinson's disease, CP, multiple sclerosis, and head injuries. "Ataxia is manifested as delayed initiation of movement, responses, errors in range and force of movement, and errors in the rate and regularity of movement.... This results in jerky, poorly controlled movements.... The client with gait ataxia has a staggering, wide-based gait with reduced or no arm swing. Step length may be uneven and the client may have a tendency to fall" (p. 478, answer A). Strength (answer C) was not identified as an area of concern for this individual. The ability to reach and bend (answer B) is of primary concern for those with limitations in range of motion. Endurance level (answer D) is a primary concern for individuals with MS, Guillain-Barré syndrome, ALS, and other neurological conditions that cause them to fatigue quickly. See Reference: Pedretti. (2013). Preston, L.A.: Evaluation of motor control.

106. (D) Hide-and-seek with clay balls in which the child "digs" for various coins and then places them in a piggy bank. Answer D is correct, as it encourages the child to work on fine motor skills. This child will most likely rely on signing as a way to communicate. "The movements of the hands of a fluent signer require opposition, finger and thumb flexion and extension, and finger and thumb abduction and adduction. The hand's coordination seems to be related to its sensory abilities, particularly tactile discrimination. The therapist can enhance kinesthetic, tactile, and visual processing through multisensory activities" (p. 771). Parachute activities (answer A) are indicated for gross motor and/or kinesthetic needs, but are not necessarily related to the child's fine motor limitations. Answer B, visually coding the child's shoes, is an appropriate choice when attempting to encourage self-care skills. "Adapting techniques or assistive devices may be needed. At times, self-care skills involve concrete concepts that require concrete cues for the child to learn" (p. 771). Although answer C, introducing the child to socialization groups, would be appropriate to address because many children with hearing impairments feel isolated from the hearing community, the goal of the OT in this scenario is to address the child's fine motor limitations. See Reference: Case-Smith & O'Brien. (2010). Russel, E. & Nagaishi, P.S.: Services for children with visual or hearing impairments.

107. (A) shoulder flexion and protraction. Answer A is correct because the infant needs to flex and protract the shoulders against gravity to reach forward and upward to grasp toys. Answer B is incorrect because shoulder extension and retraction would not be encouraged during supine activities when the toys are placed overhead. Answers C and D are incorrect because head and trunk are not working against gravity while the infant lies in the supine position.

See Reference: Case-Smith & O'Brien. (2010). Case-Smith, J.: Development of childhood occupations.

108. (C) Providing hand-over-hand assistance. "Use of hand-over-hand techniques (tactile, proprioceptive, and kinesthetic cuing),...are most commonly implemented within the context of functional task engagement (such as dressing or washing) where the OT will physically move the affected body part for the client [answer C]. Repetition is then promoted in the patterns of functional movement and frequently follow a developmental sequence" (p. 119). In this method, the caregiver places one hand over the resident's hand and provides assistance while guiding the resident's hand through the steps of the task, in this case, guiding the resident's hand from the food to the mouth. This method provides maximum assistance while still allowing the resident to feel involved and connected to the task. Given the resident's attention span deficits, the use of demonstration (answer A), verbal feedback (answer B), and even backward chaining (answer D) would be insufficient to sustain the resident's active participation. See Reference: Meriano & Latella. (2008). Proulx-Sepelak, D.: Foundational skills for functional activities.

109. (C) Divide the laundry into several small loads for carrying. Dividing the laundry into several small loads (answer C) will decrease low back strain, as opposed to one or two large loads (answer D). Folding laundry from a basket on the floor next to the chair (answer A) would require bending and twisting, two movements that people with low back pain should avoid. Pain should be avoided when possible (answer B), and therefore preventive strategies should be urged to help the person avoid getting to the point of severe pain. See Reference: Pedretti. (2013). Grangaard, L.: Low back pain.

110. (A) Grasp and release objects such as a fork or toothbrush. An orthotic device, such as "the SaeboFlex orthosis assists an individual who exhibits hypertonia in the hand to place the hand in an open, functional position. This positioning is accomplished by means of a fixed wrist support and a finger and thumb spring system of variable strength. Once the hand is open, the client can begin to retrain the finger flexors for improved motor control of the hand.... Saebo developed the FTM Arm Training Program on the basis of a distal activation model, which focused on the key point of early initiation of UE movements that incorporate grasp and release" (p. 482, answer A). Answers B, C, and D would not be the primary objective of the SaeboFlex™ dynamic orthosis, which is to address issues related to weakness in the hand. See Reference: Pedretti. (2013). Preston, L.A.: Evaluation of motor control.

111. (A) Set the atmosphere, model appropriate behavior, and develop the rules. "In the initial stage...the leader functions are usually to role-model active participation, develop the rules, assist members to establish a trusting atmosphere [answer A] and establish goals, and structure the group so that it will have the right balance, discouraging both excessive dependence and excessive floundering" (p. 679). Answers B, C, and D reflect the transition, working, and final stages of group development, respectively (pp. 679–680). See Reference: Cara & MacRae. (2013). Cara, E.: Groups.

112. (D) Encourage group members to share similar experiences and reactions with each other. "Group treatment facilitates personal growth by virtue of providing more people with whom to interact. Participants can learn about themselves through identifying with others [answer D]; observing, experiencing closeness and caring; and having opportunities to be around others in a safe or trusting context" (p. 673). This experience is designed to develop cohesiveness among members and facilitate learning new skills from others by hearing their experiences and offering feedback in a trusting environment. Defining types of behavior (answer A) and demonstrating them (answer C) is designed to impart information, not to promote group cohesion. Acting out anger or aggression (answer B) is an example of catharsis, which may not be helpful to all members. See Reference: Cara & MacRae. (2013). Cara, E.: Groups.

113. (A) Teach the child to dress in a side-lying position. Answer A is correct, as the child can "take advantage of the function that he or she possess when in a side-lying position, with the effect of gravity lessened" (p. 504) and aids independence for lower extremity dressing. Answer B is incorrect because the primary purpose of putting loops on waistbands is to help a child with limited grasp strength to pull on garments. Answer C is incorrect because using hook and loop fasteners in place of zippers also is an adaptation designed to help children with limited ability to grasp and pull, whereas answer D, teaching the child to dress in a standing position, is considered to be more difficult than dressing in a sitting position. See Reference: Case-Smith & O'Brien. (2010). Shepherd, J.: Activities of daily living.

114. (C) Use infant mesh feeder bag. Answer C is correct as the child can "practice chewing foods encased within a mesh feeding bag to experience repetitive chewing with less risk for gagging or choking" (p. 467). Answer A is incorrect because scraping off food from a spoon with the child's teeth does not encourage any voluntary oral motor control. Answer B is incorrect because it combines liquid with pieces of food (soft and chewy), and this combination of textures will be too unpredictable for a child who is having difficulty organizing oral motor skills to manage food. Answer D is incorrect because a raisin is too great a step from pureed food in terms of texture; introducing the raisin into the child's mouth may lead to choking. See Reference: Case-Smith & O'Brien. (2010). Schuberth, L.M., Amirault, L.M., & Case-Smith, J.: Feeding intervention.

115. (D) Continuous reinforcement of correct responses. "Continuous reinforcement [answer D] reinforces every instance of the behavior and is most often used at the beginning of treatment" (p. 592) or training of a task. When training individuals to complete a task, continuous positive reinforcement should be provided to promote successful completion of the task. Level of reinforcement changes as the individual becomes more confident performing the task. Answers A, B, and C are examples of intermittent reinforcement, which "is more effective at maintaining the desired response" (p. 592). See Reference: Schell, Gillen, & Scaffa. (2014). Helfrich, C.A.: Principles of learning and behavior change.

116. (D) Recommend that the girl wear an emergency alert system pendant around her neck. Answer D, an emergency alert system, would be the most likely solution for the OT to recommend to the family to enable safety and role competence for this young woman (p. 583). This intervention would be most effective because it can be placed on the client's body and does not require a great deal of dexterity to manipulate. Answer A, positioning a wireless cell phone near the girl, may be an effective solution, but would not be of much assistance if her dexterity is limited, in that she may not be able to push the buttons effectively. Answer B, establishing a quick exit routine in the event of a fire, is something that the OT and the client's family should address, but in the event that no family members are home with the client when a fire occurs is potentially hazardous. Whereas answer C, educating the client regarding fire prevention within the home, is something that should be reviewed by the OT, it does not address the immediate needs of responding to an actual fire via an emergency call system. See Reference: Case-Smith & O'Brien. (2010). Schoonover, J., Argabrite Grove, R.E., & Swinth, Y.: Influencing participation through assistive technology.

117. (A) Assemble presanded pieces of a wooden ship while standing at a high worktable for increasingly longer periods of time. Answer A is correct as "paint or stain fumes, as well as sawdust from cutting or sanding, may be detrimental for clients with respiratory illnesses" (p. 76). If not for the sanding, the birdhouse activity with wrist weights (answer B) could be a good strengthening and/or conditioning activity. A kit that can be completed in one session (answer C) could be appropriate for individuals with a need for immediate gratification. Sanding using an incline board (answer D) is a good way to increase ROM. See Reference: Tubbs & Drake. (2012). Woodworking.

118. (A) Select a picture of a calm, gentle dog, then practice mentally shifting from the image of a scary dog to the image of the gentle dog. Panic attacks are a type of anxiety disorder characterized by a period of intense fear or distress that can include "palpitations...shortness of breath, feelings of suffocation, chest pain, sensations of choking, nausea, or...dizziness" (p. 266). Cognitive-behavioral therapy (CBT) is effective with this disorder in which the individual experiences of irrational fear that does not reflect reality. In CBT, the individual confronts the fear in a safe situation and challenges negative thinking, such as learning to visualize a positive dog experience as opposed to a negative one (answer A). Making a point of avoiding parks and other areas dogs typically frequent (answer B) would be an example of environmental adaptation, not CBT. Mindfulness (answer C) is also a widely utilized intervention for anxiety that works by teaching people to respond to stressful situations reflectively in order to eliminate maladaptive strategies. Systematic desensitization utilizes "incremental exposure (answer D) that attempts to systematically diminish anxiety related to specific fears" (p. 275). See Reference: Cara & MacRae. (2013). Cara, E.: Anxiety disorders.

119. (D) Pudding. Answer D, pudding, is correct, as "foods with a smooth, even, cohesive consistency...are easier to manage when a child has oral, sensory, and oral motor impairments" (p. 462). Answers A, B, and C are incorrect, as "foods that are dense, crunchy, sticky, or uneven in consistency are more difficult to manage" (p. 462). See Reference: Case-Smith & O'Brien. (2010). Schuberth, L.M., Amirault, L.M., & Case-Smith, J.: Feeding intervention.

120. (B) Put the dried dishes away and begin to hand her wet dishes. When working with individuals with progressive memory loss, the OT must focus on "upholding the dignity of the person during each stage" (p. 236). By adapting the process (answer B), the OT is able to maximize the individual's engagement in the process. Compensating for mistakes helps to increase the sense of self-worth and integrity of individuals with dementia. This approach is preferable to drawing attention to errors, especially in situations in which safety is not an issue. Attempting to develop insight (answer D) and approaches that can undermine the client's self-confidence and contribute

to her depression (answers A and C) are all inappropriate. Answers A, C, and D all draw attention to the individual's errors. See Reference: Brown & Stoffel, 2011). Schaber, P.: Dementia.

121. (C) Include family's concerns into recommended caregiving practices. Answer C is correct and embraces principles of family-centered early intervention. Research supports the use of the infant's natural environment and approaches that "use incidental learning opportunities that occur throughout the child's typical activities and interactions with peers and adults" (p. 692). Answer A, positioning and handling to promote motor development, is incorrect, as it incorporates only one area of the infant's development and does not reflect teaching the parent how to position the infant within her regular activities and routines, such as mealtime or play. Teaching PROM (answer B) is incorrect, as family should be encouraged to help this infant actively move. Answer D is incorrect as it does not reflect therapist-parent partnership and collaboration that are features of recommended early intervention practice. See Reference: Case-Smith & O'Brien. (2010). Myers, C.T., Stephens, L., Tauber, S.: Early intervention.

122. (A) Stand back while the client pays for the ride. "Scaffolding is a method of grading an activity by providing assistance to the client at times that he or she might struggle or be unable to successfully complete this step.... Eventually, some of the support and assistance can be taken away.... As the client learns how to do the activity the clinician will provide fewer cues and less assistance to allow the client to become more independent" (p. 160). Using the scaffolding approach, the OT would allow the individual more independence in one of the components of the activity, in this case paying with a token (answer A). Getting off the bus and deciding how to get to his friend's home (answer B) is a more complex activity than paying with a token; therefore, this is not the best choice for scaffolding, but would be appropriate using a backward chaining approach. Teaching the client to read the map (answer C) is a skill development approach. Having the friend watch from the window (answer D) may enhance safety but is not a scaffolding approach. See Reference: Thomas. (2012). Grading and adapting.

123. (A) Stocking the shelves at a local grocery. Answer A is correct as it is a real-life functional activity in an actual work setting that represents an ecologic approach. "Viewed as highly functional, relevant, and contextual, ecologic approaches are considered an essential feature of effective transition practices. An ecologic approach supports the identification of student performance needs and abilities in the environments that he or she...is expected to use as an adult" (p. 820). Working in a sheltered workshop or in their own school environment (answers B and C) do not provide real-life settings for job training. Reading help wanted ads and role-playing interviews (answer D) are not considered vocational training. See Reference: Case-Smith & O'Brien. (2010). Spencer, K: Transition services: From school to adult life.

124. (D) Refer to home-delivered meal services. Answer A, continued OT services to teach the patient to use the kitchen safely, is incorrect because individuals diagnosed with Alzheimer's disease decline over time and have difficulty managing instructions that relate to memory. Volunteer companions (answer B) provide companionship to elders at home, but not skilled supervision of activities throughout the day. Transporting the patient to a community site for meals (answer C) on a daily basis could be inconvenient, overly challenging, and taxing for an elder with beginning dementia. Answer D, in-home meal delivery services such as Meals on Wheels, would be the best and safest option for providing consistent access to food in the home. See Reference: Pedretti. (2013). Schultz-Krohn, W., Foti, D., & Glogoski, C.: Degenerative diseases of the central nervous system.

125. (B) Help the child develop cognitive strategies for anxiety-producing activities. Using cognitive strategies (answer B) is correct. "Creating individualized expectations and designing the just right challenge for each child can help alleviate frustration and create a just-right match between each child's performance demands and performance abilities" (p. 439). Working with this student to devise cognitive strategies (answer B) to help engage in challenging activities and routines encourages him to use his intellect to support positive behavior and participation. Time-out periods (answer A) are not an effective match for this child's capacities, nor do they help him practice positive behavior. Children find a predictable routine helpful rather than an unpredictable routine, so answer C is incorrect. Answer D is incorrect because the parent and child need to learn mutual play in an environment that promotes positive engagement. See Reference: Case-Smith & O'Brien. (2010). Watling, R.: Interventions and strategies for challenging behaviors.

126. (B) Guide the client to position the pajama bottoms in front and insert one leg. When using the forward chaining approach, "the therapist prompts or demonstrates the first step on the first trial, the first two steps on the second trial, and continues until the whole sequence is remembered" (p. 230). The first step of this activity would be posi-

tioning the pajama bottoms in front and inserting one leg (answer B). In backward chaining, the training starts with the last step (answer C). Hand over hand guidance and having the client state the steps of the activity in advance (answers A and D) are other methods that may work but are not examples of forward chaining. See Reference: Gillen. (2009). Managing memory deficits to optimize function.

127. (B) An individual who cannot bear weight on the lower extremities. When an individual requires assistance because of decreased strength or balance, the sliding board is an appropriate device to include during transfer training. Answers A and C, the inability to follow commands and fatigue, are issues unrelated to the use of a sliding board. In answer D, when the individual is strong enough or demonstrates sufficient balance to perform a stand-pivot transfer, a sliding board would not be indicated. See Reference: Pedretti. (2013). Bolding, D., Adler, C., Tipton-Burton, M., Verran, A., & Lillie, S.M.: Mobility.

128. (C) Purchase talking books related to the student's areas of interest. Answer C, purchase talking books, is correct. "Reading contributes to play and leisure, academics and world knowledge, [and] communication . . ." (p. 612). Accommodations to enable reading "include the use of commercially available talking photo albums, specific reading software, e-text, audio recordings, screen readers, and multimedia" (p. 612). Answer A, a book holder and mouth stick, is not a practical strategy for use while the child lies in bed, as is desired for this activity. Answer B, fabricate a book holder, is incorrect as the child has limited upper extremity control to turn the pages. Answer D (parent reading to child) does not address the child's desire to independently read and instead relies on support from another person to engage in reading. See Reference: Case-Smith & O'Brien. (2010). Schoonover, J., Argabrite Grove, R.E., & Swinth, Y.: Influencing participation through assistive technology.

129. (D) Blowing cotton balls into a target. Answer D is correct. Blowing cotton balls into a target is a short-term activity with immediate reward for successful completion; therefore, it responds to the child's dual needs. Children with impaired visual attention benefit from "varied activities and time segments that are achievable.... The therapist also gradually increases the amount of sustained attention needed to complete the task" (p. 392). Answers A, B, and C require sustained visual vigilance and involve delayed gratification. They do not represent developmental expectations for a preschool-age child. See Reference: Case-Smith & O'Brien. (2010). Schneck, C.: Visual perception.

130. (C) Supervision. Answer C, supervision, is correct. At this level, the child performs the task on his own, but cannot be safely left alone, or she may need verbal cuing or physical prompts for 1% to 24% of the task. At the independent level (answer A), the child performs the complete task, including the setup. At the independent with setup level (answer B), the child performs the task after someone sets it up for her. Minimal assist (answer D) signifies that the child performs 50% to 75% of the task independently, but needs physical assistance, or other cuing, for the remainder of the task (p. 482). See Reference: Case-Smith & O'Brien. (2010). Shepherd, J.: Activities of daily living.

131. (B) Sheltered employment. Sheltered employment settings (answer B) offer work experience in a segregated environment for individuals with developmental and psychiatric disabilities. This individual would benefit from a sheltered employment setting first, in which intensive and continuing supervision is available, in order to gain work experience and skills, before moving on to an in-house job or transitional employment (answer A), which requires higher levels of skill. Income requirements (answer C) would have little bearing until the individual is qualified for mainstream employment. A job coach (answer D) may benefit the client in various work environments by providing training in skills to perform the job, but identifying a job coach would occur after placement in a vocational environment (pp. 816–829). See Reference: Cara & MacRae. (2013). Auerbach, E.S.: Vocational programming.

132. (B) Understand basic concepts related to money. Answer B, understanding basic money concepts, is correct, as children with moderate intellectual impairment "have an IQ range of approximately 40 to 55...[and] are unlikely to progress past the second grade level in academics" (p. 169). Answers A, C, and D are incorrect as they represent academic skills beyond a second-grade level and are most likely expected of a child with mild intellectual impairments. See Reference: Case-Smith & O'Brien. (2010). Rogers, S.L.: Common conditions that influence children's participation.

133. (D) Present only a few puzzle pieces at a time. Similar to other children with ADHD, this child most likely has poor impulse control and experiences great difficulty completing a task. By presenting a few puzzle pieces at a time (answer D), the OT can help the child focus on a few relevant stimuli and make it possible to complete a short-term task successfully. This experience will then help the child increase attention span. Soft foam puzzle pieces (answer A) are less likely to cause injury if thrown, but their use is not likely to help increase the child's at-

tention span. Providing puzzle pieces of only one color (answer B) may reduce visual stimulation somewhat, and using larger interlocking puzzle pieces (answer C) may make manipulation of the pieces easier, but the overwhelming stimulus caused by presenting all the puzzle pieces at once would make these strategies irrelevant. See Reference: Case-Smith & O'Brien. (2010). Parham, D. & Mailloux, Z.: Sensory integration.

134. (C) Standing kitchen activities can be performed by placing the majority of weight through both arms, using toes for balance (about 10% of weight). Teaching strategies for weight-bearing restrictions for a person with a total hip replacement is very important when planning to address ADL activities because weight-bearing can affect the healing of the hip joint. Placing the majority of weight through the arms, using toes for balance (about 10% of weight), answer C, is the correct guideline for toe-touch weight-bearing. "TTWB (toe-touch weight bearing) indicates that only the toe can be placed on the ground to provide some balance while standing—90% of the weight is still on the unaffected leg. In toe-touch weight-bearing, clients are instructed to imagine an egg is underfoot" (p. 1076). Answer A, performing all activities from a sitting position, would reflect non-weight-bearing status. Placing 50% of the body weight on the affected leg during standing activities, answer B, would be the rule for partial weight-bearing. Performing all standing activities without restriction, answer D, is another way of saying the person may be full weight-bearing. See Reference: Pedretti. (2013). Lawson, S.C. & Murphy, L.F.: Hip fractures and lower extremity joint replacement.

135. (B) detachable armrests. "Armrests come in fixed, flip-back, detachable, desk standard, reclining, adjustable height and tubular styles.... Flip-back, detachable desk and standard-length arms are removable and allow side-approach transfers" (p. 251), making answer B, detachable armrests, correct as they need to be removed to allow the individual to move sideways out of the wheelchair. Footrests (answer A) may be swung away, but do not need to be detached to perform a transfer. Antitip bars (answer C) prevent a wheelchair from tipping over backward (such as when performing a "wheelie" or when going up or down a step), but not when transferring. Brake-handle extensions (answer D) allow the brakes to be locked more easily, but would be in the way of a board transfer. See Reference: Pedretti. (2013). Bolding, D., Adler, C., Tipton-Burton, M., Verran, A., & Lillie, S.M.: Mobility.

136. (B) labels with white print on a black background. "Contrast sensitivity is the ability to detect detail when gradation between an object and the background is subtle. An example may be a white banister on a white wall in a hallway that a client is unable to see or pouring coffee into a black cup. With poor contrast sensitivity, it would be impossible to discriminate between the background and the object" (p. 1231). White print against a black background is easier to see for individuals with poor vision. Using braille labels (answer A) is not appropriate for individuals with peripheral neuropathy because they have decreased tactile sensation in their fingertips. A pill organizer box (answer C) is useful for taking pills on schedule and is particularly helpful for individuals who have memory deficits or complex medication regimens. If the pills were presorted in the box, the individual could safely take them without actually identifying them. However, using the pill organizer does not address the issue of medication differentiation. Brightly colored pills (answer D) would make it easier to identify different medications; however, the therapist has no control over how pills are manufactured and what colors are used. See Reference: Pedretti. (2013). Glover, J.S. & Wright, J.: Special needs of the older adult.

137. (A) Provide verbal cues, external aids, and opportunities to practice using the aids. This individual has a deficit in the area of orientation. "Orientation is an individual's awareness of time, person, and/or place. Deficits in orientation may typically present with memory loss and problems with new learning.... Strategies for improving orientation must be reinforced with all skills throughout the day.... Much of orientation interventions are centered on visual/verbal cuing and consistency.... Basic orientation tools may begin with only a simple calendar or sign of the day and date" (p. 158). Reducing distractions (answer B) and presenting information in short units (answer C) would be adaptive strategies to promote attention and information processing. Connecting new information to previously held knowledge and skills (answer D) is a technique to aid retrieval of information and improve memory and is a remedial, not a compensatory, strategy. See Reference: Meriano & Latella. (2008). Meriano, C. & Latella, D.: Activities of daily living.

138. (D) Recommend that a family member ride in the car when the client is driving. According to Pollard, it is unsafe for individuals functioning at Allen's Cognitive Level 4.6 or below "to drive a motorized vehicle as they do not have the functional cognitive ability necessary to do so safely" (p. 63). Individuals functioning at Allen's Cognitive Level 4.8 can benefit from cuing while driving, and having a family member in the car with him could provide that strategy (answer D). Hiding the car keys

(answer A) is not a client-centered approach. It is likely the individual has already heard from his family about the dangers he presents to himself and others (answer B), and this is not likely to make his driving any safer. Whereas he may benefit from intervention to promote memory and problem-solving skills (answer C), his cognition will nonetheless continue to decline, and he would still need someone in the car with him to provide assistance. See Reference: Pollard, 2010

139. (D) Dollhouse and dress-up clothes. Dollhouse and dress-up clothes (answer D) encourage symbolic play. The child should be exposed to toys that offer open-ended play opportunities, encourage formulation of ideas and feelings, "imagination with storytelling, fantasy; objects represent events/things" (p. 48t). Answers A, B, and C are not only representative of the younger child (answer A) or older child (answers B and C), but they also encourage more defined, closed-ended play with predictable results. See Reference: Parham & Fazio. (2007). Bryze, K.C.: Narrative contributions to the play history.

140. (B) Slide or transfer board. "Slide board transfers are appropriate for clients who have paraplegia of the LEs, bilateral amputations, severe LE weakness, or are unable to weight-bear on both LEs. The slide board is used as a bridge to transfer from one surface to another. The client must have adequate ROM and strength of both UEs, good sitting balance, and trunk mobility" (p. 183). Answer A, stand-pivot transfers, would be appropriate once pylon training begins, whereas answer C, dependent transfers, would not be indicated in a client who has good UE strength and balance. Answer D, sit to stand transfers, also would not be appropriate until pylon training begins. See Reference: Meriano & Latella. (2008). Meriano, C. & Latella, D.: Activities of daily living.

141. (B) a perception that the amputated extremity is painful, crampy, hot, or achy. Phantom sensations "are different from phantom limb in that they are detailed sensations of the limb. Individuals may describe these as cramping, squeezing, relaxed, numb, tingling, painful, moving, stuck, shooting, burning, cold, hot or achy. Phantom sensations are described as constant or intermittent" (answer B, p. 1154). Answers A and D are associated with phantom limb, but not phantom sensations. Answer C, feelings of sharp pain at the residual limb site, may be due to a neuroma, which can be related to nerve tissue issues. See Reference: Pedretti. (2013). Keenan, D.D. & Glover, J.S.: Amputations and prosthetics.

142. (C) Practicing in an actual grocery store. In addition to classroom teaching and homework exercises, practicing in an actual grocery store (answer C) is the third most important training method in grocery shopping skills training. Evidence has shown situated learning to be a more effective approach than simulation (answer A). Determining the lowest price (answer B), being able to find items (answer D), and finding the correct item are the specific skills that the training module should address (p. 669). These specific skills are taught through the use of classroom teaching, practicing in an actual grocery store, and homework. See Reference: Brown & Stoffel. (2011). Brown, C.: Activities of daily living and instrumental activities of daily living.

143. (C) Developing communication tools, as needed, and proper positioning of trunk/head and upper extremities. "The acute inflammatory phase manifests itself as acute weakness in at least two limbs that progresses and reaches its maximum in 2–4 weeks with increasing symptoms.... Developing communication tools, such a sign or picture board,...[and] positioning for trunk, head, and upper extremity stability" (p. 1097) are imperative. This should be followed by gentle, nonresistive activities and light ADLs (answer A) as tolerated. Resistive exercises and balance and stabilization activities (answers B and D) should be implemented later, during the recovery stage, after strength begins to improve. See Reference: Trombly. (2008). Forwell, S.J., Copperman, L.F., & Hugos, L.: Neurogenerative diseases.

144. (D) Weighted utensil holder. Answer D, a weighted holder, is correct. The weight increases proprioceptive (deep-pressure) feedback to the joints and muscles in the hand and wrist, adding to children's awareness of the position and movement of the hand, fingers, and wrist in relation to the pencil and paper. Use of a multisensory approach is "thought to enhance learning" (p. 571). Answers A and C, a wide pen and soft triangle grip, would assist a child with decreased grip, whereas use of a "rubber band sling [answer B]...encourages the student to use a slanted and relaxed pencil position for writing" (p. 574). See Reference: Case-Smith & O'Brien. (2010). Schneck, C. & Amundson, S.L.: Prewriting and handwriting skills.

145. (D) A long-handled reacher. A person with a total hip arthroplasty (posterior lateral approach) must avoid hip flexion of 90 degrees or greater, hip adduction, and internal rotation. A reacher (answer D) would allow the person to adhere to the precautions stated above by providing an extended reach during lower body dressing activities. A wire basket attached to the walker (answer A) would not allow the person to come close to a counter without having to step sideways, which causes hip adduction. A padded foam toilet seat 1 inch in height (answer B) or a

short-handled bath sponge (answer C) would be inadequate because they would cause the person to flex the hip past 80 degrees while performing self-care tasks. See Reference: Trombly. (2008). Bear-Lehman, J. & Maher, C.: Orthopaedic conditions.

146. (A) Power wheelchair. Answer A, a power wheelchair, would be the most appropriate choice, as the OT should consider this option when a child's upper extremity function does not enable her to "propel a manual wheelchair long distances at the same speed and efficiency as demonstrated by the average person walking" (p. 633). With greater use of her upper extremities, answer B, a standard wheelchair may have been a preferred option. Standard wheelchairs tend to be less expensive, lightweight, and portable. Answers C and D (a caster cart and powered scooter) are not considered appropriate for the child with severe cerebral palsy because adequate upper extremity function is required for use of the caster cart (p. 627) and scooter. See Reference: Case-Smith & O'Brien, 2010 Wright-Ott, C.: Mobility.

147. (C) Swing-away footrests and removable armrests. After swinging away footrests and removing armrests, the individual can perform a sliding board transfer without being blocked by the wheelchair. Answers A and B include nothing that would facilitate a sliding board transfer. One-arm drive (answer A) is useful for individuals with the use of only one upper extremity. A low backrest (answer A) is useful for those who require minimal trunk support, because it allows greater freedom of movement for the arms and shoulders. A reclining backrest (answer B) benefits individuals who are unable to sit upright for prolonged periods of time, or who need to recline for weight shifts. Elevating footrests (answer D) are desirable for individuals with lower extremity edema. Answer D is incorrect because although removable armrests may make transfers easier, elevating footrests would not. A footrest would need to be a detachable or swing-away type for it to be moved out of the way. See Reference: Pedretti. (2013). Bolding, D., Adler, C., Tipton-Burton, M., Verran, A., & Lillie, S.M.: Mobility.

148. (C) Trace lines across the page with the right index finger from the left to the right side. A person who follows a line when wheeling a wheelchair (answer A) is focusing on midline positioning, not crossing the midline. Placing objects commonly used on the unaffected side (answer B) is a compensatory technique that does not involve crossing the midline. The individual with midline problems would need cueing to avoid starting at the midline when attempting to lay cards out from the right to left side (answer C). Also, the person would have difficulty accurately completing a sequencing task on the neglected side, making it difficult to complete the midline crossing successfully. However, when tracing a line across the page, the individual receives the same proprioceptive input from the movement, and uses the same amount of space in the visual field, as when writing on paper. This task makes the transfer of skills easier when performing writing. See Reference: Trombly. (2008). Quintana, L.A.: Assessing abilities and capacities: Vision, visual perception and praxis.

149. (A) teaches parents to use firm, steady touch without rocking to help infant during feeding and diapering. Answer A is correct. The tactile system develops early and is responsive in the young NICU patient. "Early stimulations for these younger preterm infants may be safest if it replicates normal parenting activities, such as being held, listening to the caregiver's soft voice, or looking at the caregiver's face. Young infants tolerate stimulation best if it's unimodal (one sensory input at a time). Ideally, family members provide this contact" (p. 666). Playing a musical mobile (answer B) can be overwhelming in view of other visual and auditory stimulation in the NICU. Answer C can be overstimulating because it provides multisensory input to the infant. Answer D is optimal if the bond is encouraged between baby and parent. See Reference: Case-Smith & O'Brien. (2010). Hunter, J.G.: Neonatal intensive care unit.

150. (C) Wash hands between patient contacts. Washing hands between patient contacts (answer C) is the most significant way to reduce the spread of infection. "The largest source of preventable client infection is contamination from the hands of health-care workers" (p. 147). After working with a patient in the ICU or acute care, it is essential to place all linens and equipment in the correct location (answer A); however, that has nothing to do with infection control. Wearing protective clothing (mask, gown, gloves) (answer B) and disposing of any waste in proper containers (answer D) are additional examples of "standard precautions" that health-care workers must apply to prevent the spread of infection. However, hand hygiene, which can include the use of alcohol-based hand rubs, is the most important strategy of all. See Reference: Pedretti. (2013). George, A.H.: Infection control and safety issues in the clinic.

151. (D) Give the individual a rest break. Rest breaks need to be scheduled to avoid fatigue with multiple sclerosis and therefore should be encouraged (answer D). "The occupational performance assessment should include listening to the client and family describe performance patterns to identify typical daily habits, routines, and roles. Evaluating and treating the client at different times during the day will probably reflect different levels of fatigue. Under-

standing the performance patterns of rest periods, quality and amount of sleep, exercise patterns intensity of activity (activity demands) during various times of the day" (p. 939). Strengthening activities (answer C) do not need to be discontinued, but should be designed to benefit the patient without causing undue fatigue. Answers A and B would be contraindicated, as continuing the exercise could cause additional harm to the person with MS. See Reference: Pedretti. (2013). Schultz-Krohn, W., Foti, D., & Glogoski, C.: Degenerative diseases of the central nervous system.

152. (D) monitor heart rate, blood pressure, and symptoms. It is important to assess the patient's heart rate, blood pressure, ECG, and symptoms to establish the patient's tolerance for exercise when working with individuals with cardiac conditions (answer D). "During exercise, physical measurements of heart rate, blood pressure, EKG response, and symptoms are noted" (p. 1302). Shortness of breath and chest pain (answers B and C) are symptoms associated with exercise intolerance, and are subsumed within answer D. Additional symptoms may include pain referred to the teeth, jaw or ear, excessive fatigue, light-headedness and dizziness, and nausea or vomiting. MET values are units of measurement associated with how much oxygen is required to perform various activities. Light ADL activities such as eating, shaving, and standing up require approximately 1.5 to 2.0 METs. Initial ADL evaluation would usually be at this level. Dressing and undressing require about 3.0 to 4.0 METs. A MET level of 3.0 (answer A) may be too high for individuals on the first day of therapy following open heart surgery. See Reference: Trombly. (2008). Huntley, N.: Cardiac and pulmonary diseases.

153. (A) Give simple, step-by-step instructions and physical guidance. In later stages of Alzheimer disease, caregivers should be instructed to simplify communication by using "one-step commands, step-by-step verbal cues, and physical guidance [answer A]" (p. 927). Demonstration with multistep instructions (answer B) can be confusing because it provides too much stimulation. Multistep written instructions (answer C) are unlikely to be retained in the individual's working memory after reading or remembered in sequence. Also, written instructions could be lost if the individual puts them down. Verbally repeating directions over and over (answer D), or rehearsal, does not enable a person with Alzheimer disease to retain information in the memory, and he or she may not repeat the instructions properly. See Reference: Pedretti. (2013). Schultz-Krohn, W., Foti, D., & Glogoski, C.: Degenerative diseases of the central nervous system.

154. (A) Mount lever handles on doors and faucets. Answer A is correct, as lever handles on doors and faucets require less energy than knob handles and are recommended for weak grasp (p. 490). For children with reduced upper extremity strength and endurance, using less complex movements and less force results in energy conservation. Answers B and C are environmental adaptations recommended to minimize the danger of slipping and falling for children with incoordination or postural instability. Answer D is contraindicated, because work on a vertical surface against gravity requires more energy than does movement in a horizontal plane. See Reference: Case-Smith & O'Brien. (2010). Shepherd, J.: Activities of daily living.

155. (A) Brain injury and injuries as a result of fragments impacting the body. A "secondary blast injury is the result of energized fragments flying through the air; these fragments may cause penetrating brain injury" (p. 1269, answer A). Answers B and D are most representative of a tertiary blast injury, which "may occur when the individual is thrown from the blast into a solid object such as an adjacent wall or even a steering wheel. These types of injuries are associated with acceleration/deceleration forces and blunt force trauma to the brain, similar to that observed following high-speed motor vehicle accidents" (p. 1269). Whereas air, lung, and GI issues (answer C) tend to be a result of primary blast injury because of "exposure to the over pressurization wave or the complex pressure wave that is generated by the blast itself,...air-filled organs such as the ear, lung, and gastrointestina See Reference: Pedretti. (2014). Dekelboum, S. & Parecki, K.: Polytrauma and occupational therapy.

156. (B) Positive bedtime routines that are predictable. Answer B is correct. "Because children with ASD often respond to routines in general, several studies have successfully used positive bedtime routines.... Specific activities are thought to be less important than the schedule itself and the implementation of a routine" (p. 458). Jumping on a trampoline (answer A) and pulling an activity option from a bag (answer C) present unpredictable events. Quick, repetitive proprioceptive input, as experienced when jumping on a trampoline (answer A), and play with multisensory tactile media (answer D) are types of sensory input that may actually increase arousal. See Reference: Kuhanek & Watling. (2010). LaVesser, P. & Hilton, C.L.: Self-care skills for children with an autism spectrum disorder.

157. (B) Actively extending the elbow in mid-range 30 to 40 degrees with the forearm resting on the table. Actively extending the elbow in mid-range 30 to 40 degrees while the arm is resting on a table surface (answer B) is correct because muscles with poor minus strength would only be able to move a body part through partial range of motion in a gravity-eliminated position. The individual would then need assistance to complete the range of motion while using what strength is available in the body part. Answer A is incorrect because PROM would not utilize the increased strength available because the muscle does not contract. Answers C and D are incorrect because both involve resistive activities and a muscle with poor minus strength would be unable to move against gravity or to take any resistance, even with gravity eliminated. See Reference: Pedretti. (2013). Flinn, N.A., Trombly Latham, C.A., & Podolski, C.R.: Assessing abilities and capacities: Range of motion, strength and endurance.

158. (A) Provide rocking chairs, music, dimmed light, and reduced clutter. The environment should be reassuring, reminiscent, and calming, and include sensory stimulation. Rocking chairs, aviaries, manipulative tasks, music, massage, oral reading, dimmed lighting, and reduced clutter (answer A) are environmental recommendations for individuals with a diagnosis of dementia (p. 236). "The use of validation [answer B] has been found to aid caregivers in interacting with persons with disorientation" (p. 235), and is considered a communication method, not an environmental adaptation. Monitoring devices (answer C) enhance the safety of the environment, but are not directed toward agitated behavior. For individuals in the later stages of dementia, "environmental adaptations may include mealtime positioning and adaptive feeding strategies" (p. 235). See Reference: Brown & Stoffel. (2011). Schaber, P: Dementia.

159. (A) work locks and latches on doors and windows. The ability to manipulate the locks and latches is a safety concern because the individual may be unable to open them to let family members into the home or close them to keep intruders from entering. Built-up handles (answer B), energy conservation techniques (answer C), and adaptations to clothing fasteners (answer D) are not safety issues. See Reference: Trombly. (2008). Yasuda, Y.L.: Rheumatoid arthritis, osteoarthritis and fibromyalgia.

160. (D) In private, explain the nature of the client-therapist relationship. It is inappropriate for the OT to have more than a professional relationship with a client. In this case, finding a respectful way to explain why the behavior was inappropriate (answer D) is the most appropriate option. "Setting limits and professional boundaries is identifying behavior that you are unwilling to tolerate or that is inappropriate to the setting.... To the novice practitioner, it may appear that setting limits means not caring. However, establishing behavior that you are unwilling to tolerate or accept actually conveys appropriate caring because often the client behavior that one "sets limits on" is the very behavior that is a barrier to satisfying occupational performance, roles, habits, or successful relationships" (p. 646). While self-disclosing some information to clients can be a therapeutic tool, there is some information that would be misinterpreted or inappropriate, such as giving out personal information (answer A). Ignoring the client's request (answer B) constitutes avoidance on the therapist's part and is unprofessional. Though a difficult situation, the OT loses an opportunity to provide valuable feedback to her client. Whether or not the OT has a boyfriend (answer C) is immaterial; she should not use this as an excuse for not giving out her number. It might be an easy way out, but is unprofessional. See Reference: Cara & MacRae. (2013). Cara, E. & Stevenson, P.R.R.: The use of psychosocial methods and interpersonal strategies in mental health.

161. (C) Handle the child slowly and gently in warm water. Answer C is correct because the child with hypertonicity will be most relaxed and easier to handle if tone is inhibited by slow and gentle handling of the body (p. 506). Answer A is incorrect because adaptive equipment is frequently needed to provide a child with a sense of security during bathing and bathing without supports can be dangerous for the child. Answer B is incorrect because bathing the child too quickly could increase hypertonicity. Answer D is incorrect because it provides the parent with a poor model of good body mechanics; the "caregiver's positioning and handling are prime considerations in adapting bathing of children" (p. 506). The parent should kneel by the tub or sit on a low stool while bathing the child. See Reference: Case-Smith & O'Brien. (2010). Shepherd, J.: Activities of daily living.

162. (A) In the apartments, after they have moved in. Training is most effective when provided in a real-world context (answer A). "The place training perspective acknowledges the contextualized nature of learning and habit formation, particularly for major life roles, and eschews assumptions regarding the need for preparatory or transitional experiences (hence questioning the programs that train first in simulated environments [answers B and C]) for persons with disabilities" (p. 477). The clubhouse model (answer D) provides an option for daytime social participation, but would not allow for training in the natural environment. See Reference: Brown & Stoffel. (2011). Pitts, D.B.: Supported housing: Creating a sense of home.

163. (B) Prehensile function. "Each prosthesis is prescribed according to the client's needs and lifestyle and is custom made and individually fitted.... The client's lifestyle and activities determine the most appropriate TDs (terminal device). It is important to provide the wearer with certain information regarding the differences between hook-and-hand-style. The hook TD is lighter and provides better visibility when grasping objects. It is more durable and functional than prosthetic hands" (pp. 1157-1159). The fact that a hook terminal device (TD) provides better prehensile function and allows greater visibility of objects would be the most important consideration for a person whose primary concern is functioning as a carpenter (answer B). Answers A, C, and D are incorrect because although they can be important considerations for some people with UE amputations, they are not as relevant to this person's goals. See Reference: Pedretti. (2013). Keenan, D.D., and Glover, J.S.: Amputations and prosthetics.

164. (A) Use a directive approach, increase structure and repetition, and provide guidance to the client. This individual demonstrates symptoms of anxiety, which include "elevated or heightened pitch of voice, ranking or clenching hands, raised eyebrows were widened eyes, high level of need for reassurance, [and] self-doubt about performance" [p. 188]. The OT can respond in several ways, including instructing the client with "increased structuring, repetition, guidance, and leadership (answer A); encouraging the client by providing reassurance, increasing the clients sense of control, and slowing the pace of therapy" [p. 189]. It is important to validate the client's feelings of anxiety; however, prolonged validation of the client's anxiety (answer B) should be avoided. Removing the client from the work environment (answer C) would be a last resort, as the client's primary goal in this setting is to be able to work. Changing the background music to something more soothing (answer D) may be beneficial to this client, but may not be beneficial or appropriate for other workers who may need a more stimulating environment. See Reference: Taylor. (2008). Establishing relationships.

165. (D) Use deep firm pressure when holding and moving child during dressing. Using firm, deep pressure touch (answer D) is correct as "most individuals with tactile defensiveness feel comfortable with deep touch stimuli and may feel relief from irritating stimuli when deep pressure is applied over the skin areas" (p. 346). Tickling (answer A) and light stroking (answer C) represent light touch that is generally uncomfortable or intolerable for a child with tactile defensiveness (p. 346). A strong stimulus such as loud music (answer B) causes further discomfort during a time when the child is extremely vulnerable to the sensation of light touch (i.e., when clothing is being removed). See Reference: Case-Smith & O'Brien. (2010). Parham, D. & Mailloux, Z.: Sensory integration.

166. (B) Working on a mock car engine. "Work hardening includes all aspects required for the client to return to full function in employment, such as psychosocial, communication, physical, and vocational needs, and typically incorporates work simulation as part of the treatment process" (p. 876). Working on a mock car engine provides a work simulation that would be required by the client's job. This activity also would assist with increasing his endurance, strength, and productivity. Answer A, lifting weights, is not a work-hardening goal when performed in isolation from a simulated work task. Answer C, visiting the work site, would not be a work-hardening activity, but rather part of the onsite analysis that is typically completed by the practitioner and vocational retraining counselor. Answer D, meal preparation in standing position, is not considered to be a demand required by this particular vocation. See Reference: Trombly. (2008). Rice, V.J. & Luster, S.: Restoring competence for the worker role.

167. (B) Calendars. Interventions used to improve memory include restorative approaches, memory aids, and strategy training. "The most promising interventions to improve function in those with memory deficits rely at least partially on compensatory techniques" (p. 666). Calendars (answer B), memory notebooks, and alarm clocks are examples of compensatory strategies. An external memory device uses environmental adaptations or structure to assist an individual in remembering specific information. Examples include setting an alarm clock to wake up in the morning, labeling drawers according to contents, and using a log or calendar to keep track of events and activities. Visual imagery techniques (answer A), mnemonics (answer C), and repetition or rehearsal (answer D) are all examples of restorative strategies. See Reference: Pedretti. (2013). Gillen, G.: Evaluation and treatment of limited occupational performance secondary to cognitive dysfunction.

168. (A) ease the patient onto the floor. "The most important concept to remember with transfer training is that each client will be unique in his/her own assistance needs, limitations, safety issues, and frustration tolerance, to name a few" (p. 178). Whenever a situation occurs in which the OT cannot manage a transfer safely, "the therapist or caregiver should quickly consider carefully assisting the client to the floor" (answer A, p. 179). Attempting to continue or reverse the transfer of an obese patient who has already begun to slip (answers B and C) is likely to result in injury to the OT and perhaps to the client as well. Although calling for assistance (answer D) is

an appropriate action, the higher priority action is to begin easing the patient to the floor to prevent injury to the individuals involved. See Reference: Meriano & D. (2008). Meriano, C. & Latella, D.: Activities of daily living.

169. (B) Encourage staff to practice conversation skills with the client in a local market with local people. This individual is not generalizing the skills gained in the social skills training group to everyday life. Many strategies can be used to promote generalization of skills learned in treatment, including: "homework assignments, in vivo practice (meaning in the real-life/world of the person) [answer B], client's use of self reinforcement, and repeated practice and over learning," to name a few (p. 310). Watching movies (answer A) is not a focused enough activity to enable this individual benefit from it. Providing only positive feedback (answer C) and removing the opportunity to practice (answer D) would both be counterproductive. See Reference: Brown & Stoffel. (2011). Stoffel, V.C. & Tomlinson, J.: Communication and Social Skills.

170. (A) Parallel. Most of the time, individuals functioning at the parallel (answer A) level of social participation are able to "participate without interfering with others; occupy themselves within their own space and their own materials; engage in solitary activity with others in the room; minimal verbal exchange; engage in activity in the presence of others without distraction; look to the leader to select activities to meet safety, love, and esteem needs; prefer focus on activities rather than peers" (p. 46). See Reference: Cole & Donohue. (2011). Cole, M.B.: Social participation basics.

171. (A) Avoid prolonged sun exposure. Common side effects of dopamine-blocking antipsychotic medications include "sexual side effects, extrapyramidal symptoms, acute dystonia, akathisia, tardive dyskinesia...dry mouth,...sedation,...[and] photosensitivity" (p. 255). Lithium, which is a medication commonly used to stabilize mood (not a psychotropic), may cause polyuria, requiring frequent bathroom stops (answer C). Limiting access to sharp objects (answer B) is a precaution taken with individuals who are suicidal. Flashing lights (answer D) may cause seizures in individuals with epilepsy. See Reference: Bonder. (2010). Howland, R.H.: Psychopharmacology.

172. (B) Teach the child to dress her hemiparetic extremities first. Answer B is correct. A child with hemiparesis is taught to dress his or her affected extremities first (p. 503). Answer A (dressing in bed) also is considered an adapted technique, but would be most appropriate for a child with incoordination or poor balance (p. 504). While answer C, educating the child's mother regarding dressing, is something the OTA would do at some point in the occupational therapy process dependent on the child's age, it does not encourage independent dressing skills for an 8-year-old child. Finally, answer D, teaching the child to dress her nonhemiparetic extremities first, is not considered an adaptive skill because this technique will typically interfere with independent dressing skill development. See Reference: Case-Smith & O'Brien. (2010). Shepherd, J.: Activities of daily living.

173. (A) expressive aphasia. Expressive aphasia (answer A) interferes with an individual's verbal or written expression, but not comprehension of verbal or written information. An individual with expressive aphasia would be able to indicate the correct response by nodding or pointing to the stimulus used or a card marked with the correct response: "Broca's aphasia or expressive aphasia [is a condition] in which the patient can follow commands but cannot name objects, repeat phrases, or convey ideas" (p. 1020). Individuals with receptive aphasia (answer B) cannot comprehend spoken or written words and symbols; therefore, they cannot understand verbal directions or consistently respond to stimuli. Individuals with receptive aphasia may be able to imitate or follow a demonstration, but these techniques do not work for sensory evaluation. An individual who has agnosia or ataxia (answers C and D) would be able to understand directions, but be unable to accurately indicate an area because of impaired recognition of the body part or impaired coordination. The method of response may be adapted by using verbal description of an area or cue cards. See Reference: Trombly. (2008). Woodson, A.M.: Stroke.

174. (B) provide a warning tone, such as noisy bracelets on the wrist, or as a reminder to visually scan toward the affected side. Using a cue such as noisy bracelets is one technique that may be used to accomplish compensation for both unilateral neglect and absence of sensation (answer B). It is best to teach the individual visual scanning (attention training through warning tones) of the affected area and the environment, a technique that may be used anywhere. Although hazards may be removed from the environment or padded to prevent injury to an individual (answer D), use of these interventions is only feasible in a person's home. An individual may avoid using sharp tools or extreme water temperature, or use an electric razor (answers A and C), but this avoidance does not teach him or her how to monitor the affected side visually, because it is a precaution that addresses only the problem with sensation. Visual impairments that are not accompanied by sensory or perceptual deficits are more readily over-

come with retraining. See Reference: Trombly. (2008). Quintana, L.A.: Optimizing vision, visual perception, and praxis abilities.

175. (A) Assisted living. Assisted living facilities (answer A) are "housing complexes with efficiencies or one bedroom apartments in which services are included in the cost of the room, such as light housekeeping, activities, transportation, meals, laundry, medication management, and security checks" (p. 237). This is the minimum level of care this individual will require. A senior housing development (answer D) may offer meals, transportation, and light housekeeping services for a fee, but it would not be able to assist with medication management. Memory care facilities (answer B) and long-term care facilities (answer C) offer less autonomy and higher levels of skilled care than is needed at this time. See Reference: Brown & Stoffel. (2011). Schaber, P.: Dementia.

176. (C) Safety razor with extended handle. Answer C is correct. A safety razor with an extended handle is the appropriate component that allows this individual to overcome limited shoulder and elbow range of motion in order to reach his face. Attaching a safety razor or electric razor to a universal cuff (answers A and D) would benefit an individual who is unable to grasp a razor, but would not enable this individual to reach his face to shave. A safety razor with a built-up handle (answer B) would benefit an individual with limited finger flexion or strength, but it also would be ineffective in enabling this individual to reach his face (p. 490). See Reference: Case-Smith & O'Brien. (2010). Shepherd, J.: Activities of daily living.

177. (C) position the client by using a side or front hold. Using a side hold or front hold position during the swallow may be beneficial in decreasing aspiration in persons who experience a delayed pharyngeal swallow and reduced airway closure (answer C). "[There are] two different supportive positions that allow the therapist to help the client maintain head control. Correct positioning allows more appropriate muscular action, which thereby facilitates quality motor control and function of the facial musculature, jaw and tongue movement, and the swallowing process, all of which minimize the potential for aspiration" (p. 699). Full neck flexion (answer D) may make it too difficult to swallow, whereas slight neck extension (answer A) may increase the likelihood of aspiration. A sitting position, if possible, is preferable to lying down (answer B). See Reference: Pedretti. (2013). Smith, J. & Jenks, K.N.: Eating and swallowing.

178. (C) "Patient required occasional tactile cues to look to the left to compensate for visual

field deficit and was able to acquire and correctly position all 50 tiles from the container placed on the left side." "In documenting use of creative media, it is important to show that clients are learning or gaining a skill, and not that the therapist is simply 'giving' them or 'helping' them complete a project.... The therapist will be well served by emphasizing component skills and relating them to other areas of occupation" (pp. 44–45). Answer C includes the level of assistance and the skilled contribution of the therapist (occasional tactile cues, positioning of the materials), measurable data (occasional, 50), and the specific component being addressed (visual-field deficit). It would also be important for the OT to address the relationship between the craft activity and functional performance in the assessment portion of the note. A summary of the patient's progress (answer A) belongs in the assessment portion of the note, as do references to potential for progress (answer B). Answer D incorporates appropriate measurable data, but does not address the visual-field deficit, which is the focus of this question. See Reference: Tubbs & Drake. (2012). Documenting the use of crafts and other creative media.

179. (A) Phenomenological. Phenomenology, answer A, aims to "discover meaning of the lived experience...phenomenology differs from other forms of naturalistic inquiry in that phenomenologists believe that meaning can be understood only by those who experience it" (p. 129). Answer B,"Ethnography is a primary research approach in anthropology concerned with description and interpretation of cultural patterns of groups, as well as the understanding of the cultural meanings people use to organize and interpret their experiences" (p. 350). Answer C, participatory action research, is an "approach that directly involves study participants in each of the 10 research essentials; that is, it involves study participants that contribute to formulating the research questions, or query, study design, and approach to analysis" (p. 353). Answer D, grounded theory, is a method of naturalistic inquiry that is used to "generate theory, primarily employing the deductive process of constant comparison" (p. 350), whereas, answer A, phenomenology, aims to "uncover the meaning of how humans experience phenomena through the description of those experiences as they are lived by the individual" (p. 353). See Reference: DePoy & Gitlin. (2011). Naturalistic inquiry designs.

180. (A) Pretest-posttest. Pretest-posttest design, answer A, is significant "in describing what occurs after the introduction of the independent variable.... This design can answer questions about change following exposure to the independent variable in that

the pretest is given before its introduction. If subjects are tested before and after the intervention, a change in scores on the dependent variable can be reported but cannot be attributed to the influence of the independent variable" (p. 112). See Reference: DePoy & Gitlin. (2011). Experimental-type designs.

181. (C) Unacceptable because it violates the AOTA Code of Ethics. "It is critical that whatever documentation formats are chosen, they conform to federal and state laws as well as the requirements of reimbursement sources. In addition, occupational therapy documentation should adhere to professional ethical guidelines and practice standards" (answer C, p. 474). Whether or not an alternate date has been arranged (answer A) or the agency the practitioner works for allows it (answer B), stating services were provided on a day when they, in actuality, were not is falsification of documentation and violates the OT Code of Ethics. The individual's inability to participate in therapy the next day because of illness (answer D) would only serve to further complicate an already compromised situation; however, this is not the reason the action is unacceptable. See Reference: Schell, Gillen, & Scaffa. (2014). Doherty, R.F.: Ethical practice.

182. (D) Select appropriate assessment tools or screening procedures. An OT evaluation begins with the initial interview and chart review, which guide the OT in deciding on a frame of reference and the identification of specific evaluation procedures or assessments. Assessments are then performed (answer C) to gather information to identify problem areas and plan treatment. After the assessments are complete, the OTR uses clinical reasoning skills to analyze data (answer A) and to identify the person's strengths and weaknesses. The treatment plan (answer B) is developed after the individual's problems have been identified and evaluation data have been analyzed. Finally, specific interventions are selected. See Reference: Pedretti. (2013). Schultz-Krohn, W. & McHugh Pendleton, A.: Application of the occupational therapy practice framework to physical dysfunction.

183. (B) falls prevention. "Falls present a major problem in the elderly. Studies suggest that one fourth of persons aged 65 to 79 and half of those older than 80 fall every year" (p. 239). All of the answers are important to the quality of life and independence for individuals living in an ALF. However, falls are the leading cause of accidental death in people over 65 and are a major reason for nursing home placement. See Reference: Pedretti. (2013). Bolding, D., Adler, C., Tipton-Burton, M., Verran, A., & Lillie, S.M.: Mobility.

184. (C) full disclosure. Full disclosure, answer C, is the correct answer. "Any person who participates in a study, whether participatory action research, single-subject design, or randomized trial, has the absolute right to full disclosure of the purpose and procedures of the study. Full disclosure means that the investigator must clearly share with the informant, subject, or research participant the types and content of interviews, length of time of participation, types and length of observations, and other data collection procedures that will occur, as well as the scope and nature of the person's involvement. Full disclosure also means that any risk to a subject, even if the potential is rare or minimal, must be clearly identified and a plan for remediation offered for each risk to every subject" (p. 149). Answers A, B, and D are all individual components of overall full disclosure. See Reference: DePoy & Gitlin. (2011). Protecting the boundaries.

185. (B) Submit a claim including new G-code/ modifier for current status and G-code/modifier for new goals. Medicare requires providers to submit a claim including new G-code/modifier for current status and G-code/modifier for new goals (answer B) "at least once every 10 treatment days" (CMS, 12/21/12). If the therapist is not ready to discharge the patient, he or she would not "submit a claim with final status G-code/modifier and discharge the patient" (answer A). It would only be appropriate to "identify a different G-code set, such as mobility or carrying/moving/handling, and establish related goals" (answer C) if the individual's self-care goals had ALL been achieved and the patient would benefit from OT addressing a new functional performance area. Medicare employs the Medicare Physician Fee Schedule Database and does not employ the previous system requesting extensions or exemptions to continue to provide services (answer D). See Reference: http://www.cms.gov/Regulations-and-Guidance/Guidance/Transmittals/Downloads/R165BP.pdf

186. (D) There is equivalency between the study group and the control group. "In experimental-type design, procedures to establish control are implemented to minimize the influences of extraneous variables on the outcome of the dependent variable. Two basic methods of control are typically introduced: randomly assigning subjects to one group or the other, the investigator attempts to develop equivalence [answer D], or eliminate subject bias, caused by inherent differences that may occur in the two groups" (p. 90). Answers A, B, and C are incorrect and have no relation to the process of ensuring random assignment/equivalence among group mem-

bers. See Reference: DePoy & Gitlin. (2011). Language and thinking processes.

187. (B) life history. Life history (answer B) is "another important design in naturalistic inquiry, [and] uses a narrative strategy. Life history, also called 'biography of life narrative,' is an approach that can stand by itself as a legitimate type of research study" (p. 133). Answer A, ethnography, is typically used to understand a culturally related topic, whereas answer C, an phenomenological approach, examines the "lived experience" of an individual or group. Answer D, participatory action research, is "founded in the principle that those who experience a phenomenon are the most qualified to investigate it.... Participatory action research involves individuals as first-person, second-person, and third-person participants in designing, conducting, and reporting research" (p. 127). See Reference: DePoy & Gitlin. (201)1. Naturalistic inquiry designs.

188. (D) The OT and the teacher identify new strategies to help the student access and participate in classroom learning centers. Answer D is correct, as consultation is a "collaborative process that takes place between a practitioner and clients, families, other professionals, organizations or communities...to identify and solve problems with occupations, prevent future problems, and achieve identified goals" (p. 1090). Answers A, B, and C are incorrect as they represent learning and outcomes for only one person engaged in the collaborative relationship. Although each of these first three responses are likely to occur as part of the OT's service, they are not characteristics of the consultative approach. See Reference: Schell, Gillen, & Scaffa. (2014). Holmes, W.M. & Leonard, C.: Consultation.

189. (C) An OTA may contribute to the process, but not complete the task independently. "An occupational therapy assistant contributes to the transition or discontinuation plan [answer C] by providing information and documentation to the supervising occupational therapist related to the client's needs, goals, performance, and appropriate follow-up resources" (p. 5). However, because of the analytical nature of provision of discharge recommendations, the OTA does not complete this activity independently (answers A and B), regardless of level of experience. Answer D is incorrect because it does not allow for the input of data from the OTA. See Reference: AOTA Standards of Practice. (2010). http://www.aota.org//media/Corporate/Files/Practice/OTAs/ScopeandStandards/Standards%20of%20Practice%20for%20Occupational%20Therapy%20FINAL.ashx (downloaded 7/20/13).

190. (B) Achieve verbal and nonverbal communication skills. Improved verbal and nonverbal communication skills would be the most relevant behavioral outcome indicating program effectiveness in the area of social skills development. Social interaction skills include a wide variety of verbal communication skills (e.g., starting and ending conversations, questioning, disagreeing in an appropriate manner) and nonverbal communication skills (e.g., gesturing, positioning one's self, appropriate touching) (p. 254). Answers A, C, and D may all indirectly benefit as a result of improved social and communication skills, but these would not directly reflect positive outcomes for measuring effectiveness of social skill training programs. See Reference: Schell, Gillen, & Scaffa. (2014). Fisher, A.G. & Griswold, L.A.: Performance skills.

191. (B) Withhold treatment, but gather information on the course of events for documentation and consultation with the treatment team. The treatment plan may need to be revised as a result of the change in the individual's status. According to AOTA's Standards of Practice (2010), "An occupational therapist modifies the intervention plan throughout the intervention process and documents changes in the client's needs, goals, and performance" (p. 5). The OT must modify the intervention process to reflect changes in status; therefore, answer C is incorrect. Treatment cannot continue as originally planned (answer A), because of the change in status. Waiting for the OT director to return and collect information about the change in status (answer D) could delay resumption of treatment. See Reference: AOTA Standards of Practice. (2010). http://www.aota.org//media/Corporate/Files/Practice/OTAs/ScopeandStandards/Standards%20of%20Practice%20for%20Occupational%20Therapy%20FINAL.ashx.

192. (C) CARF. The Commission on Accreditation of Rehabilitation Facilities (CARF) is the regulatory agency for the provision of rehabilitation services, answer C. AOTA (answer A) was formed in March 1917, originally known as the National Society for the Promotion of Occupational Therapy. JCAHO (answer B) is the Joint Commission on Accreditation of Hospital Organizations. The NBCOT (answer D) is the agency that develops and administers the examination for registration as an OT; therefore, answers A, B, and D are incorrect. See Reference: http://www.carf.org/Accreditation/ Why does accreditation matter?.

193. (A) Reviewing charts for pertinent information. "An occupational therapy assistant contributes to the screening, evaluation, and reevaluation process by implementing delegated assessments and by providing verbal and written reports of observations and client capacities to the occupational therapist in accordance with federal and state laws, other regulatory and payer requirements, and AOTA documents" (p. 4). An identified role of the OTA is to complete data collection records such as a record review, general observation checklist, or behavior checklist (answer A). Independently completing and interpreting evaluations (answers B and C) are not tasks that are within the scope of practice of an occupational therapy assistant. A OTA can contribute to the development of a treatment plan, but it is not within the OTA scope of practice to develop treatment plans independently. See Reference: AOTA Standards of Practice. (2010).

194. (D) How many times a week do you complete a.m. care (hygiene and dressing) and transportation to school for your child? A "double-barreled question" is a one that has more than one question embedded within it. Participants may answer one but not both, or they may disagree with part or all of the question. See Reference: https://owl.english.purdue.edu/owl/resource/559/06/

195. (D) logging in and out each time an electronic entry is made. "Electronic health records are replacing paper charts in many practice settings. Because these systems are electronic, special precautions need to be taken to assure the security and confidentiality of each client's health record. These systems allow nearly instant access to updated information about the client's health care, test results, medications, and consultation reports.... Occupational practitioners (and all other health care providers) need to log in and log out of the system even if they are going to be away from their computer (or other device) for a minute or two" (answer D, p. 472). Answers A, B, and C do not pertain to electronic documentation, but serve as forms of documentation requirements (answers B and C), and answer A, legibility, refers to handwritten documentation requirements. See Reference: Schell, Gillen, & Scaffa. (2014). Sames, K.M.: Documentation in practice.

196. (B) Supported employment. Supported employment (answer B) "refers to competitive work in an integrated work environment consistent with the strengths, resources, priorities, concerns, abilities, capabilities, interests, and informed choice of the individual.... The ongoing services may include a job coach, job trainer, work-study coordinator, and/or employment counselor" (p. 692). This model provides a structure for persons with intellectual disabilities to work in actual job sites while also offering assistance from a job coach and would be more appropriate for an individual living in the community. Adult activity centers (answer A) focus on leisure rather work possibilities. Volunteer work (answer C) could be a useful form of activity, but would not address employment needs. Sheltered workshops (answer D) are designed to help individuals master basic work skills, but have been criticized for creating dependency and not preparing workers for real-life employment, and few such programs now exist outside of the institutional facilities. See Reference: Schell, Gillen, & Scaffa. (2014). King, P.M. & Olson, D.L.: Work.

197. (B) No, it violates the AOTA's Position Paper on modalities. Despite the level of training she has achieved, according to the position paper it is still necessary for the OTA to demonstrate service competency (answer B) to administer PAMs. Service competency in this area includes the theoretical background and technical skills for the safe and effective use of the modality. Although study and practice are necessary to establish service competency, they are not by themselves sufficient; an OT must determine that the OTA is competent before she can administer PAMs (answers A and C). Having an OT on duty in the facility (answer D) does not make it acceptable for a OTA to administer a modality if the OTA has not demonstrated service competency. See Reference: AOTA 2012, retrieved from: http://www.aota.org//media/Corporate/Files/AboutAOTA/OfficialDocs/Position/Physical%20Agent%20Modalities.ashx Position paper: Physical agent modalities.

198. (C) Demonstrate that a patient will perform in a consistent manner when being evaluated twice over the course of 2 weeks. An instrument is considered to be reliable when "a patient will perform in a consistent manner on a test; i.e., the test items will produce the same responses" (p. 392). An individual should achieve scores that are consistent with, but not necessarily identical to, previously achieved scores. Asking experts for their opinion (answer A) is a method for testing validity, not reliability. Determining that a new therapist is able to come up with the same results as those of an experienced therapist (answer B) is a method for demonstrating service competence. Determining an area to evaluate, assessing the need for an evaluation tool and determining an evaluation format (answer D) are the beginning steps for designing a new evaluation tool. See Reference: Hemphill-Pearson. (2008). Powell, N.J.: Research principles used in developing assessments in occupational therapy.

199. (A) The therapist who graduated 9 months ago, has taken the Fieldwork Educator Certificate Program course, and has supervised two level I students. The standards for the accreditation of OT and OTA programs require that a level II fieldwork educator be a "currently licensed or otherwise regulated occupational therapist who has a minimum of 1 year full-time (or its equivalent) of practice experience subsequent to initial certification" (p. 35). The only therapist who does not meet these criteria is the one with 9 months of experience (answer A). Although it may help to develop supervisory skills working with a level I student before taking a level II student (answer B), there is no such requirement; nor is participation in the Fieldwork Educator Certificate Program course required (answer C). The foreign-trained therapist (answer D) has both the required NBCOT certification (which would be indicated by an "R" after her name) and the required years of experience. See Reference: AOTA ACOTE Standards. (2011).

200. (D) The client asks for more beverages during meals and appears surprised when the OT practitioner indicates beverages in closed containers are on the meal tray. The subjective portion of the SOAP note should contain information gained through a chart review or communication with the patient, his or her family, or staff. This information is not measurable and therefore is considered subjective (answer D). Answer A would be in the program plan. Answers B and C would be in the objective portion of the notes because they are either measurable or based on specific observations. See Reference: Pedretti. (2013). Smith, J.: Documentation of occupational therapy services.

Simulation Examination 3

Directions: Circle the correct answer to the following questions. When you have completed this examination, check your answers against the answer key that follows. As you will see, an explanation is given for each answer along with a reference for further study. The book author is listed as well as the chapter author. See the bibliography for complete references. Study the areas in which your comprehension was low then test yourself again by taking Simulation Examination 4.

EVALUATION

1. An individual has a history of substance abuse and poor social skills and is cognitively intact. She has enrolled in a program with an emphasis on developing skills to live independently in the community. The philosophy of the facility is guided by the recovery model. Which assessment should be part of the initial evaluation?

- A. Functional Independence Measure (FIM).
- B. Assessment of Motor and Process Skills (AMPS).
- C. Canadian Occupational Performance Measure (COPM).
- D. Allen Diagnostic Module (ADM).

2. An individual requires 40% to 50% assistance from the OT to transfer from a wheelchair to a sliding board and to lift his legs from the wheelchair into and out of a bathtub. According to Functional Independence Measure (FIM) Levels, the individual will require which level of assistance to complete the transfer?

- A. Total assistance.
- B. Minimal assistance.
- C. Moderate assistance.
- D. Maximal assistance.

3. An OT working at a Veterans Administration hospital has been asked to participate in developing a new program for individuals with posttraumatic stress disorder (PTSD). The PRIMARY focus of treatment planning and intervention will most likely be on which of the following areas?

- A. Pain management and balance.
- B. Memory and concentration.
- C. Sleep and emotional regulation.
- D. Communication and social participation.

4. While developing an occupational therapy profile of a child with a autism spectrum disorder, the OT meets with the child's primary caregiver. What should the OT do as a FIRST step?

- A. Ask the caregiver about the child's typical day and nighttime routines.
- B. Explain that norm-referenced testing will be included in the evaluation.
- C. Interview the teacher to determine developmental milestones the child has reached.
- D. Observe the child in daily activities within the child's typical environment.

5. An OT wishes to identify how a patient spends his leisure time, which leisure activities he especially enjoys, and which others he has participated in that he would be interested in renewing. The MOST appropriate tool for this purpose is the:

- A. Kohlman Evaluation of Living Skills.
- B. Modified Interest Checklist.
- C. OT-Quest.
- D. Leisure Satisfaction Scale.

6. An OT observes that a 10-month-old child is able to sit alone by propping himself forward on his arms, but consistently loses his balance when reaching for a toy. What does this behavior MOST likely indicate?

- A. Developmental delay.
- B. Protective extension.
- C. Typical development.
- D. Advanced development.

7.   A toddler diagnosed with developmental delays does not finger feed and turns away when presented with food in the clinic. The BEST next step for the OT is to:

A. assume fine motor delays limit finger feeding ability.
B. observe him in his home during feeding time.
C. review his chart for food allergies.
D. repeat the observation in a quiet area to minimize distractions.

8.   Which of the following is the BEST instrument to use when assessing three-point pinch strength?

A. Aesthesiometer.
B. Pinch gauge.
C. Dynamometer.
D. Volumeter.

9.   The OT is meeting with the family of an elderly individual who has just been diagnosed with early-stage dementia. The client has had three car accidents within the past 3 months and the family does not feel that continued driving would be safe. They report difficulties with repeatedly getting lost, parallel parking, and driving more slowly than is reasonably safe. Which of the following areas would be MOST important to assess when determining this individual's ability to drive safely?

A. Cognition.
B. Problem-solving.
C. Interpersonal skills.
D. Orientation.

10.   An OT practitioner is assessing the range of motion of an individual who actively demonstrates internal rotation of the shoulder to 70 degrees. How would the OT MOST likely document this measurement?

A. Within normal limits.
B. Within functional limits.
C. Hypermobility that requires further treatment.
D. Limited mobility that requires further treatment.

11.   An individual is able to complete the full range of shoulder flexion while in a side-lying position during an evaluation. However, against gravity, the individual is not quite able to achieve 75% of the range for shoulder flexion. This muscle should be graded as:

A. good (4).
B. fair (3).
C. fair minus (3−).
D. poor plus (2+).

12.   The BEST way to screen quickly for orientation, attention, and memory in older adults is to administer which tool?

A. Loewenstein Occupational Therapy Cognitive Assessment.
B. Allen Diagnostic Module.
C. Allen Cognitive Level Test.
D. Mini-Mental State Examination.

13.   An OT is scheduled to interview an individual with a head injury about the home environment and family and child care responsibilities. Knowing the individual has an attention span of 10 to 15 minutes, which of the following strategies should the therapist utilize FIRST to obtain the most information?

A. Schedule a 30-minute treatment session.
B. Obtain as much information as possible from the chart prior to the interview.
C. Interview the individual using appropriate verbal and nonverbal communication.
D. Perform the interview in an environment where distractions can be minimized.

14.   What is the BEST method for assessing ADL performance of an individual with severe cognitive limitations and poor communication skills?

A. Self-report.
B. Observation.
C. Allen Cognitive Level Screen.
D. Allen Diagnostic Module.

15.   What is the method MOST important to apply when conducting a SEMI-STRUCTURED interview?

A. Utilize questions to influence a client's thinking and to facilitate self-reflection.
B. Follow a predetermined protocol, adjusting the process as needed.
C. Ask questions exactly as they are stated on the evaluation tool.
D. Use good timing and attention to the client's boundaries.

16. An individual with a history of homelessness, substance abuse, and mental illness has begun to participate in the OT program in a shelter for individuals in recovery. The individual indicated an interest in employment as a primary goal and reports previous work as a carpenter 10 years ago. What is the FIRST action the OT should take in assessing work potential?

    A. Observe the individual during a morning cleaning activity.

    B. Identify a low-demand volunteer job within the shelter.

    C. Conduct a readiness assessment.

    D. Determine qualifications for supported employment programs.

17. Which of the following methods is BEST for evaluating a hook grasp?

    A. Direct the individual to hold a sewing needle while it is being threaded.

    B. Observe the individual lift a tall glass half-filled with water.

    C. Have the individual hold a heavy handbag by the handles.

    D. Hand the individual a key to place in a lock.

18. Using the Model of Human Occupation as a frame of reference, evaluation of an individual should focus PRIMARILY on which of the following?

    A. Identification of problem behaviors that need to be extinguished.

    B. Clarification of thoughts, feelings, and experiences that influence behavior.

    C. Assessment of cognitive function, including assets and limitations.

    D. Evaluation of effects of values, routines, performance skills, and the environment on role performance.

19. The OT has received a referral for a patient recently admitted to the psychiatric unit. What is the BEST method to quickly screen for overall cognitive functioning?

    A. Barth Time Construction.

    B. Assessment of Motor and Process Skills (AMPS).

    C. Allen Cognitive Level Screen (ACL).

    D. Mini-Mental State Examination (MMSE).

20. An OT is performing a functional ROM assessment on an individual with arthritis. How should the OT evaluate internal rotation?

    A. Ask the individual to touch the back of his neck.

    B. Use a goniometer to measure internal rotation in a supine position.

    C. Observe the individual touching the small of his back.

    D. Interview the individual regarding areas of pain and stiffness.

21. During an initial visit with a 5-year-old child with a suspected learning disability, the OT observes the child run across the room, hop around on one foot, pick up a pencil, and draw a stick figure using a tripod grasp. When asked to complete a 10-piece puzzle, the child gives up after several unsuccessful attempts. Which type of assessment is MOST appropriate to gather additional information to understand this child's difficulty?

    A. Fine motor.

    B. Gross motor.

    C. Developmental.

    D. Visual perceptual.

22. A student working at her desk has difficulty when altering visual focus on a blackboard 20 feet away and then on items on the desktop area to complete mathematics problems. This MOST likely indicates a problem with:

    A. ocular motility.

    B. binocular vision.

    C. convergence.

    D. accommodation.

23. An individual who alternately laughs and cries without apparent provocation throughout an evaluation would be identified as exhibiting what type of behavior?

    A. Mania.

    B. Emotional lability.

    C. Paranoia.

    D. Denial.

24. An OT is evaluating a child's shoulder stability as part of an assessment of postural control. Which method is MOST likely to be used for this assessment?

    A. Child on stomach with shoulders abducted and legs extended and time how long the child can maintain this position.

    B. Child on back with arms crossed across the chest and time how long the child can maintain this position.

    C. Child in an unsupported chair and ask the child to grab the OT's thumbs, push and pull, and see whether the child can remain relatively still.

    D. Child imitates OT and raises both arms forward overhead, out to sides, return upward, and repeats for 1 minute.

25. A 6-month-old infant being seen for an OT assessment shows a strong preference for the left hand when reaching for a rattle at midline. Considering the development of dominance in normal children, what is the OT MOST likely to conclude?

    A. Further observation and evaluation of right-sided dysfunction is indicated.

    B. Development of hand dominance is proceeding in a typical manner.

    C. Hand dominance will not develop until the child is 1 year old.

    D. Unilaterality precedes bilaterality in typical development.

26. While measuring the active range of motion of a patient's metacarpophalangeal (MCP) joints, it is MOST important for the OT practitioner to provide stabilization:

    A. proximal to the MCP joints.

    B. distal to the MCP joints.

    C. at the wrist.

    D. on top of the MCP joints.

27. During which meal preparation tasks would symptoms related to deficits in executive functioning be MOST EVIDENT?

    A. Making a strawberry, banana, and mango fruit smoothie in a blender.

    B. Using a sharp knife to chop items for a salad using six ingredients.

    C. Baking and icing cupcakes using a conventional oven.

    D. Cooking hamburgers, french fries, and green beans on the stove and in the oven.

28. When measuring elbow range of motion with a goniometer, where must the axis of the goniometer be positioned?

    A. At the lateral epicondyle of the humerus.

    B. At the medial epicondyle of the humerus.

    C. Parallel to the longitudinal axis of the humerus on the lateral aspect.

    D. Parallel to the longitudinal axis of the radius on the lateral aspect.

29. The OT is working with a client who sustained an explosive-related extremity injury. Which of the following issues would the OT MOST likely be evaluating when receiving a referral for this type of injury?

    A. Tympanic membrane rupture, dizziness, and sensitivity to noise.

    B. Amputations, fractures, crush injuries, and/or burns.

    C. Hypotension, renal contusion, and failure.

    D. Hemothorax, pneumothorax, and/or sepsis,

30. The OT is considering the use of paraffin with a client who has a chronic arthritic condition. Paraffin has been shown to be most efficacious with:

    A. assisting with tumor management.

    B. assisting with tendon repair.

    C. decreasing stiffness and improving ROM.

    D. decreasing deep vein thrombosis (DVT).

31. In order to determine oxygen saturation levels during an ADL evaluation, the OT should:

    A. count respirations.

    B. measure heart rate.

    C. read the pulse oximeter.

    D. note the individual's breathing patterns.

32. Which practice should the OT follow when administering standardized tests to a 4-year-old preschool child?

    A. Test in a stimulating environment that keeps the child alert and engaged in test items.

    B. Follow the test manual directions and attend to any deviations that are made.

    C. Report testing was not possible once child fatigued during initial session and did not complete items.

    D. Use encouraging conversation and give breaks as needed to keep this young child at ease.

33. On which areas of function should an evaluation of a 3-year-old child with moderate intellectual disability be focused?

- A. Positioning and communication skills.
- B. Communication, self-care, and social skills.
- C. Reading skills and independent self-help.
- D. Developing writing skills.

34. During a coloring activity, an OT observes a preschooler stabilizing a crayon between the thumb and first two fingers. How would the practitioner MOST accurately document this grasp?

- A. Pincer.
- B. Dynamic tripod.
- C. Palmar.
- D. Lateral pinch.

35. The OT learns from reviewing the chart that an individual is exhibiting positive symptoms of schizophrenia. During the initial evaluation, what should the OT expect to encounter?

- A. A toneless voice.
- B. Very little facial expression.
- C. A false perception of reality.
- D. Difficulty concentrating.

TREATMENT PLANNING

36. An OT is fabricating a static orthotic device that will assist with the maintenance of a functional hand and finger position while keeping the soft tissues of the hand in a midrange position. Which orthotic device would the OT MOST likely select to address these needs?

- A. Bivalve.
- B. Resting.
- C. Dynamic extension.
- D. Wrist cock-up

37. A college student with neurological deficits is planning to return to independent living following discharge from therapy. The student has been working on shoelace tying, but is unable to carry over skills learned from one day to the next day. What is the most appropriate strategy to try next?

- A. Practice the same method more frequently.
- B. Replace regular shoelaces with elastic laces.
- C. Move therapy sessions to a distraction-free environment.
- D. Instruct caregivers to provide assistance for shoelace tying.

38. An OT has been working with an individual with depression who is an inpatient. Now the individual is ready to return to the job held before taking a leave of absence. Which of the following actions should the OT take next?

- A. Perform a job analysis.
- B. Request reasonable accommodation.
- C. Emphasize activities that promote a sense of self-efficacy.
- D. Encourage the individual to participate in a weekly support group.

39. An OT is evaluating an individual with a cognitive disability. The ability to complete a tile trivet following a sample is demonstrated, and an inability to utilize written instructions is observed. Which one of the following jobs would be the MOST appropriate assignment in an employment training program?

- A. Sorting plastic utensils into separate containers.
- B. Assembling packets that include a knife, fork, spoon, and napkin based on a sample.
- C. Selecting matching shoelaces from a mixed pile and lacing them into a display card.
- D. Gluing labels on cans and placing them in an appropriate container according to color.

40. An individual is recovering from digit amputations of the right hand and complains of pain when any sensation is felt on the affected hand. When implementing a program of desensitization training for the patient, the MOST appropriate sequence for grading the sensory stimuli that will be applied to the patient's hand is from:

- A. soft to hard to rough.
- B. tap to rub to touch.
- C. light to medium to heavy.
- D. rough to hard to soft.

41. When preparing a home program with the goal of independent toileting for a young child with postural balance difficulties, what is the MOST important adaptation the OT can recommend?

- A. Replacing buttons on clothes with hook and loop closures.
- B. Mounting a safety rail next to the toilet.
- C. Introducing toilet paper tongs to facilitate independence.
- D. Placing a colorful "target" in the toilet bowl.

42. An artist recently diagnosed with MS is interested in pursuing a leisure activity that will promote physical fitness. Because the individual's symptoms are limited to mild UE numbness and slight weakness in the dominant hand at this point, the BEST activity to recommend is:

    A. volleyball.
    B. painting with the dominant hand.
    C. swimming in a cool water pool.
    D. jogging on a track or treadmill.

43. Results of an occupational therapy evaluation show that a young child has many tactile defensive behaviors. What is the MOST appropriate beginning activity for intervention for this child with sensory processing difficulties?

    A. The child pretends to be part of a "sandwich" between heavy mats.
    B. The therapist applies lotion to the child's arms and legs.
    C. The child is blindfolded and guesses where he or she is touched on the body.
    D. The child and therapist play the "Duck, duck, goose" circle game.

44. When teaching children with moderate intellectual disabilities to feed, groom, and dress themselves, the OT is MOST likely to use which approach?

    A. Chaining.
    B. Sensory stories.
    C. Demonstration.
    D. Role modeling.

45. Following hospitalization for an acute schizophrenic episode, a college student in a psychosocial hospitalization program is uncomfortable in social settings, has difficulty sustaining conversations, is unable to make eye contact, and responds to others with bizarre comments. Which of the following would be the MOST effective treatment approach?

    A. Vestibular stimulation and gross motor exercises.
    B. Modification of the social environment.
    C. Activities that do not require conscious attention to movement.
    D. Social skills training.

46. A resident of a long-term care facility is in a weakened condition and has midstage dementia. Occupational therapy is requested because the resident requires assistance with dressing. What is the best way to reestablish dressing routines?

    A. Have the resident select the clothing she prefers and then have the OT dress the client.
    B. Preview each step of the process as the resident dons and doffs loose-fitting clothing in bed.
    C. Have the resident walk to retrieve clothing garments and encourage independence.
    D. Instruct resident in use of reacher, sock donner, and button hook.

47. An individual with a job installing carpeting experienced extrapyramidal syndrome side effects after being placed on antipsychotic medications in the hospital. If this individual is to continue taking the medication after discharge from the hospital, which instruction is the MOST important?

    A. Limit sun exposure as much as possible.
    B. Avoid use of power tools and sharp instruments.
    C. Get up slowly from a standing, sitting, or lying position.
    D. Be aware of the dehydrating effects of caffeinated drinks and alcohol.

48. In planning OT services using a behavioral approach, what are the BEST intervention activities to include?

    A. Opportunities for the child to express his or her interests.
    B. Play activities that encourage interaction between all children.
    C. Clear expectations and reinforcement for desired performance.
    D. Role play to rehearse and practice desired performance.

49. A long-term goal for an individual with progressive weakness is for the family to carry out his feeding program. Which statement is the MOST appropriate short-term goal?

    A. Patient will participate in feeding program.
    B. Patient will feed himself with moderate assistance.
    C. Family will feed patient safely and independently 100% of the time.
    D. Family will demonstrate independence in current positioning and feeding techniques 50% of the time.

50. A teacher in the child-care program asked the OT to help plan ways to include a preschool child with Down syndrome in parallel play. Which is the OT MOST likely to suggest?

   A. Encourage two or more children to play next to each other with a collection of books.

   B. Initiate a game of "Go Fish" with children seated in a circle on the floor.

   C. Have the child work in a distraction-free environment while coloring a picture.

   D. Encourage several of the children to play a soccer game in the center's outdoor space.

51. When planning an intervention to build self-esteem for an individual demonstrating positive symptoms of schizophrenia, what is the OT MOST likely to use as a treatment format?

   A. Projective media to facilitate expression of feelings.

   B. Work in an isolated area away from the group.

   C. Simple and highly structured activities.

   D. Discussions about the individual's delusions.

52. An OT working for an assisted living corporation needs to design programs to engage residents with dementia who wander and pace the halls throughout the day. What is the BEST type of movement-oriented programming to employ to engage these residents?

   A. Reminiscing about previous jobs.

   B. Walking as part of a walking club.

   C. Singing oldies in a group.

   D. Participating in a craft activity requiring concentration.

53. An OT is using a visual perceptual frame of reference to plan an intervention for a child with visual perceptual problems. The FIRST activities planned should address which type of visual perceptual skills?

   A. Visual memory skills.

   B. Visual attention skills.

   C. General visual discrimination skills.

   D. Specific visual discrimination skills.

54. When performing a preprosthetic evaluation of a patient who had a long above elbow amputation, the OT practitioner should measure the circumference of the residual limb at the:

   A. distal radio-ulnar joint.

   B. proximal radioulnar joint.

   C. distal humerus.

   D. proximal humerus.

55. An OT is using a sensory integration approach with a group of regressed residents on an inpatient unit who display a very low energy level, hyposensitivity to stimuli, and poor visual and tactile perception. What is the BEST activity for beginning a session focusing on identifying pleasant memories?

   A. Go around the circle and ask each patient to introduce himself or herself.

   B. Pass around a scent box and ask each patient to smell the contents.

   C. Ask each patient to select a favorite poem and read it.

   D. Discuss the lunch menu and healthy eating habits.

56. During a kitchen activity, an individual with decreased shoulder ROM demonstrates difficulty retrieving items from the higher shelves. Which of the following recommendations will BEST facilitate home management for this individual?

   A. Store the most frequently used items on shelves just above or below the counter.

   B. Use the largest joint available to move or lift items.

   C. Perform shoulder range-of-motion exercises 10 times each, twice a day.

   D. Continue reaching for items on high shelves because it will help improve range of motion.

57. A 15-month-old child is demonstrating motor performance similar to that of an 8-month-old child. In which activities would the OT MOST likely engage the child to elicit developing protective reactions?

   A. Play while prone on mat, with child reaching to grab toys suspended forward and out to child's sides.

   B. Play while floor sitting with toys placed on floor in front of child, or suspended for child's reach to front.

   C. Play while floor sitting with toys placed on floor to child's sides, or suspended for child's reach, out to child's sides.

   D. Play while in supported quadruped position, with child reaching for toys placed on floor more than arm's reach from child's body.

58. An individual who recently experienced a myocardial infarction has been evaluated by the OT and is currently receiving intervention as part of the OT. A primary concern of the cardiac team is to prevent "overexertion" in therapy. What is the BEST way to address this concern?

A. Teach the client independent medication management strategies.

B. Retrain the client in ADLs to prevent excessive strain.

C. Monitor the client's heart rate and blood pressure regularly throughout the intervention.

D. Teach energy conservation techniques to decrease stress.

59. An OT is planning a group that will include some teens who pose a suicide risk. In selecting craft media, what activity would MOST likely be the safest?

A. Leather checkbook cover with leather lacing.

B. Macramé plant hanger.

C. Ceramic vase.

D. Stenciling greeting cards.

60. Which child with neuromotor impairment would benefit MOST from using a prone scooter for exploratory play?

A. A child with cerebral palsy with predominant extensor tone.

B. A child with generalized low muscle tone who is easily fatigued.

C. A child with cognitive limitations and poor sensory awareness.

D. A child with spina bifida with lower extremity paralysis.

61. An individual who uses a wheelchair and has limited financial support is moving into a new apartment and wants to select a floor surface for easy maneuverability. Which of the following surfaces is the MOST appropriate for this situation?

A. Vinyl floor.

B. Short-pile carpeting.

C. Deep-pile carpeting.

D. Several area rugs.

62. During a meal preparation evaluation, an individual with a brain injury repeatedly cuts up the vegetables before washing them and turns on the stove before filling up the tea kettle with water. Which of the following activities MOST appropriately addresses the deficit area demonstrated?

A. Using rubber stamps in a random design to create notecards.

B. Stringing beads for a necklace, following a pattern.

C. Putting together a 100-piece puzzle and then framing it.

D. Setting a table with dishes and utensils for four people.

63. An OT in a state psychiatric hospital, using the recovery model, is working with a group of older adults with severe and persistent mental illness. They have been hospitalized for decades and will be moved into community living when the hospital closes in several months. Which of the following discharge planning activities is most appropriate for these individuals?

A. Using a map, show them where the new house will be in comparison to where the state hospital is.

B. Allow them to select their roommates.

C. Provide catalogs from which they can select bedspreads and curtains.

D. Provide collage activity to explore/express feelings about moving.

64. An OT practitioner is consulting in a long-term care setting to recommend programs for residents who seem isolated and disengaged from the other residents. Which type of group would be BEST for enhancing self-esteem, providing opportunities for socialization, and assisting residents in integrating past experiences with present life?

A. Reminiscence.

B. Meditation.

C. Grooming.

D. Movement.

65. When selecting activities for an 8-year-old child with Duchenne muscular dystrophy, which developmental issue is MOST important to consider?

A. Establishment of basic trust.

B. Freedom to use his initiative.

C. Development of self-identity.

D. Reinforcement of competence.

66. When working on cooking skills, an individual with a history of traumatic brain injury exhibits moderate upper extremity incoordination. Which of the following recommendations would be MOST beneficial for this individual?

A. Built-up utensil handles.
B. Heavy utensils, pots, and pans.
C. Use of a high stool to work at counter height.
D. Placement of commonly used items on shelves just above and below the counter.

67. In preparing a patient with a unilateral below-knee amputation for discharge from a rehabilitation facility, the MOST important adaptive equipment for the OT practitioner to recommend is:

A. lightweight cooking utensils.
B. a tub bench and toilet rails.
C. long-handled dressing devices.
D. a reacher.

68. An OT practitioner is selecting treatment activities to use with a young adult diagnosed with schizophrenia that would help to increase the ability to receive, process, and respond to sensory information. What are the MOST suitable types of activities to address this area?

A. Social skills training.
B. Gross motor exercises.
C. Life skills.
D. Expressive projects.

69. An OT is developing a pilot program to promote positive behavior in students in the local elementary school. The program will address behavior needs of students with sensory processing challenges and will provide "prevention support" for all students in the classroom. Recognizing the setting and the students' capacities, which approach is MOST likely the OT's first consideration?

A. An in-service training program for parents to help them learn about healthy limits in computer and television time at home.
B. Consultation with the physical education teacher to develop warm-up and cool-down exercises that promote self-regulation.
C. Classroom screenings to identify students who need additional occupational therapy support.
D. Instruct teacher and students to use the Alert program and include routine follow-up visits to classroom to colead sessions with teacher.

70. The OT observes that an individual's brain injury causes difficulty using a bus schedule to get to work on time. What would be the FIRST step toward developing this skill, using a problem-solving training approach?

A. Generate as many solutions as possible for the problem.
B. Identify using a bus schedule as a problem area.
C. Weigh the pros and cons of various solutions.
D. Recognize faulty solutions, self-correct errors, and develop alternate hypotheses.

71. An individual with a history of chronic obstructive pulmonary disease (COPD) has limited endurance. The long-term goal for this individual is to prepare three meals a week. The MOST relevant short-term goal for the OT practitioner to focus on is independent use of:

A. energy conservation techniques.
B. work-hardening activities.
C. graded activities to increase strength.
D. safety skills in the kitchen.

72. An individual who sustained partial-thickness burns is ready for the rehabilitative phase of treatment after 4 weeks in intensive care. The wounds have all closed and there are no open areas remaining. Prior to performing ADL training, what is the MOST important action for the OT to take?

A. Debride the wounds.
B. Remove compression garments.
C. Complete UE strengthening activities.
D. Perform skin conditioning techniques.

73. An individual has sustained a large, full-thickness burn to both upper extremities and is in the acute phase of treatment. Which of the following BEST represents a short-term rehabilitation goal in the acute stage of recovery?

A. Maintain and/or prevent loss of joint and skin mobility.
B. Issue adaptive equipment.
C. Provide compression and vascular support garments.
D. Prevent scar hypertrophy through scar management techniques.

74. Following evaluation of an elderly individual, an OT determines that the individual no longer leaves her bed primarily because of a fear of falling when moving from the bed to the wheelchair. What is the MOST important concept for the OT to remember when working with this individual?

    A. Teach the client to increase lower extremity strength.

    B. Educate the client to increase confidence in the area of functional transfers.

    C. Modify the environment to reduce safety risks.

    D. Reduce the use of medications that may be contributing to falls.

75. The OT is thinking ahead to a child's rehabilitation following a traumatic brain injury. His current program, while he is in acute care, is focused on positioning and movement to maintain joint movement, sensory stimulation, and family education. Which is the OT MOST likely to consider to help identify when the child's awareness increases to a point at which his occupational therapy program can shift its focus?

    A. The child's muscle tone increases.

    B. Child's visual disturbances have diminished.

    C. Parents have prioritized ADL independence as a goal.

    D. Scores on the Ranchos Los Amigos Cognitive Recovery Scale.

76. An individual is about to be discharged to home following a brief hospitalization for substance abuse. The family asks the OT what they should do the first weekend at home. Which of the following suggestions is MOST appropriate?

    A. Throw a welcome home party for some close friends.

    B. Go out to hear a favorite band.

    C. Go on a minivacation.

    D. Attend an AA meeting.

77. In a social skills group, members have learned about social skills and their components, and the OT practitioner has spent time in modeling and demonstrating ways to perform social skills. Based on a Social Skills Training approach, which of the following would be the NEXT step in the process of developing social skills?

    A. Self-evaluating one's social behavior.

    B. Independently practicing in real-life situations.

    C. Role-playing of social situations.

    D. Providing feedback on the client's hygiene.

78. An OT who is employed by a senior center has been asked to develop groups to address the motor needs of people with Parkinson's disease. Which of the following activities would be MOST appropriate to include?

    A. A game of rhythmic exercises performed to music.

    B. Creating time capsules for their grandchildren.

    C. Wheelchair races performed in pairs.

    D. Taking turns reading out loud from the newspaper.

79. A 4-year-old child with spina bifida has a lesion at the lumbar level resulting in a flaccid bladder. The parents are requesting a bladder-training program. What is the OT's MOST appropriate response?

    A. Explain to the parents that toilet training is not a feasible option.

    B. Recommend waiting until the child is 5 years old.

    C. Develop a toilet-training program together with the parents.

    D. Assess the child's ability to remove lower extremity garments.

80. When planning services for a preschool child using the Model of Human Occupation to guide the intervention, what is the OT is MOST likely interested in learning about the child?

    A. Teacher's report of how the child spends classroom free play time and choices made during outdoor recess.

    B. How the child's posture and seating positions impact visual-motor control and use of hands during learning activities.

    C. Instructions, assistance, and cues child is given in preparation for transition between activities, and response following attempts to change activities.

    D. Child's preferences among activities that require movement, such as playground activity, "move and sing" activities, and sand and water play.

81. When designing and implementing an assertiveness training program, what should be the focus of the FIRST session?

    A. Strategies for making a direct request for a desired change.

    B. How to make I statements using the "when you _____, I feel _____" format.

    C. How to stand up for yourself in order to have more control in your life.

    D. Defining the three types of responses: passive, assertive, and aggressive.

82. Which activity should the OT suggest to promote handwriting readiness skills for children in a preschool classroom?

A. Hammering dowels into a Styrofoam board.

B. Creating buildings with wooden blocks in the block center.

C. Rolling clay into many different-sized balls.

D. Drawing lines and shapes using shaving cream or sand.

83. Based on review of evaluation results, the OT believes that school-based services to support a student with autism spectrum disorder should include education for the teaching staff concerning ways to promote positive behavior throughout the school day. In preparation for the IEP meeting, what is the BEST plan to address this concern?

A. Collect handouts with strategies teachers can use to help alert the child in the classroom and distribute them at the meeting.

B. Recommend the staff attend an in-service programs to learn ways to help all students promote self-regulation.

C. Demonstrate for the teacher how the student can use fidget toys and other sensory strategies to help him stay focused during seat work.

D. Discuss the benefit of OT provision of staff education and determine how this can be implemented and documented in the student's IEP.

84. One of the key positioning strategies an OT practitioner plans to provide for a patient with a hip replacement while the patient is sitting or supine is to:

A. place pillows on the lateral side of the hips.

B. elevate the foot on the side of the hip surgery.

C. use a foam wedge between the legs of the patient.

D. insert a roll under the patient's knees.

85. A treatment plan for a child with a visual discrimination problem would MOST likely include which adaptation of visual materials?

A. Low contrast and defined borders.

B. High contrast and defined borders.

C. High contrast and shaded borders.

D. Low contrast and shaded borders.

86. The OT is planning intervention to promote developmental skill acquisition for an infant in the neonatal intensive care unit. Which action will have the MOST therapeutic impact?

A. Adjust infant's positioning to promote physiological development.

B. Recommend early intervention referral to assess the infant when home following discharge.

C. Complete the neurobehavioral assessment and identify interventions.

D. Create a comfortable collaborative relationship with parents and promote parenting skills.

87. An OT hypothesizes that a child's handwriting difficulty is related to a writing posture and posture ergonomics that limit automaticity in handwriting skill. Which option does the OT MOST likely pursue?

A. Promote work habits such as positioning paper in midline area of table/desk, use of nondominant hand to stabilize paper, use of eraser when needed.

B. Implement activities to refine grasp and manipulation of writing tool, gauge speed of work, avoid fatigue when writing.

C. Help student learn strategies to ensure correct spacing, orientation, uniform size of letters drawn.

D. Recommend student work station arrangement that supports pelvis/shoulder/head alignment and optimizes arm/hand position for endurance in writing tasks.

88. An OT is seeing a home health-care client who is in the moderate stages of Alzheimer's disease and whose memory loss is now interfering with the performance of daily self-care activities. What is the MOST relevant OT intervention for this client?

A. Memory-retraining activities for the client.

B. ADL-retraining program for the client.

C. Caregiver instructions in problem-solving.

D. Leisure activity planning.

89. An individual covered by Medicare who has been receiving OT and PT in the home is now able to transfer in and out of the car with supervision of a caregiver and visit friends 30 minutes away. OT services are still required to improve mobility, upper extremity function, and home management skills. Which of the following actions should the OT practitioner take FIRST?

    A. Provide a home program and discharge the individual.

    B. Explain to the individual and caregiver that one must be "homebound" in order to be eligible for home care services.

    C. Refer the individual for outpatient therapy and provide a comprehensive discharge summary to the outpatient setting.

    D. Inform the PT of the individual's status.

90. While developing an occupational therapy program for an adolescent with significant learning disabilities, the OT MOST likely includes which strategies to promote the developmental changes associated with adolescent development?

    A. Opportunities to explore new areas of interest, helping to identify strengths and needs.

    B. Encouragement to join clubs in high school to meet new friends.

    C. Recommendation that the family pursue OT outside of school to prevent negative peer pressure.

    D. Intervention in private area of the school to protect privacy.

91. An individual diagnosed with Guillain-Barré acute syndrome exhibits good upper extremity strength. The activity MOST appropriate for further strengthening and endurance building would be:

    A. peeling potatoes.

    B. bed making.

    C. polishing furniture.

    D. washing windows.

92. When transferring an individual from one seat to another, OT practitioners can BEST protect themselves from injury by:

    A. stepping back from the individual.

    B. keeping the back in a flexed position.

    C. keeping the knees bent.

    D. maintaining a narrow base of support.

93. When treating individuals in the acute phase of cardiac rehabilitation post-myocardial infarction (MI), it is important for the OT practitioner FIRST to select activities that:

    A. prompt dyspnea.

    B. decrease the effects of prolonged inactivity.

    C. promote strength and ROM.

    D. assist with independence in relearning daily activities.

94. An OT observes that an individual who had been doing well on a pureed diet has demonstrated a gurgle, or wet voice, after swallowing a second time. What is the MOST appropriate recommendation for the OT to make?

    A. Videofluoroscopy.

    B. Diet change to include thin liquids.

    C. Tracheostomy tube.

    D. Advancement to a regular diet.

INTERVENTION

95. When fabricating an orthotic device for an individual with swan-neck deformities, the orthotic should be designed to prevent what positions?

    A. Hyperextension of the PIP and DIP joints.

    B. Hyperextension of the PIP joint and flexion of the DIP joint.

    C. Flexion of the PIP joint and hyperextension of the DIP joint.

    D. Hyperextension of the MP joint and flexion of the PIP joint.

96. An OT is developing a retirement planning protocol for a group of older adults at a community senior center, based on the transtheoretical model. Which activity would be MOST appropriate for individuals in the precontemplation stage?

    A. "Identify one life role you wish to continue after retirement."

    B. "List five potential changes you will face following retirement."

    C. "List the steps you need to take to accomplish one of your goals."

    D. "Choose one goal to address for this session."

97. An OT is working as part of a multidisciplinary team that contributes to an Individualized Education Program (IEP). How is an IEP MOST ACCURATELY described?

    A. A contract that lists the student's goals and services intended to help achieve those goals.

    B. A document that outlines the district's educational curriculum together with the state's learning standards.

    C. A process and legal document that outlines strengths, needs, and educational services for a student with disability.

    D. A plan of services and supports for families and their infants and toddlers with disabilities.

98. A patient with a fractured radial head has the arm immobilized from above the elbow to below the wrist. The patient has requested exercises that will help maintain strength in the elbow and forearm muscles while awaiting permission to move the arm. In response, what types of exercises should the OT provide instructions to perform?

    A. Isometric.

    B. Isotonic.

    C. Progressive resistive.

    D. Passive.

99. An individual with a below-elbow amputation lacks sensation in the residual limb. What is the MOST appropriate intervention for the OT to teach the patient?

    A. Techniques of tapping, rubbing, and application of textures to the residual limb.

    B. Routinely inspect the skin closely for signs of skin breakdown.

    C. Deeply massage the residual limb.

    D. Perform proper skin hygiene.

100. After several months of working with an OT, a client with severe and persistent mental illness has obtained a job cleaning empty offices for 4 hours a day. While taking public transportation to the job site, the client experiences ridicule from school-age children taking the same bus to school in the morning. Using an environmental adaptation approach, what is the BEST action for the OT to take so that this client can keep this job?

    A. Negotiate work hours that would allow the client to travel at times that children are less likely to be on the same bus.

    B. Have the client take a taxi rather than a city bus.

    C. Work with the client on coping skills so that the schoolchildren's taunting is more manageable.

    D. Volunteer to offer a mental health awareness day for the local school district.

101. The OT is observing a 3-year-old child during toothbrushing. The child demonstrates good bilateral upper extremity/hand strength, but decreased dexterity. Which piece of equipment would the OT MOST likely encourage the child to use during toothbrushing?

    A. A small soft bristle toothbrush.

    B. A toothbrush with universal cuff.

    C. An electric toothbrush.

    D. A soft sponge-tipped toothette.

102. An individual with a history of anger self-control issues has met the goals of independently identifying anger-provoking stressors in his home and work life and identifying his typical behaviors in anger-provoking situations. What action should the OT take NEXT?

    A. Initiate training in conflict resolution strategies.

    B. Utilize creative media to explore situations that trigger anger.

    C. Implement use of journaling to identify stressors and responses.

    D. Recommend discontinuation of occupational therapy services.

103. A child who has had a traumatic brain injury (TBI) demonstrates tongue thrust. What should the OT do FIRST, prior to feeding?

A. Position the child's trunk, head, neck, and shoulders in proper alignment.

B. Recline the child's seat backward and position neck in slight extension.

C. Place the OT's digits directly under the child's chin, facilitating tongue retraction.

D. Provide upward pressure under the child's lower jaw prior to chewing.

104. The OT is working individually with a client who has demonstrated anger and aggression on several occasions. When the OT observes the client becoming increasingly restless, then yelling, what is the FIRST action the OT should take?

A. Remove himself/herself from physical proximity of the client altogether.

B. Provide the client with the choice to talk about it or end the session.

C. Call for help to escort the client to the emergency room.

D. Leave the door to the treatment room open.

105. An individual reports that back pain during sexual activity is so severe that it prevents any enjoyment. The BEST strategy to recommend is to:

A. use a side-lying position.

B. time sexual activity for periods of high energy.

C. avoid discussing pain with the sexual partner because it may be a "turn off."

D. encourage client to identify alternative methods with the partner for meeting sexual needs that do not cause pain.

106. An OT consults with the parents of a child with anxiety disorder and challenging behavior that interfere with homework completion. They consider modifications to the child's bedroom and homework routine. What recommendation would BEST help the child with self-organization skills?

A. Providing open storage space for clothing and school supplies for easy access.

B. Painting walls and furniture in bright colors to create a cheerful environment and hanging-a-picture schedule.

C. Adding cabinets with labeled compartments to store items out of sight and creating a consistent nightly routine.

D. Giving the child a choice about when he wants to complete homework.

107. An OT making a bedside visit finds the patient poorly positioned with an edematous upper extremity caught between the mattress and the bed rail. The MOST appropriate intervention to address the edema in the upper extremity is to:

A. elevate the arm on pillows so it rests higher than the heart.

B. massage the arm gently, stroking toward the fingers.

C. instruct the patient to avoid active range of motion.

D. suggest the patient avoid passive range of motion

108. An OT is working with the family of a 3-year-old child who lacks sitting balance in the bathtub. The family's insurance does not cover durable medical equipment costs. What should the OT recommend for this child who loves bath time?

A. Place a foam-lined plastic laundry basket in the tub for use with direct adult supervision at all times.

B. Wrap a horseshoe-shaped inflatable bath collar around the child's neck while bathing.

C. Utilize a bath hammock in the tub while bathing.

D. Suggest that the child shower in a standing position instead of bathing in the tub.

109. An OT is advising the parents of a 5-year-old child with athetoid cerebral palsy about the type of toy they might buy to facilitate their child's construction play. What is the BEST type of toy to recommend for this child?

A. Large magnetized shapes and blocks.

B. Blocks that are small and have a firm surface.

C. Soft, nonhardening modeling clay in a variety of colors.

D. Colorful books with heavy paper or laminated pages.

110. An individual with Parkinson's disease has particular difficulty with both starting and stopping movements. What is the BEST strategy for the OT to teach the individual and their caregivers?

A. Perform a deep-breathing exercise when movement is "frozen."

B. Practice the starting phase of the movement repeatedly.

C. Encourage the client to mentally identify the series of steps needed to initiate the movement.

D. Avoid crowds and potential distractions, and perform tasks slowly while walking.

111. An individual who is functioning at Allen's Cognitive Level 4 has difficulty remembering to take his medication twice daily. Which of the following is the MOST appropriate recommendation?

    A. Instruct the client to take medication at 9 a.m. and 9 p.m.

    B. Place a card near the refrigerator showing the blue pill with a picture of breakfast and a white pill with a picture of lunch.

    C. Teach the caregiver to remind the client to take medication twice daily.

    D. Teach the caregiver to place pills into client's hands at the designated times.

112. A sixth grader with poor upper extremity control due to fluctuating muscle tone needs an adapted computer for communication. What is the BEST adaptation to allow for computer use?

    A. Single pressure switch, firmly mounted within easy reach.

    B. Lightweight keyboard placed at midline.

    C. Low-resistance mouse and pad.

    D. Mercury switch headband set to respond to minimal movement.

113. An OT working with adults with serious persistent mental illness is planning a weight management program. Based on a lifestyle redesigned model, the OT will begin with a didactic component. Which of the following is most appropriate for the first session?

    A. Participants share stories about past experiences, challenges, and successes when trying to lose weight.

    B. Participants identify one meal that has personal meaning to them and list substitutes for the least healthy ingredients.

    C. Participants form a cooking group in which they make low-calorie snacks.

    D. The OT presents information on nutrition, diet, and their impact on health and occupations.

114. Following the use of a hand-over-hand approach with accompanying verbal cues to help a child practice bringing the spoon with food to her mouth, the OT is ready to reduce cuing. Which is the BEST method that represents the next step in cue reduction?

    A. Using an index finger on child's wrist, OT guides hand with spoon to child's mouth.

    B. OT cuts child's food into pieces for easier spearing.

    C. As child brings spoon to her mouth, OT reinforces by saying "spoon in."

    D. OT implements a sticker chart to reinforce child's successful eating.

115. An individual who previously worked as a cashier in a clothing store has been referred to a work-hardening program following knee surgery. Limitations are present in standing tolerance and balance. The simulated activity that BEST prepares this individual to return to work is:

    A. moving piles of clothing from one end of the clinic to the other.

    B. folding clothing and putting it in a basket while standing.

    C. washing dishes while standing.

    D. putting price tags on clothing while seated.

116. An OT is considering seating options for a student with extensor tone triggered through LE weight-bearing. What should the therapist recommend to inhibit the child's extensor tone and enable his participation during seat work in the classroom?

    A. Provide lateral trunk supports and a headrest during all seat work periods.

    B. Install a chest seat belt on the chair to maintain upper body support.

    C. Sit on a wedge-shaped seat cushion that is higher in the front and include an abduction post between the knees.

    D. Use a wheelchair with custom-molded seat cushion and lap tray for all seat work.

117. An OT practitioner is planning to introduce constraint-induced movement therapy (CIMT) for an individual who recently experienced a left CVA as she meets the "motor" criteria suggested in the hospital's protocol. What is the suggested motor control inclusion criteria for CIMT?

   A. 15 degrees of wrist extension and 10 degrees of extension for each digit.

   B. 5 degrees of wrist extension and 10 degrees of individual digit extension.

   C. 20 degrees of wrist extension and 10 degrees of extension for each digit.

   D. 30 degrees of wrist extension and 20 degrees of extension for each digit.

118. An OT is fabricating an orthotic device for an individual who has carpal tunnel syndrome. Which of the following orthotic devices fabrication techniques BEST describes the position of the trim lines to allow for adequate digit motion?

   A. Distal to the MCP crease.

   B. Proximal to the DIP joint.

   C. Proximal to the MCP crease.

   D. Distal to the ulnar fifth MCP crease.

119. An individual is learning how to perform transfers into a bathtub 2 weeks after a total knee replacement, but is still unable to extend or flex the knee more than 20 degrees. Which of the following would MOST likely allow for safe tub transfers?

   A. Wait another 2 to 4 weeks, because this activity is contraindicated until 4 to 6 weeks after surgery.

   B. Use a handrail attached to the side of the tub.

   C. Obtain a tub-transfer bench and leg lifter.

   D. Use a low kitchen stool with rubber tips.

120. An OT is working with a fifth-grade child with spina bifida who will need to self-catheterize twice a day. What will this child need in order to perform the self-catheterization?

   A. Assistance with self-awareness, set up and sequencing.

   B. Good hand strength, range of motion, and perceptual awareness.

   C. A powered bidet.

   D. Reducer rings.

121. A child has difficulty sitting due to inadequate postural reactions. What is the FIRST activity the OT would use to promote the development of independent sitting?

   A. Swinging on a playground swing with a bucket seat.

   B. Wide-base sitting on the floor while reaching for a suspended balloon.

   C. Straddling a bolster swing while batting a ball.

   D. Bouncing on a ball with a handle using only one hand for support.

122. An individual who demonstrates compulsive behaviors is repeatedly late for work and in danger of job loss as a result of spending so much time on morning grooming activities. Upon observing this, how should the OT respond?

   A. Explain that washing and brushing so many times is unnecessary.

   B. Encourage speaking about his fear one-on-one.

   C. Acknowledge the use of rituals to cope with anxiety.

   D. Discontinue group work and provide individual treatment.

123. A child with cerebral palsy tends to flex forward while riding her adapted tricycle, even though her lower extremities are correctly positioned. Which adaptations should the OT recommend to BEST enable the child to maintain an upright position while riding?

   A. Raise the seat height.

   B. Raise the handlebars.

   C. Lower the seat height.

   D. Lower the handlebars.

124. Following a hip replacement, a patient is limited to "toe-touch" weight-bearing (TTWB) on the operated extremity. While performing a transfer, the OT should instruct the client to do which of the following?

   A. Attempt to bear 90% of their weight onto the unaffected leg.

   B. Attempt to place 50% of their weight on the affected side.

   C. Try to judge how much weight they can tolerate when standing.

   D. Prompt the client to put 100% of their weight on the affected leg.

125. An OT is simulating cylindrical grasping activities with an individual who desires to work on the skills necessary to be a carpenter. Which of the following activities would MOST likely address these needs?

    A. Positioning a nail on a piece of wood.

    B. Hammering a nail into a piece of wood.

    C. Carrying a pail of bolts.

    D. Unscrewing a lunchbox thermos.

126. A resident of a long-term care facility is receiving OT because of difficulties with eating. The FIRST step the OT practitioner should perform at mealtime is to:

    A. provide skid-proof placemats, plate guard, and utensils with built-up handles.

    B. observe for swallowing after each bite of food.

    C. instruct the caregivers about a special eating setup for the resident.

    D. position the person in an upright posture, making sure head is flexed slightly and in midline.

127. An individual with depression finishes making a poorly constructed Christmas tree ornament and tells the OT to throw it away because it is "such a sorry-looking thing." What is the BEST way for the therapist to respond?

    A. Suggest giving the ornament to a family member.

    B. State that it is beautiful and ask to keep it.

    C. Ask whether it is okay to hang it on the tree on the unit.

    D. Emphasize the importance of participation rather than the end product.

128. An individual with an eating disorder attends a partial hospitalization program as part of an agreement to use a harm-reduction approach to avoid hospitalization. However, at the conclusion of the "Healthy Eating" group that day, the client refuses to eat any of the food. Which is the BEST action for the OT to take in response to the situation?

    A. Set limits by reinforcing the inability to return to the group unless there is an agreement to eat.

    B. Explain the importance of menu planning and meal preparation as key elements of recovery.

    C. Accept her choice and support the decision to, at a minimum, avoid diet pills, laxatives, and/ or diuretics.

    D. Encourage attendance at the stress management group that will be offered later that day.

129. An OT is educating a caregiver regarding manual wheelchair mobility. Which of the following is the BEST way to teach the caregiver to propel a wheelchair down a steep ramp?

    A. Angle the wheelchair backward and guide it down the ramp backward.

    B. Tip the wheelchair backward and guide it down the ramp forward.

    C. Allow the patient to propel the wheelchair independently.

    D. Obtain the assistance of a second individual.

130. An individual has been referred to OT following open heart surgery and a period of prolonged bedrest. After the individual is able to tolerate sitting unsupported at the edge of the bed, and according to MET levels, the NEXT activity the OT practitioner should introduce is:

    A. knitting while seated.

    B. seated sponge bathing.

    C. engaging in sexual intercourse.

    D. taking a hot shower.

131. The OT is educating the parents of a young child with sensory defensiveness regarding hair grooming. The parents report that each time they shampoo their child's hair she becomes anxious, restless, and agitated. What would the OT MOST likely recommend to the parents?

    A. Wash the child's hair with water only and avoid shampoo.

    B. Have the child's hair washed thoroughly at each haircut.

    C. Use a calm voice and explain each step of the hair wash prior to doing it.

    D. Use cool water when shampooing the child's hair.

132. An OT provided information about adaptations that will assist in resuming sexual activity to a patient with a spinal cord injury. Afterward, the patient confides to the OT that there are serious personal issues affecting the sexual relationship with his spouse. What is the BEST action for the OT to take?

    A. Encourage the patient to explain further about the problems.

    B. Explain that this is normal and that divorce rates are actually higher after serious injuries.

    C. Direct the patient to speak with a physiatrist about the concerns.

    D. Encourage the patient to speak with the rehabilitation psychologist.

133. An individual is receiving OT to promote independence in meal preparation and cleanup activities. Which method of structured activity practice would BEST promote retention of learning and generalization of meal preparation skills?

A. Preparing a variety of foods using different cooking methods and recipes.
B. Cooking one meal from beginning to end in the same kitchen setting several times.
C. Mastering one part of a meal at a time.
D. Performing each step of the food preparation process, such as cutting vegetables.

134. A 10-year-old child with a diagnosis of athetoid cerebral palsy would like to be able to dress herself independently. Which clothing features could the OT recommend that would be MOST useful in facilitating self-dressing?

A. Mini T-shirts made of elasticized fabric.
B. Dresses with side zippers and zipper pulls.
C. Oversized T-shirts and elastic-top pants.
D. Front-opening shirts with snaps or buttons.

135. A child has difficulty controlling food in her mouth when swallowing. In helping the parents plan snacks, what type of nipple would the OT MOST likely recommend?

A. Habermann.
B. Single hole.
C. Broad-based.
D. Long, thin.

136. The OT is observing dressing skills in an individual with COPD. While putting a shirt, the individual becomes short of breath, stops to rest before finishing with the shirt, and frequently elevates his shoulders while dressing prior to attempting to put on pants. This behavior MOST likely indicates he is experiencing issues in which areas?

A. Postural control.
B. Muscle tone.
C. Strength.
D. Breathlessness.

137. An client with Parkinson's disease reports recently having "an accident" when unable to make it to the bathroom in time. When the home health OT recommends a bedside commode, the idea is immediately rejected by the client. Which of the following actions should the OT take FIRST?

A. Discuss options and the consequences of each option.
B. Document the reasons for rejection of the adaptation.
C. Practice transferring to a chair at the bedside.
D. Allow time for the individual to think about the options.

138. An individual with moderate cognitive limitations lives in a group home and shares a bathroom with two other clients. He is able to open the toothpaste, apply it to the toothbrush, and brush his teeth independently, but he has difficulty identifying which toothbrush is his, and occasionally uses someone else's toothbrush by mistake. What modification would BEST meet this individual's needs?

A. Using an electric toothbrush.
B. Having the only red toothbrush.
C. Putting a built-up handle on his toothbrush.
D. Requesting a caregiver brush his teeth twice a day for him.

139. The OT is instructing the parents of a child with strong lower extremity extensor tone in dressing techniques. What is the BEST way to position the child to make putting on shoes and socks less difficult?

A. Extend the child's hips and knees.
B. Flex the child's hips and knees.
C. Adduct the child's lower extremities
D. Flex the child's shoulders.

140. An individual who had a stroke is copying a picture of a clock. The drawing appears as a lopsided circle with a flat side on the left. The numbers 1 through 8 are written in numerical order around the right side of the clock. The hands are correctly drawn on the clock to represent three o'clock. The individual's performance appears to demonstrate:

A. right hemianopsia.
B. hemi-inattention.
C. cataracts in the left eye.
D. bitemporal hemianopia.

141. The OT has completed an evaluation on an individual with severe and persistent mental illness while observing the individual in a horticulture group. The client was able to share gardening tools for brief periods of time and participate in the planting activity for a few minutes. Occasional cuing was required from the group leader to allow her to interact appropriately with others. Which group level would BEST enable social participation for this individual?

A. Parallel.
B. Associative.
C. Cooperative.
D. Mature.

142. An individual demonstrates the ability to pick up a penny from a flat surface. The OT practitioner would document this as which type of prehension?

A. Lateral.
B. Palmar.
C. Tip.
D. Spherical.

143. An OT observes a child move from a completely prone position to a prone-on-elbow position. In reporting the child's progress, the OT documents the child is gaining control in the midline position through the development of what type of reactions?

A. Amphibian.
B. Prehensile.
C. Righting.
D. Equilibrium.

144. An OT is employed by a school district to provide consultation to vocational instructors in a high school program for students with intellectual disabilities. Which approach is MOST appropriate for the OT to provide?

A. Developing an in-house prevocational work program.
B. Bringing in outside speakers from different job settings.
C. Teaching the vocational instructor different assessment tools and scoring procedures.
D. Meeting the vocational instructor weekly to discuss adaptations to work tasks.

145. An OT is performing an assistive technology intervention with an individual who demonstrates severely impaired motor performance. What should the OT do FIRST?

A. Research the most appropriate commercially available forms of assistive technology.
B. Identify the individual's abilities, needs, and goals.
C. Select the appropriate method of accessing the technology.
D. Modify the assistive technology device to meet the needs of the client.

146. A young mother is s/p TBI and demonstrates deficits in sequencing and problem-solving. She will need to resume cooking for her family. In her most recent OT session, she successfully made a peanut butter sandwich. What is the NEXT meal preparation activity that should be planned?

A. A cold cheese sandwich.
B. A lettuce, tomato, and cucumber salad.
C. A casserole.
D. A spaghetti dinner with salad and garlic bread.

147. The OT is introducing a new member to a group at a day program for individuals with dementia. Using an errorless learning approach, which one of the following is the BEST way to begin teaching the new group member the names of the other group members?

A. Each group member holds up a sign with his or her name on it, and the new member reads the names of each.
B. Group members create an association between group members' names and characteristics.
C. Each group member introduces him- or herself, and the new group member is then asked to identify one or two names he or she remembers.
D. Each group member states his or her name while tossing a balloon to another group member.

148. An OT is fabricating a dynamic orthosis for an individual who sustained a low-level radial nerve injury while slicing lunchmeat. How should the orthosis be designed?

A. Provide wrist extension, MCP flexion, and thumb flexion.

B. Prevent wrist extension, MCP extension, and thumb extension.

C. Prevent wrist extension, MCP flexion, and thumb flexion.

D. Provide wrist extension, MCP extension, and thumb extension.

149. A patient diagnosed with Parkinson's disease is being seen by an OT to develop a routine for performing self-care activities. How should the OT instruct the patient about the performance of self-care activities?

A. Coordinate with consistent timing of medications.

B. Complete before medications are taken.

C. Only attempt with the assistance of others.

D. Complete at intervals throughout the day until completed.

150. A school-based OT is working on hand function with a school-age child diagnosed with juvenile rheumatoid arthritis. To prevent hand fatigue, what piece of adaptive equipment should the OT recommend?

A. Reacher.

B. Jar opener.

C. Wide-barreled pencil.

D. Plate guard.

151. An OT is performing a home evaluation for an individual with paraplegia who uses a standard manual wheelchair and notes that the entrance to the bathroom is 32 inches wide and the toilet is 15 inches high. Which of the following recommendations will BEST facilitate use of the bathroom for this individual?

A. Widen the doorway.

B. Raise the toilet.

C. Widen the doorway and raise the toilet.

D. Widen the doorway and lower the toilet.

152. An individual diagnosed with substance abuse experiences difficulty gluing two pieces of a birdhouse together, becomes increasingly agitated, and finally storms out of the room. Which approach would be best for the OT to use to facilitate occupational performance?

A. Provide a project with larger pieces.

B. Encourage the individual to take a relaxation break.

C. Make sure each piece of the birdhouse is clearly labeled.

D. Move the individual to an area with fewer distractions.

153. The OT is working with an individual with mental illness and cognitive deficits who has expressed interest in learning to cook in order to move into a less restrictive environment. The OT observes as the client prepares macaroni and cheese from a box. The individual is able to open the box and combine the ingredients but is unable to turn on the heat or recognize when the food is ready. The OT decides to downgrade the activity for the next session. What is the MOST appropriate way to downgrade the activity?

A. Baking chicken and mashed potatoes.

B. Assembling a peanut butter and jelly sandwich.

C. Preparing a frozen dinner.

D. Making instant pudding.

154. On arrival to the neonatal intensive care unit, the OT finds the infant's parents present. Which is the OPTIMAL intervention to assist the parents in responding to their infant's behaviors?

A. Review the chart to complete birth history information and speak to the infant's primary nurse.

B. Introduce yourself as their OT, explain your role in their child's developmental care, and leave to review the medical record.

C. Provide "parent-friendly" written positioning recommendations for the parents to review.

D. Discuss parents' concerns and provide appropriate information and resources.

155. An individual with a C6 spinal cord injury is unable to button his shirt. The OT would be MOST likely to select which type of adaptive equipment to assist the individual with buttoning?

    A. A buttonhook with an extra-long, flexible handle.

    B. A buttonhook with a knob handle.

    C. A buttonhook on a 0.5-inch diameter, 5-inch-long wooden handle.

    D. A buttonhook attached to a cuff that fits around the palm.

156. During the evaluation, an OT observes that an individual is able to place dentures in his mouth, but has difficulty applying denture cream to the appropriate place on the dentures and attempts to place the cap on the tube backward or on the wrong end of the tube. How would the OT MOST LIKELY interpret this observation?

    A. Constructional apraxia.

    B. Ideomotor apraxia.

    C. Constructional impairment.

    D. Unilateral neglect.

157. An OT for a school-age child with visual perceptual deficits is making recommendations to compensate for visual figure-ground challenges in the classroom. Which activities would the OT MOST likely recommend to the child's teacher?

    A. Place a red line on the left side of the page.

    B. Use a timer for certain activities.

    C. Teach the child to use lists and color coding of books and folders.

    D. Block out areas of a page to expose material that is the immediate focus.

158. The OT is instructing the client in tendon gliding exercises. Which of the following is MOST representative of a potential immediate outcome of performing a twice-daily tendon gliding exercise program?

    A. Increased independent use of adaptive equipment.

    B. Decreased edema and prevention of tendon adhesions.

    C. Increased ability to engage in fine motor coordination tasks.

    D. Increased ability to perform resistive tasks.

159. An OT is leading a discussion with a group of individuals who are diagnosed with major depressive disorder. What is the MOST helpful therapeutic communication approach for the practitioner to take?

    A. Be upbeat, positive, and cheerful when encouraging the individuals to discuss their feelings.

    B. Offer even-tempered acceptance, reflection, and assurance that they will get better.

    C. Remain silent and still while the individuals are describing their feelings.

    D. Allow the individuals to structure and lead the group discussion.

160. A preteen with intellectual disability enjoys independent use of his computer-assisted technology, but engages for brief periods and then complains of general fatigue. How can the OT BEST assist the student?

    A. Reassess the physical environment and location of AT.

    B. Increase the size of the computer screen to reduce visual exertion.

    C. Encourage the student to request assistance when feeling fatigued.

    D. Take turns with the student while typing homework assignments.

161. An individual with an SCI has an indwelling catheter and is participating in a group trip to a movie. He is self-conscious about the catheter bag and wants to be sure it is not obvious during the trip. What is the BEST action for the OT to take?

    A. Use a condom catheter for the duration of the trip.

    B. Place the catheter bag in a backpack hung from the handles of the wheelchair.

    C. Utilize a leg-bag for the trip.

    D. Hide the catheter bag under a backpack on the individual's lap.

162. Using an evidence-based approach, how will an OT use Constraint-Induced Movement Therapy with a preschool child with hemiplegic cerebral palsy?

    A. As an adjunct to intervention to promote child's function.

    B. To promote hand dominance.

    C. To restrain the child's dominant hand.

    D. In an attempt to diminish hypersensitivity in the affected limb.

163. A school-based OT works with a classroom teacher to develop strategies that promote good handwriting habits and readiness for written seat work. What is the MOST likely recommended strategy for postural and arm preparation (strength and stability)?

A. Provide physical education instructor with upper body strengthening activities for use in class.

B. Begin writing periods with students completing "chair push-ups" and elastic band stretches.

C. Include paper and pencil tracing games just prior to written seat work periods.

D. Have students trace letters in shaving cream smeared across the tabletop.

164. An OT is positioning a child with low muscle tone and postural instability into a prone stander so she can participate in activities in the art studio. The child rapidly fatigues. How can the OT BEST adjust the stander to promote head righting and enable the student to participate in the class?

A. Place the child in prone on the floor.

B. Position the stander at 45 degrees from the floor.

C. Position the stander at 75 to 80 degrees from the floor.

D. Position the child upright in a prone or supine stander.

165. A client who is diagnosed with depression participates in the group activity for 10 minutes and then states she is just too tired to continue. How would the OT document this in the subject portion of a SOAP note?

A. "Fatigue limits client's participation in the therapy process."

B. "Low level of motivation will limit client's progress in therapy."

C. "Client stated she was too tired to continue."

D. "Client appears unmotivated."

166. A member of a discussion group frequently monopolizes the discussion and interrupts others. The OT has tried to give the client various indirect cues to decrease the disruptive behavior, but the client continues to monopolize discussion. Which direct intervention should the OT implement NEXT to modify the individual's behavior?

A. Sit beside the individual who is monopolizing the discussion and touch his or her hand or arm as a reminder not to interrupt others who are talking.

B. Confront the individual's behavior and ask, "Are you aware that your frequent interruptions prevent others from having a chance to contribute?"

C. Redirect the individual and say, "Now let's hear what others have to say about this."

D. Restructure the task by selecting a group activity that requires sequential turn taking.

167. The OT is working with an older adult diagnosed with diabetes and peripheral neuropathy, following a LE amputation. The client has indicated interest in doing a craft activity while increasing standing tolerance with the new prosthesis. Activities of interest include needlepoint, scrapbooking, woodworking, and painting. Which activity is MOST appropriate for the OT to recommend first?

A. Scrapbooking.

B. Woodworking.

C. Painting.

D. Needlepoint.

168. A parent of four who was diagnosed with a right CVA is receiving home care OT services to improve left upper extremity function and sitting and standing balance. What is the MOST appropriate activity for the OT to recommend?

A. Stacking cones.

B. Manipulating a door pulley.

C. Folding laundry.

D. Throwing a ball.

169. The hospital-based OT is working with a 6-year-old child who has upper extremity weakness and incoordination sustained after a recent head injury. The child wishes to put on and take off her pants independently. What would the OT MOST likely recommend?

A. Pants with Velcro inserts placed in the zipper area.

B. Pants with an elastic waistband.

C. Cotton pants with large buttons inserted where the zipper area is located.

D. Pants with an enlarged zipper-pull attachment.

170. A 13-year-old boy with paraplegia wants to take a bath without assistance from his mother. What would the OT MOST likely recommend to increase independence in bathing?

   A. A transfer bench with a handheld shower.
   B. A hydraulic lift with a sling seat.
   C. An inflatable tub and a bath mitt.
   D. A wheeled shower chair.

171. Which of the following is the MOST important adaptation to recommend to an individual returning home following a total hip replacement?

   A. Move items from high cabinets to lower locations.
   B. Obtain a raised toilet seat.
   C. Place high-contrast tape at the edge of each step.
   D. Install a handheld shower head.

172. What is the appropriate level of involvement for an OT within a parallel group in order to address the psychosocial needs of the group members?

   A. Provide verbal encouragement to support participation.
   B. Observe from the sidelines and refrain from taking a directive role.
   C. Participate as an active member, allowing the participants to run the group.
   D. Assist clients in the selection of simple, short-term tasks.

173. What is the MOST appropriate adaptation for gardening for an individual with a back injury?

   A. Ergonomically correct hand tools.
   B. A wheelbarrow with elongated handles.
   C. A 12-inch-high seat with tool holders.
   D. A raised-bed garden.

174. The OT is encouraging playfulness in a 7-year-old girl with developmental coordination disorder. The child experiences difficulties with motor tasks and often complains that no one likes her. After establishing rapport with the child, what activity would the OT MOST likely introduce?

   A. Playing a game of "Go Fish."
   B. Playing a game of checkers.
   C. Jumping rope.
   D. Role-playing with dolls.

175. Which scar management technique is MOST appropriate to utilize during the rehabilitative phase of treatment with an individual who sustained a partial-thickness burn 6 months ago?

   A. Preventing scar development through static use of orthoses.
   B. Controlling edema to prevent loss of range of motion.
   C. Minimizing scar hypertrophy through compression garments and proper skin care.
   D. Promoting self-care skills in order to resume the role of homemaker.

176. An OT provides consultation to a school district to help maximize the learning environment for students with attention deficit-hyperactivity disorder. Which environmental adaptation recommendation would BEST promote optimal learning for students with ADHD without affecting other students?

   A. Use dim lighting and reduce glare by turning down lights.
   B. Remove all posters and visual aids to reduce visual distractions.
   C. Provide a screen to reduce peripheral visual stimuli.
   D. Restructure classroom activities into a series of short-term tasks.

SERVICE MANAGEMENT AND PROFESSIONAL PRACTICE

177. At the end of an outpatient treatment session, a patient states that his Medicare cap has been reached and he does not want to continue occupational therapy services because he cannot afford to pay for the treatment. Which of the following actions would be MOST appropriate for the OT practitioner to take?

   A. Treat the individual per the physician's order and notify the office manager about the patient's refusal.
   B. Based on his refusal, do not treat the individual and document the interaction in the chart.
   C. Treat the individual, but do not charge or document the services.
   D. Do not treat the individual and only charge for the time spent completing the chart review.

178. An OT is part of a team developing a policy for discontinuation of services to students in school-based settings. When is the MOST appropriate time to end school-based OT services?

   A. Failure to achieve long-term objectives by the end of the school year.

   B. Inability to accomplish short-term goals within one marking period.

   C. Transition from middle school to high school.

   D. Participation in all classroom activities and routines with agreed upon adaptations.

179. An OT is filling out an incident report regarding a patient who was seen on the rehabilitation unit. Which of the following scenarios is the MOST likely to be the subject of an incident report?

   A. The patient complained of nausea during a standing activity.

   B. A patient with a spinal cord injury indicated that his hand orthoses were uncomfortable.

   C. A patient who had a total hip replacement did not follow precautions while completing dressing activities but did not complain of discomfort.

   D. A patient with the diagnosis of CVA and left neglect caught his left arm in the wheel of the wheelchair, resulting in a cut and bruise.

180. An OT in a psychosocial setting is documenting a client's responses to an activity. Which of the following should the therapist write in the chart in order to relay the objective portion of the note?

   A. The client did not want to finish her stenciling activity.

   B. The client was hostile to another client in the activity group.

   C. The client independently selected one of six craft designs presented.

   D. The client demonstrated an appropriate level of frustration tolerance.

181. An OT clinician is teaching her colleagues about survey development and various forms of survey design. A survey is considered to be which of the following?

   A. Non-experimental.

   B. Quasi-experimental.

   C. Pre-experimental.

   D. Time series tool.

182. The OT has just observed a child eating lunch in the school lunch room. Which statement BEST describes an objective observation?

   A. The child did not appear to like the food presented.

   B. The child demonstrated tongue thrust with food presented in five of 10 trials.

   C. The child was uncooperative and unhappy.

   D. The child was apparently not hungry at the time.

183. The OT is seeking a noncompetitive employment environment for a client with an intellectual disability who wants to develop basic work skills. What would be the MOST appropriate community environment?

   A. A clubhouse program.

   B. Supported employment.

   C. A shop with job-coach assistance.

   D. Sheltered workshop.

184. The goal of a work program for homeless youths is to develop job skills that will improve housing status. Which must occur FIRST?

   A. Help clients feel safe and supported, and explore the meaning of the worker role.

   B. Develop work skills, habits, and appropriate interpersonal and work behaviors.

   C. Emphasize quality and identify realistic work interests.

   D. Evaluate participants' performance strengths and weaknesses.

185. The family of a client receiving OT services asks the OT to write a recommendation to terminate the client's driver's license. The OT is uncomfortable taking this action and perceives it as an ethical dilemma. Which principle of the AOTA Code of Ethics could such an action most clearly conflict with?

   A. Social justice

   B. Veracity

   C. Fidelity

   D. Autonomy

186. A parent refuses to allow a level II field-work student to lead his son's therapy session, stating he only wants "someone who's qualified." He insists the OT student must observe the OT lead the session. What action should the OT take FIRST under these circumstances?

- A. Attempt to persuade the parent to allow the occupational therapy student to lead the session.
- B. Advise the parent that the occupational therapy student is finishing her fieldwork next week.
- C. Cancel the session for that day and document that the parent refused occupational therapy.
- D. Comply with the parent's request and allow the OT student to observe the treatment session.

187. At an initial IFSP meeting for a 1-month-old infant with Down syndrome, the team determines that the OT will serve as the primary therapist implementing home visits and interacting with the family. Which team approach for young children does this represent?

- A. Unidisciplinary.
- B. Multidisciplinary.
- C. Interdisciplinary.
- D. Transdisciplinary.

188. The OT program manager of a local hospital must determine the cost-effectiveness of services provided. Which of the following methods would MOST effectively obtain this information?

- A. Outcomes measurement.
- B. Utilization review.
- C. Program evaluation.
- D. Benefit or cost center analysis.

189. The parent, child, and OT worked collaboratively to develop a short-term goal: "demonstrate increased manipulation skills by opening a 3-inch-wide thermos jar independently." The MOST important tool for determining the child's progress is a:

- A. goniometer.
- B. 3-inch screw-top jar.
- C. dynamometer.
- D. developmental fine motor assessment.

190. An OT is attempting to determine the best model to support the idea related to a falls prevention program in a well elderly setting. During the planning, the OT reviews the ethical principles of the Belmont Report to be sure which of the following is adhered to in relation to the participants?

- A. HIPAA and guidelines.
- B. Completion of annual review to maintain approval of participants.
- C. Respect, beneficence, and justice.
- D. The Nuremberg Code, confidentiality, and privacy.

191. An OT practitioner is developing a factory on-site work-hardening/work-conditioning program protocol for workers returning to light duties following musculoskeletal work-related injuries. Which of the following would be MOST relevant to include in the design of the program?

- A. Pain management techniques.
- B. Achieving a balance between work and leisure.
- C. Energy-conservation techniques.
- D. Vocational counseling.

192. A manager of an OT department is attempting to increase the visibility of an OT practice within a community setting that provides services for recipients of Medicare. In order to market the program, the OT manager would MOST likely market via:

- A. a community newsletter.
- B. a presentation to local physicians with flyers and business cards.
- C. a local community workshop.
- D. a presentation to staff at a local hospital.

193. OT and PT are working with an individual with Medicare benefits in outpatient OT following a total hip arthroplasty. The OT's initial evaluation identifies limitations in lower body dressing and moving around the kitchen safely to make meals. Which G-code(s) should the OT use when identifying goals?

- A. G8988—Self-care.
- B. G8979—Mobility.
- C. G8988—Self-care; and G8985—Moving, handling and carrying objects.
- D. G8979—Mobility; and G8988—Self-care

194. A homebound individual has been receiving OT for self-care and home management training and PT for ambulation and stair training following a stroke. The individual reported to the OT that since the last visit she walked to the bus stop independently by herself. This statement is significant in that it indicates that the individual:

    A. is making progress toward her goals and home therapy should be continued.

    B. has achieved her PT goals.

    C. has achieved her OT goals.

    D. is no longer homebound.

195. A third grader's readiness for direct occupational therapy as a related service has been determined on the basis of:

    A. whether occupational therapy services support participation in the education program.

    B. the degree of functional skills possessed by the child.

    C. the level of independence in ADL.

    D. the degree of accessibility of the learning environment.

196. An OT and an OTA work in a collaborative relationship. The teamwork between the two professionals is BEST exemplified by which of the following?

    A. The OT completes the assessment and instructs the OTA to provide a specific intervention.

    B. The OTA updates the OT on the progress a patient has made in the past week, and both provide information to update the goals.

    C. The OTA gives a progress note to the OT and the OT writes the discharge summary based on the progress note.

    D. The OT tells the OTA what type of equipment to order for a patient and the OTA orders the equipment from a medical equipment company.

197. A team composed of an experienced OT and an experienced OTA have worked closely together for 5 years. Of the following, which task(s) MUST be performed by the OT?

    A. Activity programming, environmental adaptations, and caregiver and staff education.

    B. ADL training and running feeding and leisure activity groups.

    C. Interpreting results of assessments for the purposes of treatment planning.

    D. Positioning, providing adaptive devices, and instructing in use of orthotic devices.

198. An occupational therapist has just been hired by an organization with locations in two states and is about to begin seeing patients in both states. When working with patients covered by Medicaid, what must the therapist be sure to do?

    A. Obtain preauthorization.

    B. Understand how Medicaid coverage varies from state to state.

    C. Perform and document monthly reevaluation.

    D. Apply to the federal government for reimbursement.

199. A lead OT researcher is selecting a sample for a study on the effects of a healthy diet and its influence on health and wellness. For the design, the researcher has relied on volunteers pulled from their own OT practice office as a way to recruit clients into the study. This form of sampling is MOST commonly referred to as what type of sampling?

    A. Convenience.

    B. Quota.

    C. Snowball.

    D. Purposive.

200. An OT is writing a job description for an aide position in the OT department. According to AOTA guidelines, which of the following is BEYOND the scope of practice of an aide?

    A. Cue an individual with schizophrenia to maintain attention to task during a weekly cooking group led by an OT.

    B. Practice use of a sock aid and shoehorn in the OT department with a patient who has had a hip replacement and is able to perform the task safely but takes an excessive amount of time.

    C. Help place food on the spoon for a patient learning how to use a universal cuff in the patient's room at lunchtime, while the OT supervisor runs a lunch group in the dining room.

    D. Help a child maintain correct positioning during paper and pencil activities next to the OT who is working with another client.

Answers for Simulation Examination 3

1. (C) Canadian Occupational Performance Measure (COPM). The recovery model emphasizes empowerment of the individual by providing opportunities for self-determination, access to resources, and attention to the individual's values and goals. The COPM (answer C) is consistent with the recovery model because it is "self-directed and person centered and assists the individual in determining what life areas are important to focus on. It also allows the client to indicate his or her level of satisfaction with current performance in the previously identified life areas," allowing "intervention to be guided by what the client finds meaningful" (p. 551). The FIM (answer A) evaluates performance of self-care tasks and was designed for physical rehabilitation populations. The AMPS (answer B) measures ADL and IADL performance, but is not meant to be used with individuals having underlying psychosocial impairments. The ADM (answer D) is a cognitive evaluation used to determine cognitive disability the needed accommodations. See Reference: Brown & Stoffel. (2011). Exley, S.M., Thompson, C.A., & Hays, C.A.: State hospitals.

2. (C) Moderate assistance. Moderate assistance (correct answer, C) is defined as having the ability to complete the task with supervision and cuing, while requiring physical assistance for approximately 50% of the task. The individual who requires minimal assistance (answer B) is able to complete a task with supervision and cuing, while the person completes 75% or more of the task. An individual who performs less than 25%–50% of the task is performing at the maximum assist level (answer D). An individual is rated total assist (answer A) when he or she performs less than 25% of the task. See Reference: Pedretti. (2013). Smith, J.: Documentation of occupational therapy services.

3. (C) Sleep and emotional regulation. Individuals with PTSD have been exposed to a traumatic event and then persistently reexperience the event, often in the form of flashbacks or dreams. The DSM-IV identifies five areas of persistent symptoms: "difficulty falling or staying asleep; irritability or outbursts of anger; difficulty concentrating; hypervigilance; exaggerated startle response." (p. 169). Two of these symptoms are found in answer C—sleep and emotional regulation. Problems with concentration may occur, but not necessarily with memory (answer B), pain, or balance (answer A). Social participation may be impacted by a sense of disconnection from others

or diminished interests, but the ability to communicate (answer D) is not typically an issue. See Reference: Brown & Stoffel. (2011). Davis, J.: Anxiety disorders.

4. (A) Ask the caregiver about the child's typical day and nighttime routines. Asking the caregiver about the child's daily activities (answer A) is the first thing the OT should do when compiling an occupational therapy profile. "Family members can report on the child's functional abilities in various contexts, and situations, the contexts within which the child functions, and the features in those contexts that serve as supports or barriers to the child" (p. 288). A caregiver can provide valuable information about how his or her child with ASD participates in home and community-based activities. Answers B and D, performing testing on the child and observing the child in the home, are something the OT would most likely do after speaking to the child's parent/primary caregiver. Answer C, meeting with the child's teacher, is not considered to be part of the interview with the primary caregiver. See Reference: Kuhanek & Watlin. (2010). Watling, R.: Occupational therapy evaluation for individuals with an autism spectrum disorder.

5. (B) Modified Interest Checklist. The Modified Interest Checklist (answer B) is frequently used to initiate discussion of how a patient usually spends his leisure time and to identify areas of specific interest. It asks respondents "to identify if they currently participate in the activity or if they hope to participate in the activity in the future" (p. 730). Although the Kohlman Evaluation of Living Skills (answer A) addresses the area of leisure, it is used primarily to assess skills in personal care, safety and health, money management, transportation, use of the telephone, and work. The OT-Quest (answer C) was designed specifically for occupational therapists to assess spirituality. There are five key factors, including spiritual, being, meaning, intention, and expression. The Leisure Satisfaction Scale (answer D) measures a client's level of satisfaction in leisure activities in six categories: psychological, educational, social, relaxation, psychological, and aesthetic. See Reference: Brown & Stoffel. (2011). Howells, V.: Leisure and play.

6. (A) Developmental delay. This child demonstrates delayed development (answer A), as typically developing children should be able to sit unsupported for several minutes by the age of 6 to 7 months (p. 68). Protective extension (answer B) is a postural reflex that appears as arms reach out (around 6 months) to protect against falling when the child is pushed or lowered to the floor (p. 255). Sitting unsupported earlier than 6 months may indicate advanced development (answer D). See Reference: Case-Smith & O'Brien. (2010). Case-Smith, J.: Development of childhood occupations.

7. (B) observe him in his home during feeding time. Answer B is correct. Considering the context that surrounds a child's performance is a critical process in occupational therapy assessments (p. 207). The reason he does not feed himself may be environmental; for instance, his parents may have taught him not to touch food with his fingers or he may not have learned to feed himself because his grandmother always feeds him. In addition, the child may not be able to transfer skills learned at home to the clinic; that is, he may believe that the place to eat is home, not the clinic. Although answers A and C provide useful information for treatment planning, they do not address feeding skills. Answer D does not put the skill to be assessed into an environmental context. See Reference: Case-Smith & O'Brien. (2010). Stewart, K.B.: Purposes, processes, and methods of evaluation.

8. (B) Pinch gauge. A pinch gauge is used to measure the strength of "a three-point pinch (thumb tip to tips of index and middle fingers)" (p. 1048), in addition to key (lateral) pinch and tip pinch. These tests are performed with three trials that are averaged together and then compared with a standardized norm. Answer A, the aesthesiometer, measures two-point discrimination. Answer C, the dynamometer, measures grip strength. Answer D, the volumeter, measures edema in the hand. See Reference: Pedretti. (2013). Kasch, M.C. & Walsh, J.M.: Hand and upper extremity injuries.

9. (A) Cognition. This individual appears to be functioning no higher than Allen's Cognitive Level 4.8. Older individuals at this level tend to drive too slowly and reaction time is affected. They may experience repeated collisions and have increasing difficulty with double parking. They "may argue with authorities and their family's assessment that they are unsafe to drive" (p. 79). Therefore, cognition (answer A) is the most important area to assess. The therapist would not want to limit cognitive assessment to the area of problem-solving (answer B). Difficulty in interpersonal skills (answer C) may arise as cognition declines; however, that is not the focus of the situation, nor is orientation (answer D). See Reference: Pollard, 2010

10. (A) Within normal limits. Normal range of motion for internal rotation is 70 degrees (answer A).

Rotation can be assessed with the humerus adducted against the trunk or with the shoulder abducted to 90 degrees. If the humeral movements for internal or external rotation are observed during the performance of activities and found to be adequate for performance of functional activities, range of motion may be noted as WFL (answer B). The OT practitioner may choose not to perform a formal joint measurement if the joint is WFL, even though the end of the range may be lacking a few degrees, because the loss of movement may not be significant to the individual. Hypermobility (answer C) at a joint is motion past the average range of motion, which at the shoulder would be past 70 degrees of internal rotation. If hypermobility is caused by an unstable joint as might occur after a surgical repair or a disease process, then use of orthoses or another form of stabilization or immobilization can be used to correct the problem. If the practitioner observes hypermobility during range of motion, he or she should compare the range of motion to that on the individual's opposite side in order to assess normal range. A limitation of internal rotation (answer D) at the shoulder would be less than 70 degrees of motion. If a limitation is apparent, the rehabilitation team may choose not to treat it unless it interferes with the function of the upper extremity. See Reference: Trombly. (2008). Flinn, N.A., Trombly Latham, C.A., & Robinson Podolski, C.: Assessing abilities and capacities: Range of motion, strength, and endurance.

11. (C) fair minus (3−). The definition of fair minus (3−) is the grade given when an individual moves a part through incomplete range of motion (50% or less) against gravity or through complete range of motion with gravity eliminated against slight resistance. A grade of good (4), answer A, indicates ability to move through full range of motion against gravity and to take moderate resistance. A fair grade (3), answer B, would be the ability to move through the full range of motion against gravity, but not take any additional resistance. A grade of poor plus (2+), answer D, would move through full range of motion with gravity eliminated and take minimal resistance before suddenly relaxing. See Reference: Pedretti. (2013). Phillips Killingsworth, A., Williams Pedretti, L., & McHugh Pendleton, H.: Evaluation of muscle strength.

12. (D) Mini-Mental State Examination. The Mini Mental State Examination (answer D) "is a widely used screening tool for assessing cognitive function in older adults. The MMSE assesses orientation, registration, attention, recall, and language" (p. 250) and takes approximately 10 minutes to administer. The Loewenstein Occupational Therapy Cognitive Assessment (answer A) takes much longer to administer (30 to 50 minutes) and is a more comprehensive assessment of "orientation, visual and spatial perception, visuomotor organization and thinking operations" (p. 249). The Allen Cognitive Level Test (answer C) screens for cognitive level, but does not specifically assess orientation, attention, and memory. The Allen Diagnostic Module (answer B) provides more in-depth information about cognitive level. See Reference: Brown & Stoffel. (2011). Brown, C.: Cognitive skills.

13. (B) Obtain as much information as possible from the chart prior to the interview. An individual who has difficulty sustaining attention demonstrates inability "to consistently engage in an activity over time such as reading for 15 min. without losing concentration" (p. 794). This individual will most likely have difficulty with a lengthy interview or evaluation. By reviewing the individual's medical records before the interview (answer B) the OT can determine what information has already been obtained. This will enable the therapist to make the best use of the available time. With such a limited attention span, it would probably be more efficient to schedule two 15-minute sessions rather than one 30-minute session (answer A). Using good communication skills (answer C) and providing an environment where distractions are minimized (answer D) are both important to a successful interview. These techniques would optimally be applied after the therapist reviews the chart. See Reference: Schell, Gillen, & Scaffa. (2014). Toglia, J.P. et al: Cognition, perception, and occupational performance.

14. (B) Observation. "Observational assessment [answer A] is particularly useful with people with communication difficulties...limited mental capacity...or younger clients" (p. 630). It "allows a degree of flexibility that enables therapists to use judgment and improvisation when moving from theory and hypothesis generation to an understanding of the person's unique experience and performance in a particular context" (p. 631). Self-Report (answer A) "helps the therapist to identify what clients want to do...and the things they need or are expected to do" (p. 630), facilitating a client-centered approach. However, this would not be an appropriate approach for an individual with poor communication skills. The Allen Cognitive Level Screen and the Allen Diagnostic Module (answers C and D) evaluate cognitive level and assist with treatment planning and intervention, but do not assess ADL performance. See Reference: Cara & MacRae. (2013). Laver-Fawcett, A.: Assessment, evaluation, and outcome measurement.

15. (B) Follow a predetermined protocol, adjusting the process as needed. "Generally, occupational therapists administer two basic types of interviews. The first type includes a semi-structured interview in which a therapist follows a predetermined protocol and asks a set of questions designed to probe for specific kinds of information...the interview the therapist conducts is adjusted as the interview progresses to allow the interview to feel more like a naturally unfolding conversation" (p. 195). Skillful interviewing also involves using good timing and attention to boundaries (answer D) and utilizing questions to influence a client's thinking and to facilitate self-reflection (answer A), regardless of the type of interview. Standardized assessments require the therapist to follow the protocol exactly (answer C). See Reference: Taylor. (2008). Interviewing skills and strategic questioning.

16. (C) Conduct a readiness assessment. This individual has a history of chronic mental illness, chronic substance abuse, and chronic unemployment. According to the transtheoretical model, a person will not change until his is ready to change. "Readiness assessment [answer C] is an important first step in any rehabilitation assessment process, and...must come before conducting functional and resource assessments" (p. 701). Behavioral observation (answer A), identifying volunteer opportunities (answer B), and determining whether the individual qualifies for any type of work program (answer D) would all occur later. See Reference: Brown & Stoffel. (2011). Pitts, D.B.: Work as occupation.

17. (C) Have the individual hold a heavy handbag by the handles. The hook grasp is strongly based on the use of digits two to five. "Hook grasp is the only prehension pattern that does not include the thumb to supply opposition.... This is the attitude the hand assumes when holding a shopping bag, a pail, or a briefcase" (p. 767). A needle would be held with a two-point pinch while being threaded (answer A). A glass would be held with a cylindrical grasp (answer B). Finally, a key being placed in a lock would be held by a lateral pinch (answer D). See Reference: Pedretti. (2013). Lashgari, D. & Yasuda, L.: Orthotics.

18. (D) Evaluation of effects of values, routines, performance skills, and the environment on role performance. The concepts that make up the theory of this model "address (1) the motivation for occupation, (2) the routine patterning of occupations, (3) the nature of skilled performance, and (4) the influence of environment on occupation" (p. 506); therefore, these are the areas that would be addressed in the evaluation process. Evaluation according to the Behavioral frame of reference identifies problem behaviors that need to be extinguished (answer A). The Object Relations frame of reference attempts to clarify thoughts, feelings, and experiences that influence behavior (answer B). An OT using the Cognitive Disability frame of reference should evaluate cognitive function, including assets and limitations (answer C). See Reference: Schell, Gillen, & Scaffa. (2014). Forsyth, K. et al: The model of human occupation.

19. (D) Mini-Mental State Examination (MMSE). The Mini Mental Status Examination (answer D) "is a widely used screening tool for assessing cognitive function.... The MMSE assesses orientation, registration, attention, recall, and language. It is a quick measure that takes approximately 10 min. to administer" (p. 250). The Barth Time Construction (answer A) requires an individual to complete a color-coded chart to demonstrate how the individual spends their time during the day. The AMPS (answer B) assesses ADL performance, scoring the individual on both motor and process abilities. The ACL (answer C) uses a leather lacing activity to assess problem-solving skills. See Reference: Brown & Stoffel. (2011). Haertl, K. & Christiansen, C.: Coping skills.

20. (C) Observe the individual touching the small of his back. Touching the small of the back requires shoulder abduction and internal rotation. Reaching the back of the neck (answer A) requires external rotation. Functional evaluations are best performed by observing movements during functional activities. A goniometer would be used when formal joint measurement is required (answer B). An interview (answer D) will provide useful information concerning pain, stiffness, and limitations in occupational performance, but it is not a reliable method for assessing ROM. See Reference: Trombly. (2008). Flinn, N.A., Trombly Latham, C.A., & Podolski, C.R.: Assessing abilities and capacities: Range of motion, strength and endurance.

21. (D) Visual perceptual. Visual perception (answer D) contributes to a child's ability to "relate materials to one another" (p. 384) and visual perceptual deficits may result in "problems with cutting, coloring, constructing with blocks or other construction toys, doing puzzles..." (p. 384). Running, hopping, using a tripod grasp, drawing a stick figure, and putting together a 10-piece puzzle are all developmentally appropriate skills for a 5-year-old child (p. 74). Although this child cannot put together the 10-piece puzzle, the gross and fine motor skills required to assemble the puzzle are observed. No fine motor evaluation (answer A) is indicated because the child demonstrates the expected tripod grasp. No gross motor evaluation (answer B) is necessary because running and hopping skills are evident. Because the child's abilities appear developmentally appropriate, developmental evaluation (answer C) is not indicated. See Reference: Case-

Smith & O'Brien. (2010). Case-Smith, J.: Development of childhood occupations; Schneck, C.: Visual perception.

22. (D) accommodation. Answer D, accommodation, is correct. "Accommodation refers to the process used to obtain clear vision. Focusing must take place efficiently at all distances, and the eyes must be able to make transition from focusing at near point to far point and vice versa" (p. 357). Answer A, ocular motility, refers to the ability to pursue an object visually in an efficient and smooth manner. Answer B, binocular vision, is the ability to focus the eyes on an object at varying distances and on seeing a single object clearly. Answer C, convergence, is the ability to move the eyes inward or outward with continued focus on the object. See Reference: Hinojosa & Kramer. (2009). Schneck, C.: A frame of reference for visual perception.

23. (B) Emotional lability. "Lability is a state of unstable emotions.... [O]ne individual may swing rapidly between laughter and tears, while another person may cry uncontrollably yet be unable to identify the reason for the tears" (p. 181). Emotional lability may be one of the symptoms observed in individuals experiencing mania (answer A). Paranoia (answer C) describes enduring beliefs about being harmed. Denial (answer D) is not acknowledging the presence of information. See Reference: Cara & MacRae. (2013). MacRae, A.: Diagnosis and psychopathology.

24. (C) Child in an unsupported chair and ask the child to grab the OT's thumbs, push and pull, and see whether the child can remain relatively still. The correct response is answer C. Stability results from the "ability of opposing muscle groups to contract at the same time to provide stability around joint" (p. 248), known as co-contraction. The approach given in answer C enables the therapist to observe if muscles around the glenohumeral joint contract together so the left and right shoulder girdles provide stability to the upper torso, enabling the child to resist the therapist's force and retain the upright seated position. Answer A is the ability to maintain the prone extension position, while answer B is an example of supine flexion. Answer D may be used to examine range of motion, strength, and symmetry of both upper body sides; however, it incorrectly assesses shoulder stability. See Reference: Mulligan. (2014). Mulligan, S.: Conducting interviews and observations.

25. (A) Further observation and evaluation of right-sided dysfunction is indicated. Answer A is correct because infants usually use a bilateral approach at this age. Research reflects that "60% of the children...(and in the infants 6 to 24 months of age) were inconsistent in hand use for a simple grasp task" (p. 289). "It is worrisome and atypical when infants (less than 7 months old) consistently use one hand, and these infants should be further evaluated for possible neurological impairment" (p. 289). Answer B is incorrect because unilaterality at age 4 months is not typical development. Answer C is incorrect because research has shown that consistent hand preference is seen from 2 to 4 years. "Inconsistency was noted in some children in the 2.5- to 3-year-old group but not in the 4-year-old group" (p. 289). Answer D is incorrect because bilaterality precedes unilaterality in the course of infant development. See Reference: Case-Smith & O'Brien. (2010). Exner, C.: Evaluation and intervention to develop hand skills.

26. (A) proximal to the MCP joints. Stabilization is applied proximal to the MCP joints to isolate the joint movement being measured and to eliminate any combined movements. Answers B, distal to the MCP joints, and C, at the wrist, would allow combined movements of the joints and would invalidate the individual joint measurements. Answer D, on top of the MCP joints, would block joint movement and make any individual joint measurements incorrect. See Reference: Trombly. (2008). Flinn, N.A., Trombly Latham, C.A., & Podolski, C.R.: Assessing abilities and capacities: Range of motion, strength and endurance.

27. (D) Executive functioning refers to higher-order mental capacities such as "decision making, problem solving, planning, task switching, modifying behavior in light of new information, self-correction, generating strategies, formulating goals, and sequencing complex actions" (p. 245). Cooking the hamburgers, fries, and green beans (answer D) requires planning, sequencing, timing, and judgment to make sure the items, which all need to be cooked in different ways and for different amounts of time, are all ready at the same time. All of the other tasks are cognitively less complex and require the individual to follow straightforward directions that are not sensitive to a particular order (answers A and B) or only require timing for one item (answer C). See Reference: Gillen. (2009). Managing executive function impairments to optimize function.

28. (A) At the lateral epicondyle of the humerus. The "lateral epicondyle of the humerus" is the axis at which goniometer placement would occur as this is the bony prominence on the lateral side of the elbow. The medial epicondyle (answer B) is the bony prominence on the medial side of the elbow. The stationary arm of the goniometer should be positioned parallel to the longitudinal axis of the humerus on the lateral aspect (answer C). The movable

arm of the goniometer should be positioned parallel to the longitudinal axis of the radius on the lateral aspect (answer D). See Reference: Trombly. (2008). Flinn, N.A., Trombly Latham, C.A., & Podolski, C.R.: Assessing abilities and capacities: Range of motion, strength and endurance.

29. (B) Amputations, fractures, crush injuries, and/or burns. An explosive-related extremity injury (answer B) can present as "traumatic amputations, fractures, crush injuries, compartment syndrome, burns, cuts, lacerations, infections, arterial occlusion, air embolism-induced injury." Answer A typically results from an auditory or vestibular explosive-related injury, whereas answer C results from a renal injury and answer D from a respiratory related explosive injury. See Reference: Pedretti. (2013). Dekelboum, S. & Parecki, K.: Polytrauma and occupational therapy.

30. (C) decreasing stiffness and improving ROM. "Paraffin is primarily used to decrease stiffness and improve ROM. It is frequently used to treat chronic arthritic conditions and also offers pain control.... A primary advantage of paraffin is that it allows for an even distribution of heat to the treatment surface, which is effective in reducing stiffness and pain" (answer C, p. 118). Answer A, B, and D are situations in which "superficial heat agents should not be used" (p. 110). See Reference: Bracciano. (2008). Thermotherapy: Superficial heat agents.

31. (C) read the pulse oximeter. Oxygen saturation levels may drop during activity in individuals with compromised lung capacity. The use of oxygen may be required if oxygen saturation falls below 90% during activity. The instrument used to measure oxygen saturation is the pulse oximeter (answer C). Increased respirations and heart rate (answers A and B) may indicate the individual is not receiving enough oxygen, but they also occur normally with increased activity levels. It is important to note breathing patterns (answer D) when working with individuals with compromised lung capacity, such as fast and shallow breathing, holding the breath, or shoulder elevation. Although any of these behaviors may be indicative of decreased oxygen saturation, specific information about the saturation levels cannot be ascertained. See Reference: Trombly. (2008). Huntley, N.: Cardiac and pulmonary diseases.

32. (B) Follow the test manual directions and attend to any deviations that are made. Answer B is correct. When administering a standardized test, directions from the test manual should be followed closely to ensure reliability of test results. The test environment should be free of visual or auditory distractions or the child may have difficulty concentrating; therefore, answer A, "test in a stimulating environment," is incorrect. Answer C is incorrect because there are times when "a child's fatigue, behavior, or time constraints" make it impossible to give the complete test in one session, and "most tests provide guidelines about how the test can be administered in two sessions" (p. 239). Answer D is incorrect because although the overall success of an evaluation can depend on the OT's ability to establish a rapport with the child and the family, too much conversation with the child may be distracting and prevent optimal performance. See Reference: Case-Smith & O'Brien. (2010). Richardson, P.K.: Using standardized tests in pediatric practice.

33. (B) Communication, self-care, and social skills. Answer B is correct. "Early programs for children with intellectual impairment usually focus on facilitating the attainment of developmental milestones; enriching the environment; developing self-help, language and motor skills" (p. 170). Answer A is a more appropriate focus for a child with significant intellectual disabilities who relies on caregiver for assistance with all daily activities and care. Answer C is incorrect, as individuals with moderate intellectual disabilities can develop independence in ADLs, and can achieve academic performance at the third- to seventh-grade level. However, these areas are not a focus in early preschool programs. Answer D is incorrect because it is focused on skills expected in kindergarten programming. See Reference: Case-Smith & O'Brien. (2010). Rogers, S.L.: Common conditions that influence children's participation.

34. (B) Dynamic tripod. Answer B, dynamic tripod, is correct. In this grasp, the writing tool "rests against the distal phalanx of the radial side of the middle finger while the pads of the thumb and index finger control it" (p. 58). A pincer grasp (answer A), or tip pinch, is characterized by opposition of the thumb and index fingertips to allow the child to make a circle with the fingers. The palmar grasp (answer C) is a power grasp in which the individual flexes the fingers around an object while stabilizing it against the palm. In a lateral pinch (answer D), the individual places the pad of the thumb against the radial side of the index finger near the DIP joint. This pattern is used as a power grip on small objects. See Reference: Case-Smith & O'Brien. (2010). Schneck, C. & Amundson, S.L.: Prewriting and handwriting skills.

35. (C) A false perception of reality. The symptoms of schizophrenia can be divided into two categories: negative symptoms resulting in trait loss, such as flat affect, impoverished thought process, lack of interest or energy, inability to experience pleasure, and inability to sustain attention (p. 203), and positive symptoms that add traits, such as delusions, hallucinations, disorganized or pressured speech, and

disturbed sleep patterns (p. 199). Answer C, a false perception of reality, or hallucinations, is representative of a positive symptom. Negative symptoms (answers A, B, and D) tend to persist after the positive symptoms, which are treated with medications. See Reference: Cara & MacRae. (2013). MacRae, A. & Andonian, L.: Schizophrenia; Hoppes, S., Bryce, H.R., & Peloquin, S.M.: Substance abuse and occupational therapy.

36. (B) Resting. A resting orthotic device is the most appropriate orthosis to fabricate for the maintenance of a functional hand position. "A resting or functional position splint [orthotic device] is one that is worn when the client is not involved in active movements or functional tasks. Once the splint [orthotic device] has been fitted, a wearing schedule must be established" (p. 901). Answer A, a bivalve cast, is typically used when circumferential pressure of a body part is required to maintain a desired position. Areas that commonly benefit from bivalve casts are digits, wrists, and knees. Answer C, dynamic extension orthosis, is not considered to be a static orthosis, but an orthosis with moving parts (dynamic). This incorporates outriggers to maintain a position of function. Answer D, a wrist cock-up orthosis, does not impact the position of the entire hand owing to the orthotic device's distal aspect terminating at the MCP crease. See Reference: Pedretti. (2013). Lashgari, D. & Yasuda, L.: Orthotics.

37. (B) Replace regular shoelaces with elastic laces. A patient who exhibits no capacity for new learning will be unable to benefit from therapy interventions that require the ability to transfer learning (answers A, C, and D). Inability to carry skills over suggest the individual is not capable of new learning, and more practice (answer A) would not be a useful approach. A compensatory approach of adapting the environment and recommending assistance for safe performance of daily activities is the most appropriate intervention. Using elastic laces (answer B) is a compensatory approach, appropriate when "a disability is considered permanent" or when "underlying client factors or performance skills are not expected to improve" (p. 331). A distraction-free environment (answer C) would be useful for individuals with attention deficits. If the student's goal is to live independently, caregiver assistance (answer D) is not an appropriate solution. See Reference: Schell, Gillen, & Scaffa. (2014). Gillen, G.: Occupational therapy interventions for individuals.

38. (A) Perform a job analysis. "A job analysis [answer A] provides an objective basis for hiring, evaluating, training, accommodating, and supervising people with disabilities" (p. 683) and identifies essential functions of a particular job. Based on the results, the OT can then work with the individual to maximize performance or request reasonable accommodation (answer B). Activities that promote self-efficacy (answer C) can be beneficial for individuals with depression, but would have been used earlier in the intervention process. A weekly support group (answer D) may be an effective way for the individual to obtain support and can be recommended, but the job analysis is more relevant to the individual's immediate needs. See Reference: Schell, Gillen, & Scaffa. (2014). King, P.M. & Olson, D.L.: Work.

39. (B) Assembling packets that include a knife, fork, spoon, and napkin based on a sample. This individual's abilities suggest a functional level of Allen's Cognitive Level 4. At this level of functioning, an individual is able to copy demonstrated directions presented one step at a time and may find it easier to copy a sample than to follow directions or diagrams, as would be the case for the activity of assembling packets that include a knife, fork, spoon, and napkin based on a sample (answer B). Answer A reflects functioning at Allen's Cognitive Level 3, at which individuals are capable of using their hands for simple, repetitive tasks and sorting tasks, but are unlikely to produce a consistent end product. The individual could do this, but it would not be the most appropriate choice because he is capable of performing at a higher level. The shoelace task (answer C) is more appropriate for those functioning at Allen's Cognitive Level 5, because these individuals can identify the relationships between objects and generally perform three-step tasks. Gluing labels on cans (answer D) and placing them in an appropriate container according to color describes a task that can be performed by an individual who has the ability to anticipate errors and plan ways to avoid them. This is also a generally more complex task and requires attention to detail, all of which requires that an individual be able to function at Allen's Cognitive Level 6 (pp. 203–208). See Reference: Cole. (2012). Allen's cognitive disabilities group.

40. (A) soft to hard to rough. The desensitization process involves applying a sequence of graded texture and force stimuli to the skin to reduce tactile hypersensitivity. Texture begins with soft, progresses to hard, and moves to rough stimuli. "These surfaces are graded from very resilient, such as soft foam, to variously resistant and textured, such as layers of felt, rice, and clay...and increase the contact time and pressure as tolerated" (p. 1269). Answer B is incorrect because the force of the stimuli begins at the level of touch, progresses to rub, and moves to tapping as tolerance for sensation increases. Light, medium, and heavy (answer C) do not specify what the texture and force of the stimuli would be during

training. Answer D is incorrect because a person with hypersensitivity would be unable to tolerate stimuli beginning with a rough texture. See Reference: Trombly. (2008). Stubblefield, K. & Armstrong, A.: Amputations and prosthetics.

41. (B) Mounting a safety rail next to the toilet. The safety rail (answer B) is the best option; to be able to sit independently on the toilet and relax sufficiently to control muscles needed for elimination, the child has to feel posturally secure (p. 500). Safety rails next to the toilet, low toilets that allow the child to put both feet on the ground, and reducer rings to decrease the size of a toilet seat all help to provide maximal stability for the child with unstable posture. Answers A, C, and D describe adaptations used for other needs. Replacing zippers and buttons with Velcro closures (answer A) is helpful for a child with reduced strength or fine motor coordination. Introducing toilet paper tongs (answer C) helps increase reach in a child with limited range of motion. Placing a colorful "target" (answer D) helps boys aim into the bowl, a difficulty associated with perceptual or cognitive limitations. See Reference: Case-Smith & O'Brien. (2010). Shepherd, J.: Activities of daily living.

42. (C) swimming in a cool water pool. Swimming is an excellent activity for promoting physical fitness, and the cool water pool (temperature cooler than 84F) will prevent the overheating that is contraindicated for individuals with MS. Jogging and volleyball (answers A and D) are both likely to result in overheating, and volleyball would probably also fatigue weak hand muscles. Painting (answer B) is a lightweight activity that would probably appeal to an artist, but would do very little to promote physical fitness. See Reference: Pedretti. (2013). Schultz-Krohn, W., Foti, D., & Glogoski, C.: Degenerative diseases of the central nervous system.

43. (A) The child pretends to be part of a "sandwich" between heavy mats. The sandwich activity (answer A) is correct. This provides heavy touch pressure over the body, and "most individuals with tactile defensiveness feel comfortable with deep touch stimuli" (p. 346). Answer B is incorrect because "[g]enerally, tactile stimuli that are actively self-applied by the child are tolerated much better than stimuli that are passively received" (p. 346) and the cool temperature of the lotion may be uncomfortable. Answer C, touch while blindfolded, is incorrect because "[t]actile stimuli may be especially threatening if the child cannot see the source of touch" (p. 346). Answer D is incorrect as it includes light touch provided by others and touch that is unseen (touch from behind). See Reference: Case-Smith

& O'Brien. (2010). Parham, D. & Mailloux, Z.: Sensory integration.

44. (A) Chaining. Backward and forward chaining are among the behavioral approaches frequently used with children with cognitive limitations (p. 502). Sensory stories (answer B) are frequently used with children whose sensory processing interferes with their participation in occupation. Answers C and D may be used together with other approaches; by themselves, they do not address the cognitive and perceptual deficits and limited processing performance skills that are characteristic of children with intellectual disabilities (p. 501). See Reference: Case-Smith & O'Brien. (2010). Shepherd, J.: Activities of daily living.

45. (D) Social skills training. Social skills training (answer D) is the correct answer because it can be used to develop the ability to relate appropriately and effectively with others. "Social skills training uses behavioral demonstrations, role play activities, feedback, prompting, coaching, modeling, shaping, and out of session assignments to help participants develop the skills necessary for communication, social adaptation, and interpersonal relationships" (p. 1175). The sensory integration treatment approach, which aims to improve the reception and processing of sensory information within the central nervous system, uses vestibular stimulation and gross motor exercise (answer A). This approach involves the use of pleasurable activities that do not require conscious attention to movement (answer C), and is best suited to individuals with chronic schizophrenia who have proprioceptive deficits. Modification of the social environment (answer B) will not help in developing social skills and is most appropriate for individuals with cognitive disabilities. See Reference: Schell, Gillen, & Scaffa. (2014). Appendix 1: Common conditions, resources, and evidence.

46. (B) Preview each step of the process as the resident dons and doffs loose-fitting clothing in bed. Because of her cognitive deficits, a compensatory strategy will be more effective than teaching her to do things differently by using adaptive equipment (answer D). "Activity performance can be enhanced through modifications that compensate for activity limitations rather than restore previous capacities" (p. 639). This individual has low endurance as well as cognitive deficits so they would most likely benefit from an adapted, structured approach. Dressing in bed will require less energy initially, and the larger, stretchy garments (answer B) will make dressing easier. Reviewing each step before it occurs will provide cognitive cues. Having the client only select clothing (answer A) does not provide enough participation to be therapeutic. Answers C and D are too demanding and do not provide the structure necessary to ensure safety and successful performance. See Reference: Schell, Gillen, & Scaffa. (2014). Gillen, G. & Schell, B.A.B.: Introduction to evaluation, intervention, and outcomes for occupations.

47. (B) Avoid use of power tools and sharp instruments. Extrapyramidal symptoms are "a set of possible neurological side effects most often associated with psychotropic medication. Common symptoms associated with EPS include extreme restlessness and involuntary muscle movements" (p. 967). Individuals experiencing extrapyramidal syndrome, which may cause muscular rigidity, tremors, and/or sudden muscle spasms, should avoid or take care when using power tools or sharp instruments (answer B). Photosensitivity, an increased sensitivity to the sun, is another side effect often associated with antipsychotic medications that can be addressed by limiting sun exposure (answer A), but is less of a concern because this individual works indoors. Answer C is a strategy that can be used to avoid postural hypotension, a sudden drop in blood pressure resulting in feeling faint, or loss of consciousness when moving from lying or sitting to standing. Dry mouth is a common side effect of many drugs and can be intensified by the dehydrating effects of caffeinated drinks and alcohol (answer D). Of all the above possible side effects of neuroleptic medications, answer B is the most important precaution because it relates to the only side effect the client has experienced. See Reference: Cara & MacRae. (2013). Cara, E. & MacRae, A.: Glossary.

48. (C) Clear expectations and reinforcement for desired performance. Positive behavior is facilitated when children understand expectations and simple rules and are reinforced for desired performance, so answer A is correct. "A core concept in the behavioral perspective is that all behavior is learned; this learning is based on the child's capacities, ...drive to engage or perform, the situation or environment, the demands for learning and performance, and the feedback or support for the behavior or performance" (p. 61). Answers B, C, and D do not reflect these concepts and are incorrect. See Reference: Dunn. (2011). Dunn, W.: Using frames of reference and practice models to guide practice.

49. (D) Family will demonstrate independence in current positioning and feeding techniques 50% of the time. Goals should be functional, measurable, and objective. In addition, short-term goals must relate to the long-term goal being addressed. Answer D meets those criteria. Answer A does not provide measurable criteria, nor does it directly relate to the long-term goal of family training. Answer B, although measurable, does not relate to the long-term goal. Answer C describes the long-term goal of family independence in the feeding program. See Reference: Schell, Gillen, & Scaffa. (2014). Sames, K.M.: Documentation in practice.

50. (A) Encourage two or more children to play next to each other with a collection of books. Parallel play is evident when a child "plays beside others but play remains independent" (p. 60). Encouraging the child to play next to another child while assembling a puzzle and looking at books (answer A) is most representative of a parallel play situation. Answers B and D are most representative of cooperative play in which children in small groups are "organized to achieve a goal...[of] group games with simple rules" (p. 61). Answer C is a form of solitary play, in which the child is simply playing in isolation of other children. See Reference: Parham & Fazio. (2007). Knox, S.: Development and current use of the revised Knox Preschool Play Scale.

51. (C) Simple and highly structured activities. "Structured tasks...provide habit training, diversion, coping skills, and time management training potential for leisure skill development, may also build self-esteem through successful completion" (p. 201). Projective media, isolation, and discussing delusions are all contraindicated for people with schizophrenia. Projective activities (answer A) are most useful for encouraging expression of feelings. It may be appropriate to separate individuals (answer B) who are violent or unable to tolerate the presence of others nearby, but this would not be desirable as part of a regular group routine. Discussing delusions (answer D) is undesirable because it is likely to reinforce them. "People who display positive symptoms, especially hallucinations, benefit from activities that divert attention from their symptoms" (p. 213). See Reference: Cara & MacRae. (2013). MacRae, A. & Andonian, L.: Schizophrenia.

52. (B) Walking as part of a walking club. Walking as part of a walking club throughout a facility can provide an outlet for the movement needs of some people with dementia. Walking in a structured way can be calming, provide an activity of exploration, and help to refocus the resident. Additional strategies to prevent wandering may include creating a safe area in which to walk, setting up simple alarms, and using barriers to make doorways less obvious (p. 494). Answers A, C, and D are good activities, but would not provide the element of movement to the same degree. See Reference: Cara & MacRae. (2013). MacRae, A. & Smith, J.: Mental health of the older adult.

53. (B) Visual attention skills. Building on oculo-motor control and visual acuity, "the next level is vi-sual attention according to Warren's model" (p. 353). "First the child needs to have good attention to the task, which allows the visual information to be stored in memory" (p. 380). Answer A is incorrect because visual memory skills can only be developed after visual attention skills are established. Answers C and D are incorrect because general and specific visual perceptual skills develop after visual memory. See Reference: Hinojosa and Kramer. (2009). Schneck, C.: A frame of reference for visual perception.

54. (C) distal humerus. An individual who has undergone a long above elbow amputation has lost the limb at the level of the distal humerus, answer C. This results in loss of hand and wrist function. See Reference: Pedretti. (2013). Keenan, D.D. & Glover, J.S.: Amputations and prosthetics.

55. (B) Pass around a scent box and ask each patient to smell the contents. Sensory integration theory holds that individuals can learn by receiving, processing, and responding to sensory stimulation. Starting a group for regressed individuals with sensory stimuli such as touch and smell helps to get an individual's attention and arouse interest. "Smell is the only sense that connects directly to the amygdala and hippocampus before going to the thalamus. The amygdala and hippocampus have functions that are associated with emotional responses and the consolidation of memories" (p. 282). Asking individuals in this type of a group to introduce themselves (answer A) can be confusing and time consuming, especially when dealing with regressed individuals with limited attention spans. Reading favorite poems (answer C) and discussing lunch menus (answer D) are activities more suited to patients functioning at higher levels than the group described here. See Reference: Brown & Stoffel. (2011). Brown, C. & Nicholson, R.: Sensory skills.

56. (A) Store the most frequently used items on shelves just above or below the counter. When an individual experiences difficulty reaching because of limited range of motion, convenient placement of commonly used items will facilitate home management. Using the largest joint available (answer B) is an important principle of joint protection, and although it may be an appropriate suggestion for an individual with arthritis, it would not address the specific problem of reaching high shelves. Although it is possible that range-of-motion exercises and reaching for high shelves (answers C and D) may eventually improve this individual's shoulder function, neither provides a home management solution. See Reference: Pedretti. (2013). Foti, D. & Koketsu, J.S.: Activities of daily living.

57. (C) Play while floor sitting with toys placed on floor to child's sides, or suspended for child's reach, out to child's sides. Answer C is correct. Protective extension is an automatic response in which the child's "(a)rm extends and places on the supporting surface to prevent falling" (p. 151). A child with motor development at an 8-month-old level has typically developed protective extension responses in a forward direction and is developing these responses to a sideward direction. Answer A is incorrect, as a child with motor development skills at an 8-month-old level has already developed protective extension forward in a sitting position, a higher level skill than elicited in prone. Answers B and D are incorrect, as explained by rationale for answer A, above. See Reference: Mulligan. (2014). Mulligan, S.: Typical child development.

58. (C) Monitor the client's heart rate and blood pressure regularly throughout the intervention. For the safety of the client, "precautions to prevent overexertion of the client should be taken, and the OT should monitor heart rate and blood pressure regularly and alert the appropriate members of the rehab team of any changes" (p. 1126) (answer C). Answers A (medication management), B (retraining in ADLs), and D (energy conservation techniques) all pertain to typical OT interventions introduced by the cardiac rehab OT that must be monitored to prevent overexertion. See Reference: Schell, Gillen, & Scaffa. (2014). Vaughn, P.: Cardiac conditions.

59. (D) Stenciling greeting cards. The stenciling activity (answer D) is the safest craft choice, because it is free of sharp, toxic, and cordlike materials. When planning craft activities, it is important for the OT to consider "whether there are any items that could be used in a suicide attempt or injurious behavior,...performing sharps counts and limiting the length of string or ribbon provided are ways for ensuring safety" (p. 397). A ceramic object (answer C) could be broken into sharp pieces that individuals could use to harm themselves. Craft projects that contain rope or cordlike materials that can be used for hanging (answers A and B) also should be avoided. See Reference: Cara & MacRae. (2013). Lambert, W.L.: Mental health of children.

60. (D) A child with spina bifida with lower extremity paralysis. Answer D is correct. "Prone scooters require the use of the arms and the ability to lift the head while moving" (p. 626). Typically, children who have spina bifida have enough upper extremity coordination and strength to propel themselves on a scooter that supports their lower extremities. A child with spina bifida will usually have the cognitive and sensory awareness to negoti-

ate a scooter within the environment. Prone scooters may be contraindicated for the children described in answers A, B, and C. The neck hyperextension required for exploratory play on a prone scooter could cause further increase in the abnormal extensor tone of the child with cerebral palsy (answer A). A child with low tone who is easily fatigued (answer B) may be unable to maintain this very exhausting position for very long and is likely to become even more tired. The child with cognitive limitations and poor sensory awareness (answer C) is at risk of injury owing to lack the sensory feedback and cognitive skills. See Reference: Case-Smith & O'Brien. (2010). Wright-Ott, C.: Mobility.

61. (A) Vinyl floor. Vinyl floors are the easiest and least expensive surface over which to maneuver a wheelchair. Although it is possible to find inexpensive short-pile carpeting (answer B), a smooth, uncarpeted surface is still the easiest over which to maneuver. The friction provided by deep-pile carpets (answer C) makes them difficult to push a wheelchair across, and wheeling over the edge of an area rug (answer D) also increases the level of difficulty for wheelchair users. See Reference: Pedretti. (2013). Foti, D. & Koketsu, J.S.: Activities of daily living.

62. (B) Stringing beads for a necklace, following a pattern. The individual should have washed the vegetables prior to cutting them and filled the tea kettle before turning on the stove, demonstrating a deficit in the area of sequencing (p. 246). Stringing beads for a necklace following a pattern (answer B) is the only activity that addresses the skill of sequencing. Rubber-stamping in a random design (answer A) utilizes a random approach, which eliminates the need to sequence. Putting together a jigsaw puzzle (answer C) is a good activity for developing problem-solving skills, but does not target sequencing skills. Setting a table (answer D) is a good activity for developing organizational skills. See Reference: Gillen. (2009). Managing executive function impairments to optimize function.

63. (C) Provide catalogs from which they can select bedspreads and curtains. "Interventions centered on the recovery model provide individuals with choice, support them in achieving self-identified goals, address all aspects of life, and empower them to make decisions and do for themselves" (p. 548). Providing them with an opportunity for choice regarding the decor in their new bedrooms (answer C) is consistent with the recovery model. In addition, it is at an appropriate cognitive level for people with severe and persistent mental illness, who will benefit from information that is presented in a concrete manner, such as a catalog. Understanding a map (answer A) requires a higher level of cognition than most of these individuals would have. Considerable judgment and safety considerations need to go into roommate selection (answer B), and this would not be left up to the patients to choose, although their input would be sought. A collage activity (answer D) could facilitate exploration and expression of feelings, but does not address choice or empowerment of the individuals. See Reference: Brown & Stoffel. (2011). Exley, S.M., Thompson, C.A., & Hays, C.A.: State hospitals.

64. (A) Reminiscence. The focus of a reminiscence group (answer A) is on providing social opportunities for sharing life stories and feelings, expressing pride in past life experiences, and gaining support for past life difficulties, all of which would enhance self-esteem and help the residents achieve acceptance of past and present life. "Reminiscence may be defined as the act or process of recalling the past.... Older adults need to reminisce as part of their preparation for death.... Reminiscence has four interdependent parts—remembering...recall...review...reconstruction.... Elders tend to reminisce as a natural part of group interaction.... The resulting cohesiveness facilitates greater self-disclosure and greater courage to explore significant but more painful memories" (p. 286). Answers B, C, and D would address some of the goals stated, but not as comprehensively as a reminiscence group. See Reference: Cole & Donohue. (2011). Cole, M.B.: Older adult interventions to facilitate social practice the patient.

65. (D) Reinforcement of competence. An 8-year-old child is usually at the stage of industry versus inferiority, during which time he or she develops a sense of competency. For a child who is expected to lose motor function gradually, a treatment plan that will provide an ongoing sense of competence (possibly in other areas) is especially relevant. Answers A, B, and C describe other developmental issues identified by Erikson that are typically achieved at other ages: basic trust (answer A) in infancy; initiative (answer B) during the toddler years; and self-identity (answer C) during adolescence (p. 90). See Reference: Case-Smith & O'Brien. (2010). Vroman, K.: In transition to adulthood: The occupations and performance skills of adolescents.

66. (B) Heavy utensils, pots, and pans. Using heavy kitchen items (answer B) increases stability for individuals with incoordination. Other suggestions include using prepared foods, nonskid mats, easy-open containers, serrated knives, and tongs. Built-up handles (answer A) are useful for individuals with limited grasp. A high stool (answer C) benefits those who fatigue easily. Placing the most commonly used items on shelves just above and below the counter

(answer D) is a useful way to adapt the environment for individuals with limited reach. See Reference: Trombly. (2008). James, A.B.: Restoring the role of the independent person.

67. (B) a tub bench and toilet rails. A tub bench and toilet rails (answer B) make bathroom transfers easier and safer, and allow the person with a unilateral LE amputation to transfer independently. Lightweight cooking utensils (answer A) are recommended for those individuals with weakness or joint involvement of the upper extremities. Answers C and D are incorrect because long-handled dressing devices and reachers are more likely to be recommended when compensation for hip or trunk flexion is needed, and use of these devices might discourage the normal bending activity in the person with LE amputation. See Reference: Pedretti. (2013). Keenan, D.D. & Glover, J.S.: Amputations and prosthetics.

68. (B) Gross motor exercises. The sensory integration treatment approach, which aims to improve the reception and processing of sensory information within the central nervous system, uses gross motor exercises (answer B). "The interventions recommended by the theory are based on the premise that the integration of the tactile, vestibular, and proprioceptive systems is not adequate to develop organization in the nervous system, which can result in postural instability, gravitational insecurity, oculomotor dysfunction and oral motor difficulties. Subsequent levels of intervention involved the development of body perception, bilateral coordination, motor planning, activity level, attention to task, emotional responses, and visual motor integration" (p. 290). From the choices given, gross motor activities (answer B) most effectively address the individual's needs. Social skills training (answer A) could also be appropriate for the purpose of developing interpersonal skills. Answer C, life skills, would be used for addressing self-care skills and independent living goals. Excessive projects (answer D) might be used when an individual needs opportunities for nonverbal communication and outlets for emotion and creativity. Although these interventions may be a part of the overall treatment program, this type of individual would benefit from being able to receive and process sensory information before embarking on more complex treatment formats. See Reference: Brown & Stoffel. (2011). Brown, C. & Nicholson, R.: Sensory skills.

69. (D) Instruct teacher and students to use the Alert program and include routine follow-up visits to classroom to colead sessions with teacher. The Alert Program (answer D) is a cognitive intervention that is well suited for use with a whole classroom. The program "likens arousal levels to an engine running.... Children and caregivers also explore methods for changing engine levels, allowing the child to function more frequently at an optimal level" (p. 520). Answer A, providing this in-service program to parents, does not have a direct connection with the students' classroom behavior and does not give the students any strategies they can implement when they need help to focus/remain alert during the day. Answer B, consulting with the physical education teacher, may provide some limited benefit; however, the resulting strategies would be used only when the students are in the physical education class and therefore are not available for their use as needed. Answer C, implementing screenings, is not an appropriate activity in this pilot program. See Reference: Lane & Bundy. (2012). Cronin, A.: Emotional and behavioral disorders.

70. (B) Identify using a bus schedule as a problem area. Gillen describes a systematic approach to problem-solving training involving five steps: (1) problem orientation/identifying and analyzing the problem (answer A); (2) problem definition and formulation; (3) generating alternatives and solutions (answer D); (4) decision-making (answer B); and (5) solution verification and evaluation (answer C) (p. 265). See Reference: Gillen. (2009). Managing executive function impairments to optimize function.

71. (A) energy conservation techniques. Energy conservation techniques reduce the amount of energy expenditure an individual requires to perform various activities. For a client with COPD and limited endurance, energy conservation techniques should be taught early so they can be implemented and reinforced while performing other activities, such as preparing meals. Work hardening (answer B) and graded activities to increase strength (answer C) would not address the need to perform meal preparation in the most energy-efficient manner. Safety in the kitchen (answer D) would be more relevant to individuals with sensory or balance loss rather than limited endurance. See Reference: Pedreitti, 2013. Huntley, N.: Cardiac and pulmonary diseases.

72. (D) Perform skin conditioning techniques. "Skin conditioning techniques are used to improve scar integrity and durability against minor trauma caused by pressure or shearing forces, decrease hypersensitivity, and moisturize dry, newly healed skin. These techniques should be used for any burned areas or surgical sites that took longer than 2 weeks to heal. Lubrication and massage with a water-based cream or lotion should be performed three to four times a day or whenever the skin feels excessively dry, tight or itchy" (p. 1132). Wound debridement (answer A) begins in the acute phase of treatment, and does not necessarily need to be performed prior

to ADL training. Compression garments (answer B) are worn constantly after wounds are healed, not prior, and should not be removed for anything other than bathing and skin care. Compression garments are beneficial for desensitization, general skin conditioning, edema control, and early scar compression. Upper extremity strengthening (answer C) may be part of the treatment plan, but does not need to be performed prior to ADL activities. See Reference: Pedretti. (2013). Reeves, S.U. & Deshaies, L.: Burns and burn rehabilitation.

73. (A) Maintain and/or prevent loss of joint and skin mobility. During the acute stage, when burn wounds are partial or full thickness in nature, maintenance of joint range of motion and skin mobility is the primary goal of intervention. "In the acute phase, splinting and positioning are used in combination with exercise and activity. Exercise is especially important to control edema and prevent muscle atrophy, tendon adherence, joint stiffness, and capsular shortening. Exercise types include passive range of motion, active range of motion, active assistive range of motion, and functional activity. If the patient cannot participate in active exercise or activity because of poor medical status or impaired level of alertness, passive range of motion is indicated" (p. 1251). Providing adaptive equipment (answer B) is typically performed during the subacute, surgical, or postoperative stage, and wearing compression and vascular garments (answer C) and the prevention of scarring (answer D) are goals most commonly implemented during the rehabilitation phase. See Reference: Trombly. (2008). Pessina, M.A. & Orroth, A.C.: Burn injuries.

74. (B) Educate the client to increase confidence in the area of functional transfers. "The most important concept to remember with transfer training is that each client will be unique in his/her own assistance needs, limitations, safety issues, and frustration tolerance.... Adaptations must be made for each situation and physical context, as well, while keeping generalization of skills in mind" (p. 178). Strategies to achieve confidence in safe transfers may include reducing factors that contribute to risk of falls such as increasing lower extremity strength (answer A) and balance, eliminating environmental hazards (answer C), and reducing the use of medications that may be contributing to the fear of falls (answer D). See Reference: Meriano & Latella. (2008). Meriano, C. & Latella, D.: Activities of daily living.

75. (D) Scores on the Ranchos Los Amigos Cognitive Recovery Scale. Answer D is correct. "Assessments are used commonly to determine extent of (traumatic brain) injury; these include the...Rancho Los Amigos Cognitive Recovery Scale.... The Ranchos

Scale lists ten levels of cognitive performance, with I being 'no response' and X being 'purposeful, appropriate; modified independent'" (p. 579). Answers A and B are incorrect, as each change is not necessarily evident in all children with traumatic brain injury, and further, each does not signal increased awareness nor the point at which to begin intervention to develop ADL performance. Family priority for their child's return to independence (answer C) is important for all families and may be stressed immediately after the child's accident and throughout the acute care phase. However, this priority itself does not enable a child to begin rehabilitation when medical concerns are paramount or the child's awareness and level of activity prevent participation in subsequent rehabilitation steps. See Reference: Lane & Bundy. (2012). Tomcheck, S. & Aberli, L.: Multitraumatic injuries.

76. (D) Attend an AA meeting. An individual who has recently been discharged from drug/alcohol rehabilitation is likely to need support (such as Alcoholics Anonymous) her first weekend at home (answer D). "Frequently, conscious and deliberate choices about the people and places where one engages in social and community participation need to be considered, as continuing to spend time in drinking or using environments with former drinking and using friends might place the person with a substance use disorder at high risk for relapse" (pp. 204–205). People in recovery should avoid situations, people, and places that lead to abuse of substances. Parties and clubs/concerts (answers A and B) are often closely associated with access to substances and should be avoided. A minivacation with the kids (answer C) would probably be too stressful for her first weekend at home. See Reference: Brown & Stoffel. (2011). Sells, C.H., Stoffel, V.C., & Plach, H.: Substance-related disorders.

77. (C) Role-playing of social situations. "This highly structured approach to teaching skills involves breaking skills into discrete steps, rehearsing the behaviors through role-plays, and providing feedback and reinforcement to participants regarding their effectiveness" (pp. 307–308). The first step in social skills training is to identify interactional challenges, followed by teaching skills, practicing and developing those skills, then feedback and reinforcement of the skills. The first two steps in this process, identifying needs (answer A) and teaching about social skills, have been addressed in the group. The group members are now ready for practice through role-playing (answer C). This will be followed up with independent practice (answer B) and feedback (answer D). See Reference: Brown & Stoffel. (2011). Stoffel, V.C. & Tomlinson, J.: Communication and social skills.

78. (A) A game of rhythmic exercises performed to music. Rhythmic activities facilitate motor performance in individuals with Parkinson's disease, especially when performed to music. Time capsules (answer B) are a meaningful activity for those who are approaching the end of life, but the description of the activity provides no rationale for why it would benefit the motor skills of those individuals with Parkinson's disease. Races (answer C) are generally not a good idea for this population because of the difficulty they often have stopping during ambulation. Reading out loud (answer D) is an effective intervention for addressing the communication, not motor deficits, frequently experienced by these individuals. Group activities are particularly beneficial because of the added advantage of social interaction. See Reference: Trombly. (2008). Forwell, S.J., Copperman, L.F., & Hugos, L.: Neurogenerative diseases.

79. (A) Explain to the parents that toilet training is not a feasible option. Answer A is correct because "when the lesion is in the lumbar region or below, the reflex arc is no longer intact and the bladder is flaccid (lower motor neuron bladder).... Bladder training will be ineffective because the bladder has insufficient tone and requires assistance in emptying" (p. 496). These children are commonly provided with some type of catheterization after medical testing is performed. As toilet training is not appropriate, answers B and C are incorrect. Independence in lower extremity dressing (answer D) is an appropriate goal for this child, but it is not relevant to the issue at hand. See Reference: Case-Smith & O'Brien. (2010). Shepherd, J.: Activities of daily living.

80. (A) Teacher's report of how the child spends classroom free play time and choices made during outdoor recess. The correct answer is A because the Model of Human Occupation includes an emphasis on "occupational adaptation" through "motivation," "routines and patterns," "nature of skills and performance," and the "influence of context on occupations" (p. 44). Core concepts in this model include a person's motivations and habits. By learning from the teacher about the choices this child makes and his play preferences, the OT gathers information that helps develop intervention plans using MOHO's constructs. Answer B includes areas related to postural control as a foundation for skilled distal motor performance, and this suggests a Biomechanical Practice Model (p. 51). Answer C suggests a Behavioral Practice Model (p. 61), as it references variables that may be antecedents and reinforcers related to the child's learned behavior/performance. Answer D considers activities that are rich in vestibular, proprioceptive, and tactile input, suggesting a Sensory Processing Model (p. 47) See Reference: Dunn.

(2011). Dunn, W.: Using frames of reference and practice models to guide practice.

81. (D) Defining the three types of responses: passive, assertive, and aggressive. "Assertiveness training programs begin by defining three basic types of behavior in social situations: passive, assertive, and aggressive" (p. 56). In order to understand their own behavior and the behavior of others, group members will first need to understand the difference between passive, assertive, and aggressive behaviors (answer D). The ability to act in one's own best interest (answer C), identify one's own feelings (answer B), and ask another person to change his behavior (answer A) are all skills that the group can begin to practice once they understand the different types of responses. See Reference: Cole & Donohue. (2011). Cole, M.B.: Social participation basics.

82. (D) Drawing lines and shapes using shaving cream or sand. Activities to develop handwriting readiness skills aim at "improving fine motor control and isolated finger movements, promoting prewriting skills, enhancing right-left discrimination" (p. 557). Drawing lines and shapes in these media enables the child to practice drawing forms and isolated finger skills. Answers A, B, and C, hammering dowels, building with wooden blocks, and rolling clay into a ball, emphasize whole-hand skills, use of two hands together, and regulating pressure during hand activity. None of these three activities emphasizes isolated finger movements. See Reference: Case-Smith & O'Brien. (2010). Schneck, C. & Amundson, S.L.: Prewriting and handwriting skills.

83. (D) Discuss the benefit of OT provision of staff education and determine how this can be implemented and documented in the student's IEP. IDEA 2004 regulations include services "on behalf of the child" and "[i]n the school setting, it may be more appropriate for the OT to provide services to the teacher of a student with ASD on behalf of that student, rather than to work directly with the student" (p. 649). "To do this, the OT may need to work with the team in establishing how services are documented on the IEP" (p. 651). This is especially important if the recommended service delivery approach is different from what the team has typically experienced. Answers A, B, and C may be components of the OT's service delivery; however, in isolation, they do not represent approaches that promote a collaborative approach to program development for this student. See Reference: Kuhanek & Watling. (2010). Swinth, Y.: Occupational therapy in school-based settings for children with an autism spectrum disorder.

84. (C) use a foam wedge between the legs of the patient. A key aspect of the OT practitioner's plan when working with patients who have had hip replacement surgery is to provide positioning strategies to prevent postsurgical complications and maintain function. Patients who have had either posterolateral or anterolateral surgical approaches for hip replacement must be avoid leg adduction past the midline (p. 919), as it is a position of instability for the healing joint. Placing a foam wedge between the legs of the patient (answer C) in sitting or supine position is the correct answer because this positioning method helps to prevent hip adduction. Answer A, placing pillows on the lateral side of the hips, would not prevent hip adduction; elevating the foot on the side of the surgery, answer B, would increase hip flexion, which is contraindicated; and placing a roll under the patient's knees, answer D, would also increase hip flexion. See Reference: Pedretti. (2013). Lawson, S.C. & Murphy, L.F.: Hip fractures and lower extremity joint replacement.

85. (B) High contrast and defined borders. Visual material that is adapted using high contrast and defined borders provides "specific attention to the distinctive features of a visual stimulus through highlighting...to enhance visual discrimination learning" (p. 380) and provides the only combination of features that assist children with visual discrimination problems. High contrast of the stimuli (shape, letter, number, and so on) in relation to the background, and defining important areas of the stimuli with a border, attract the eye, and provide clear input. Answer A is incorrect because low contrast of the stimuli, such as blue ditto lettering, is difficult for the eyes to discriminate. Vague borders around the important stimuli (answer C) make for less clear input. Answer D, both low contrast and vague borders, would make visual discrimination difficult. See Reference: Hinojosa & Kramer. (2009). Schneck, C.: A frame of reference for visual perception.

86. (D) Create a comfortable collaborative relationship with parents and promote parenting skills. "Development support with NICU families is relationship-based,...evolved to family-centered mutual collaboration,...[and] facilitates the family's active role with their infant and the NICU team.... Recognizing parental skills, celebrating successes, and facilitating parent's expertise are invaluable" (p. 659). This approach provides the parents with effective tools to best nurture and care for their infant at any time and in any environment and has a permanent impact on the developmental outcome for the infant. Answer A, adjusting the infant's positioning has an impact on the infant only until the baby is moved for care and changing. Answer B, recommending an early intervention referral, and answer C, identifying interventions to support the infant's development, are strategies that can impact the infant when they enhance the parents' capacity to nurture their child. See Reference: Case-Smith & O'Brien. (2010). Hunter, J.G.: Neonatal intensive care unit.

87. (D) Recommend student work station arrangement that supports pelvis/shoulder/head alignment and optimizes arm/hand position for endurance in writing tasks. A functional writing posture considers both body position and fatigue. Students who have difficulty with this postural control express writing difficulties while trying to sustain optimal postural ergonomics/adjustments or they have difficulty using "increased physical effort, including moving the upper extremity fluidly and easily across the page, or displaying a loss of balance or weight bearing on the writing surface" (p. 439). Answer A is incorrect as it represents concerns related to difficulty in using writing tools. Answer B is incorrect as it represents concerns related to difficulty in writing grasp. Answer C is incorrect as it represents concerns related to difficulty with writing legibility. See Reference: Hinojosa & Kramer. (2009). Roston, K.: A frame of reference for the development of handwriting skills.

88. (C) Caregiver instructions in problem-solving. The most appropriate intervention at a moderate to moderately severe stage of decline in cognition is to "help the caregiver problem-solve and recognize the degree of need for initiation, verbal cues, and physical assistance in performing ADLs; provide time orientation, [and] simplify the environment" (p. 927). Instructing the client's caregivers in task breakdown, or breaking down tasks into simple steps and then providing step-by-step instructions, will allow the client to perform activities as capabilities decline. At this stage of the disease, memory retraining (answer A) and ADL retraining (answer B) will probably not be effective. Leisure activities (answer D) structured to meet the needs of the client with Alzheimer's disease could be helpful, but will not address the primary problem of performance of self-care activities. See Reference: Pedretti. (2013). Schultz-Khron, W., Foti, D., & Glogoski, C.: Degenerative diseases of the central nervous system.

89. (B) Explain to the individual and caregiver that one must be "homebound" in order to be eligible for home care services. To be eligible for home care services, the individual must be defined by Medicare as "homebound." The individual need not be bedridden, but leaving the residence must require a considerable or taxing effort. Absences from the home are permitted, but must be infrequent in nature, short in duration, or for the purpose of receiving medical treatment. Given that this individual is able to leave the home for a social visit and tolerate riding in a car for 30 minutes, he is not considered homebound. The OT practitioner would first inform and explain this criteria to the individual and caregiver (answer B). After this has been explained, the OT practitioner would communicate with the PT (answer D) and refer the individual for outpatient therapy (answer C). Simply providing a home program and discharging the individual would not meet the individual's needs because he continues to require therapeutic intervention. See Reference: Centers for Medicare and Medicaid Services, 2010. Medicare and home health care. Retrieved from: http://www.medicare.gov/Publications/Pubs/pdf/10969.pdf Medicare PDF.

90. (A) Opportunities to explore new areas of interest, helping to identify strengths and needs. Answer A is correct, as the OT provides the student with "exploration and experimentation [that] provide teens with experiences of success and failure, both of which are required if they are to develop a sense of the boundaries of their competence" (p. 101). Answers B, C, and D remove the teen from his peer group and reduce the opportunities he has to self-advocate and develop positive interactions with his peers. See Reference: Case-Smith & O'Brien. (2010). Vroman, K.: In transition to adulthood: The occupations and performance skills of adolescents.

91. (D) washing windows. Washing windows (answer D) is a repetitive activity that involves resisted, elevated upper extremity activity. Rests can be taken as needed. Making the bed, peeling potatoes, and polishing furniture (answers A, B, and C) do not provide adequate resistance to achieve upper extremity strengthening. See Reference: Pedretti. (2013). Southam, M., Schmidt, A., & George, A.H.: Disorders of the motor unit.

92. (C) keeping the knees bent. Keeping the knees bent is the only correct choice. All of the other answers could potentially contribute to injury. For prevention, the OT practitioner should stand close to the individual, keep the back in a neutral position, and maintain a wide base of support. See Reference: Pedretti. (2013). Bolding, D., Adler, C., Tipton-Burton, M., Verran, A., & Lillie, S.M.: Mobility.

93. (B) decrease the effects of prolonged inactivity. Some of the main objectives of inpatient cardiac rehabilitation include decreasing the effects of prolonged inactivity, answer B. "During the first 1 to 3 days after MI, stabilization of the patient's medical condition is usually attained. This acute phase is followed by a period of early mobilization. Phase 1 of treatment, inpatient cardiac rehabilitation, includes monitored low-level physical activity, including self-care; reinforcement of cardiac and postsurgical precautions; instruction in energy conservation and graded activity; and establishment of guidelines for appropriate activity levels at discharge. Through monitored activity, the ill effects of prolonged inactivity can be averted while medical problems, poor responses to medications, and atypical chest pain can be addressed" (p. 1202). Prompting dyspnea, answer A, is contraindicated. "Look for shortness of breath with activity or rest.... Dyspnea at rest with a resting respiratory rate of greater than 30 breaths per minute is a sign of acute congestive heart failure. The patient may require emergency medical help" (p. 1203). Activities that promote strength are beneficial, but ROM (answer C) is not usually an area of concern. Most individuals do not need to relearn activities, other than applying energy conservation techniques; therefore, independent performance (answer D) is not a primary concern. See Reference: Pedretti. (2013). Huntley, N.: Cardiac and pulmonary diseases.

94. (A) Videofluoroscopy. "A videofluoroscopic swallow study (VFSS) is the most commonly used instrumental assessment tool to examine oropharyngeal swallowing disorders. This assessment uses fluoroscopy to capture the client's swallow with a variety of foods and textures.... Videofluoroscopy, in conjunction with clinical assessment, may be used to select appropriate intervention techniques and assist the therapist in determining the safest diet level to help the client achieve a safe swallow" (p. 696). A videofluoroscopy should be performed when it is suspected that the individual is aspirating. An individual who suddenly has a wet voice when there was no prior difficulty may have had a sudden change in medical status causing aspiration. He or she should be reevaluated to determine whether there is aspiration into the larynx or trachea. Answers B, a change to thin liquids, and D, a regular diet, would be inappropriate for an individual who does not have a normal swallow or who may be aspirating, because they are too difficult to control. Answer C, a tracheostomy tube, is usually in place prior to the initiation of a feeding program, because the individual was having difficulty with breathing, not swallowing or wet voice qualities. See Reference: Pedretti. (2013). Smith, J. & Jenks, K.N.: Eating and swallowing.

95. (B) Hyperextension of the PIP joint and flexion of the DIP joint. Answer B is the only answer provided that describes a swan-neck deformity. The orthotic should minimize the continued deformity. The pattern of hyperextension of the PIP and DIP joints (answer A) may be seen in lower motor-neuron palsies. Flexion of the PIP joint and hyperextension of the DIP joint (answer C) is descriptive of a boutonniere deformity. An individual who has overstretched the volar plates at the PIP and DIP joints would have hyperextension of the MP joint and flexion of the DIP joint (answer D). See Reference: Pedretti. (2013). Deshaies, L.: Arthritis.

96. (B) "List five potential changes you will face following retirement." Individuals in the precontemplation stage have "only a vague awareness of the need for change" (p. 274). Identifying potential changes (answer B) is the beginning of developing awareness of a need to change. This would be followed by identifying roles the individual would wish to continue after retirement (answer A), an activity appropriate for the contemplation stage. Choosing a goal (answer D) is representative of the preparation stage, and identifying the steps needed to achieve the goal (answer C) is representative of the action phase. See Reference: Cole & Donohue. (2011). Cole, M.B.: Older adult interventions to facilitate social participation.

97. (C) A process and legal document that outlines strengths, needs, and educational services for a student with disability. The IEP is both a summary document and a collaborative team process that includes evaluation, planning, and program implementation for students with disabilities that impact their participation in the curriculum and activities in the educational setting. See Reference: Schell, Gillen, & Scaffa. (2014). Swinth, Y.L.: Education.

98. (A) Isometric. "During an isometric contraction, no joint motion occurs and the muscle length remains the same. The limb is set or held taut as agonist and antagonist muscles are contracted at a point in the ROM to stabilize a joint" (p. 742). Isotonic exercises (answer B) shorten muscle length, which results in joint movement. Progressive resistive exercises (answer C) are a type of isotonic exercise in which resistance is increased during exercise repetitions. With the arm immobilized, the individual would be unable to perform isotonic exercises. Passive exercises (answer D) are performed by an outside force. Passive range-of-motion (PROM) exercise, for instance, results in joint motion, but does not involve any active muscle contraction. Passive exercises could not be performed by an individual whose joint is immobilized. See Reference: Pedretti. (2013). Breines, E.B.: Therapeutic occupations and modalities.

99. (B) Routinely inspect the skin closely for signs of skin breakdown. Teaching a patient with a residual limb to compensate for the lack of sensation with visual inspection is essential to prevent injury from skin breakdown. Answer A is incorrect because tapping, rubbing, and application of textures are used when a residual limb is hypersensitive. Answer C, deep massage, is a technique used to loosen and prevent scar adhesions. Answer D, teaching procedures of skin hygiene, is important, but would not, by itself, prevent skin breakdown, which is the primary concern when the residual limb lacks sensation. See Reference: Pedretti. (2013). Keenan, D.D., & Glover, J.S.: Amputations and prosthetics.

100. (A) Negotiate work hours that would allow the client to travel at times that children are less likely to be on the same bus. "Fear of harm or ridicule is often a major factor in a client's poor performances in negotiating public transportation" (p. 40). In this case, the OT would want the most cost-effective and expedient environmental intervention to enable the client to continue with the job. Negotiating a change in work hours (answer A) could occur quickly and would not cost anything. Taking a taxi (answer B) is a viable option but would be more expensive, so would not be the first choice. Volunteering to speak to children in the local school district (answer D) is a good example of advocacy, but would probably take some time to arrange. Working with the client on coping skills (answer C) may ultimately be necessary, but it is not an environmental adaptation. See Reference: Cara & MacRae. (2013). MacRae, A. & Boggis, T.D.: Environmental and cultural considerations.

101. (C) An electric toothbrush. According to Shepherd, "for the child who independently brushes, an electric toothbrush...allows more thorough cleaning. This is a good solution for children with limited dexterity, although for children with weakness, an electric toothbrush may be too heavy to manage" (p. 506). Answer A, using a soft bristle brush, would most likely assist a child with tongue thrust (p. 506), whereas answer B, attaching a universal cuff to the toothbrush, would assist a child who has decreased grip strength in the hand (p. 506). Answer D, encouraging the child to use a soft sponge-tipped toothette, is typically indicated in the child with oral hypersensitivity or defensiveness (p. 506). See Reference: Case-Smith & O'Brien. (2010). Shepherd, J.: Activities of daily living.

102. (A) Initiate training in conflict resolution strategies. Anger management programs typically address "perspective taking, problem solving, recognizing emotions that lead to anger, and conflict resolution strategies" (answer A) (p. 352). Beginning instruction in anger-management techniques would be the next step in a plan to address anger management, because the individual is already able to identify his key stressors and typical responses to these stressors

(answer C). Creative media (answer B), which can include writing, art, drama, and other forms of creative expression, is "designed to provide a means for the client to express feelings and come to self realization" (p. 321). Though the individual has made some progress toward his goals, he has not achieved competence in anger management skills. Therefore, discontinuation of services (answer D) is also incorrect. See Reference: Brown & Stoffel. (2011). Scheinholz, M.: Emotion regulation; Haertl, K. & Christiansen, C.: Coping skills.

103. (A) Position the child's trunk, head, neck, and shoulders in proper alignment. Proper positioning is the first thing the OT must address prior to feeding the child. "A strong tongue thrust movement pattern may also be present.... A well-supported and slightly flexed position reduces the severity of this abnormal movement pattern" (p. 461). Answer B, hyperextending the child's head and reclining the child's seat, is contrary to recommended practice. Answers C and D are techniques commonly employed to facilitate proper feeding techniques, but they should not be initiated until after the child is appropriately positioned. See Reference: Case-Smith & O'Brien. (2010). Schuberth, L.M., Amirault, L.M., & Case-Smith, J.: Feeding intervention.

104. (B) Provide the client with the choice to talk about it or end the session. "When clients' anger escalates, it is often a reaction to a perceived loss.... [R]estoring control is an effective means of compensating for feelings of loss and intervening in the client anger" (pp. 186–187). Providing the client with a choice (answer B) is one way of restoring a sense of control to the individual. Leaving the door to the room open (answer D) is something the therapist should have done before beginning a session with an individual with aggressive tendencies. Leaving the room (answer A) and calling for assistance (answer C) are actions that might be necessary if attempts to deescalate the client's behavior are not effective. See Reference: Taylor. (2008). Establishing relationships.

105. (D) encourage client to identify alternative methods with the partner for meeting sexual needs that do not cause pain. "Sexual activities require positions that place the lower part of the back in the neutral position. Clients with back pain may be most comfortable taking a passive position on their back.... In addition, the client is advised to start slowly and gradually work up to more vigorous movements.... A bit of planning will allow enjoyment of sexual activity" (p. 1104). Because the individual's pain cannot be seen or felt by the sexual partner, communication is particularly important. The couple can discuss alternate positions and methods for achieving sexual fulfillment that are acceptable to them and do not cause pain, such as alternate positions, masturbation, and fantasy. Good communication will ensure the needs of both partners are met and will prevent misunderstandings (answer D). Therefore, answer C is inappropriate. A pain-free position is important for successful sexual expression, but there is insufficient information to determine whether answer A, a side-lying position, is a pain-free position for this individual. Timing sex for periods of high energy (answer B) is an appropriate strategy for individuals with low endurance. However, timing sex for periods of lessened pain, such as after taking pain medication, may be a useful strategy for individuals with severe pain. See Reference: Pedretti. (2013). Grangaard, L.: Low back pain.

106. (C) Adding cabinets with labeled compartments to store items out of sight and creating a consistent nightly routine. A "consistent context in relation to schedule, environment, people, and demeanor helps to allay a child's anxiety about what is going to happen next" (p. 435). Placing unused items out of sight reduces visual distraction and labeling compartments helps the child retrieve items. Answers A and B add visual distraction. Answer D, giving the child a choice about homework schedule and behavior, is contrary to recommendations to provide consistency and predictability. See Reference: Case-Smith & O'Brien. (2010). Watling, R.: Interventions and strategies for challenging behaviors.

107. (A) elevate the arm on pillows so it rests higher than the heart. Elevating the arm would be the first thing to do to address edema (answer A). "Early elevation with the hand above the heart is essential.... Resting the hand on pillows while seated or lying down is effective" (p. 1059). When massaging an edematous extremity, stroking should be performed from the distal area to the proximal, not the reverse (answer B). Because active ROM and PROM can both be beneficial to managing edema, instructing the patient to avoid range-of-motion activities (answers C and D) would be incorrect. See Reference: Pedretti. (2013). Kasch, M.C., & Martin Walsh, J.: Hand and upper extremity injuries.

108. (A) Place a foam-lined plastic laundry basket in the tub for use with direct adult supervision at all times. Answer A, a laundry basket with a foam-lined bottom, would be the most appropriate item for the OT to recommend because this piece of equipment addresses both cost and positioning concerns. The laundry basket also will permit the child to continue to submerse herself in the tub, an activity that was stated as enjoyable to the child. Answer B, a

horseshoe-shaped bath collar, would be indicated for a child with "severe motor limitations who is lying supine in shallow water" (p. 516). Whereas answer C, a bath hammock, might be considered as an alternative choice for this child because "bath hammocks fully hold the body and enable the parent to wash the child thoroughly" (p. 516), this type of equipment would not be as cost effective as the laundry basket. Answer D, suggesting that the child stand in the shower versus bathing, does not address the parent's or child's immediate needs of bathing in the bathtub. If the child lacks sitting balance, it is likely that they also will lack standing balance, thus indicating the need for durable medical equipment, such as a shower bench and/or grab bars. See Reference: Case-Smith & O'Brien. (2010). Shepherd, J.: Activities of daily living.

109. (A) Large magnetized shapes and blocks. The child with athetosis has fluctuating muscle tone, and difficulty grading and timing movements, insufficient force, and inadequate isolation of movements (p. 291) interfere with hand function. Efforts should be made to provide a means of stabilizing toys and equipment. Magnetic blocks and shapes will provide some stability and their attraction to each other will enable the child to "build" despite hand skill challenges. Small or lightweight blocks (answers B and C) are more challenging to manipulate, and therefore are not recommended for constructive play for a child with coordination difficulties. Colorful books with rugged pages (answer D) may be enjoyed by this child, but have no direct bearing on the child's ability to engage in construction efforts. See Reference: Case-Smith & O'Brien. (2010). Exner, C.: Evaluation and intervention to develop hand skills.

110. (D) Avoid crowds and potential distractions, and perform tasks slowly while walking. It is important to educate the client who is experiencing "freezing" with ambulation to avoid crowds and potential distractions and to perform tasks slowly while walking. Strategies to address "freezing" while walking include "avoiding crowds, narrow spaces, and room corners; reduce distractions such as not carrying items while walking; reduce clutter in pathway; doing one activity at a time; not hurrying to answer the phone; focusing when changing directions; rhythmic beat or counting to maintain momentum" (p. 1093), answer D, can help the person with Parkinson's disease change the motor program in which they are engaged. Deep-breathing exercises (answer A), practicing movements (answer B), and mentally reviewing steps in the sequence of movement (answer C) will not provide the sensory information needed at the moment to evoke movement or change a "frozen" movement pattern. See Reference: Trombly. (2008). Forwell, S.J., Copperman, L.F., & Hugos, L.: Neurogenerative diseases.

111. (B) Place a card near the refrigerator showing the blue pill with a picture of breakfast and a white pill with a picture of lunch. Allen's Cognitive Levels of Disabilities distinguish the types of assistance an individual needs to safely complete everyday tasks. An individual at Cognitive Level 4 can carry out familiar routines and is able to attend to visual cues. The best therapeutic response for individuals at this level is to "make all objects clearly visible, provide visual comparisons so the individual knows what he or she is working toward, [and] situation-specific training is useful" (p. 255). Linking medications with meals helps the goal become routine and linking the visual cues on the card (answer B) to the routine also assists with training at this level of functioning. Providing the individual with a verbal timeline (answer A) is consistent with Cognitive Level 5. The need for a caregiver to remind the individual to take his or her medication (answer C) is consistent with Level 3. Individuals requiring the caregiver to place the pill in their hands and instruct them to take it (answer D) is most consistent with Level 2. See Reference: Brown & Stoffel. (2011). Brown, C.: Cognitive skills.

112. (A) Single pressure switch, firmly mounted within easy reach. Answer A is correct. A child with fluctuating muscle tone lacks stability and demonstrates extraneous movement; therefore, deliberate motor action is most effectively executed on a securely mounted device using simple movement patterns. Answers B, C, and D involve devices that would respond to slight touch, and therefore would not be effective for a person with extraneous movement and difficulty grading motor action (p. 607). See Reference: Case-Smith & O'Brien. (2010). Schoonover, J., Argabrite Grove, R.E., & Swinth, Y.: Influencing participation through assistive technology.

113. (D) The OT presents information on nutrition, diet, and their impact on health and occupations. Lifestyle redesign programs emphasize the power of occupations by educating participants about the "health relevant consequences of their occupations" (p. 376). Each module begins a didactic presentation (answer D) and "occupational analysis." In addition, modules include peer exchange (answer A)—using stories to share personal experiences; direct experience (answer C)—applying their newly acquired information and skills; and personal exploration—opportunities to reflect on the meaning that the didactic content has to them personally (answer B). See Reference: Meriano & Latella. (2008). Cole, M.B.: Retirement/volunteer and end of life issues.

114. (A) Using an index finger on child's wrist, OT guides hand with spoon to child's mouth. Researchers described a "hierarchical approach to presenting artificial cues from least intrusive (verbal and gestural cues), to most intrusive (verbal and physical cues)" (p. 486). Using a finger to guide the child's hand represents less physical guidance and also eliminates the verbal cue. Answer B is incorrect. Although it may help the child to spear food once it is cut into larger pieces, the focus of the intervention is to enable the child to bring the utensil to her mouth with reduced intensity of cues. Answer C is incorrect as all physical and verbal cues have been eliminated until the endpoint of the movement when the spoon nears the child's mouth. While providing the child with a sticker chart (answer D) may help to reward her success and motivate her to improve her results during the next meal, it is focused on the outcome and not changing the cue level during the meal. See Reference: Case-Smith & O'Brien. (2010). Shepherd, J.: Activities of daily living.

115. (B) folding clothing and putting it in a basket while standing. Work-hardening programs prepare individuals to return to work by combining work simulation, strengthening, and behavioral components. "Work hardening is a multidisciplinary structured, graded return-to-work treatment program that progressively introduces greater rehabilitation requirements on the client-worker to achieve full capability of the worker to meet the demands of the job" (p. 876). A cashier stands during the job, removes clothing from a hanger, folds it, puts it in a bag, runs price tags through a scanner, operates a cash register, and makes change. Putting price tags on clothing while seated (answer D) does not include standing, a critical component of the job. Washing dishes while standing (answer C) incorporates the standing aspect of the client's job, but not the other aspects. Moving piles of clothing from one end of the clinic to the other (answer A) involves walking, not standing. The activity that incorporates the most components of the client's job is folding laundry and putting it in a basket while standing (answer B). See Reference: Trombly. (2008). Rice, V.J. & Luster, S.: Restoring competence for the worker role.

116. (C) Sit on a wedge-shaped seat cushion that is higher in the front and include an abduction post between the knees. Answer C is correct, as the angle of the hip joint is key to limiting extensor tone while sitting. "Children with extensor tone may have a reduction of muscle tone with less than 90° of hip flexion combined with hip abduction" (p. 641). Answer A is incorrect because trunk support from lateral trunk supports prevents sideward movement only. Seat belts promote "stability...above the pelvis to reduce sliding in an upward and forward direction" (p. 641). Answer B would be addressed following the support of the child's pelvis. Although the child's wheelchair with custom-molded seat cushion (answer D) provides individualized positioning, using this with a lap tray for all seat work limits the student's inclusion with peers in the classroom. See Reference: Case-Smith & O'Brien. (2010). Wright-Ott, C.: Mobility.

117. (C) 20 degrees of wrist extension and 10 degrees of extension for each digit. Answer C is correct as "motor inclusion criteria. Control of the wrist and digits is necessary to engage in this type of intervention. Current and past protocols have used the following inclusion criteria: 20 degrees of extension of the wrist and 10 degrees of extension of each finger" (p. 870). Answers B, C, and D are not indicative of the necessary motor control required of the involved extremity postinjury to suffice for CIMT intervention. See Reference: Pedretti. (2013). Gillen, G.: Cerebrovascular accident/stroke.

118. (C) Proximal to the MCP crease. Trim lines of an orthosis that extend proximal to the MCP crease allow for adequate MCP digit extension and flexion. Answers A, B, and D fall distal to the MCP crease, thus restricting full extension and flexion of the digits at the metacarpal heads. See Reference: Pedretti. (2013). Lashgari, D. & Yasuda, L.: Orthotics.

119. (C) Obtain a tub-transfer bench and leg lifter. The use of a tub transfer bench (answer C) would allow the client "to back up to the tub chair or tub transfer bench using the walker or crutches for support.... The legs can then be lifted into the tub bench...using a leg lifter" (p. 1084). Answer A, postponing bathing, is not considered a standard course of treatment. Answer B, use of a handrail, would assist with transfers, but would not address the limitation of knee motion. Answer D, use of a low kitchen stool in the tub, even one with rubber tips, would not be considered a safe or stable selection for transfer training. See Reference: Pedretti. (2013). Lawson, S.C. & Murphy, L.F.: Hip fractures and lower extremity joint replacement.

120. (B) Good hand strength, range of motion, and perceptual awareness. According to Shepherd, children performing catheterizations or bowel programs "may have difficulty in...maintaining a stable yet practical position; hand dexterity (praxis and speed); perceptual awareness; strength, range of motion and stability; and accuracy in emptying collection devices" (p. 497). Answer A is typically indicated for a child with intellectual disabilities, whereas answers C and D (bidets and reducer rings) are toileting adaptations commonly used to assist with cleansing and positioning on the toilet. See Reference: Case-Smith & O'Brien. (2010). Shepherd, J.: Activities of daily living.

121. (B) Wide-base sitting on the floor while reaching for a suspended balloon. The child first practices skills in unsupported sitting on a stable surface, using a wide base of support (answer B). As skills improve, the wide base is reduced to a more narrow one. Reaching activities are used to promote postural reactions, because they involve displacement of the center of gravity and weight shifting. "Infants use ring-sitting...which provides a wide base of support and low center of gravity.... As the pelvis becomes more stable, the wide base is no longer necessary and long sitting is possible" (p. 498). Answers A, C, and D are activities involving unstable support surfaces, typical of more advanced skills. See Reference: Hinojosa & Kramer. (2009). Colangelo, C.A. & Shea, M.: A biomechanical frame of reference for positioning children for functioning.

122. (C) Acknowledge the use of rituals to cope with anxiety. Obsessive-compulsive disorder (OCD) is a type of anxiety disorder in which individuals perform unnecessary and meaningless actions repeatedly. The OT practitioner should recognize that no matter how unnecessary the ritual may appear, it is one the patient uses to cope with anxiety. Demonstrating empathy and acknowledging the challenges the individual faces (answer C) are "essential component[s] of the therapeutic relationship" and the most appropriate response. Explaining that the behavior is unnecessary (answer A) will not help to modify the behavior. Talking about their fears (answer B) is useful for individuals with phobias. Individual treatment (answer D) is indicated when an individual cannot tolerate a group environment. See Reference: Cara & MacRae. (2013). Cara, E. & Stevenson, P.R.R.: The use of psychosocial methods and interpersonal strategies in mental health.

123. (B) Raise the handlebars. The correct answer is B because raising the handlebars demands that the arms are raised, thus bringing the child to an upright posture. "Adapted vertical handgrips that place the forearm in a neutral position also encourage an erect trunk, provided there is enough forearm mobility" (p. 554). Answers A and C are incorrect because the hips and lower extremities are already positioned correctly. Answer D is incorrect because the arms would be lowered, and trunk forward flexion would be increased. See Reference: Hinojosa & Kramer. (2009). Colangelo, C.A. & Shea, M.: A biomechanical frame of reference for positioning children for functioning.

124. (A) Attempt to bear 90% of their weight onto the unaffected leg. As encouraging the client to bear 90% of their weight onto the unaffected leg is appropriate. "In toe touch weight bearing, clients are instructed to imagine that an egg is under the foot' (p. 1076). Answer B, attempting to place 50%

of their weight on the affected side is representative of partial weight-bearing precautions (PWB). Answer C, suggesting the client "judge" how much weight they can tolerate when standing is typically associated with weight-bearing as tolerated (WBAT) precautions, while answer D, prompting the client to put 100% of their weight on the affected leg if considered to be full weight-bearing status (FWB). See Reference: Pedretti, 2013. Lawson, S.C. & Murphy, L.F.: Hip fractures and lower extremity joint replacement.

125. (B) Hammering a nail into a piece of wood. "Cylindrical grasp, the most common static grasp pattern, is used to stabilize objects against the palm and the fingers, with the thumb acting as an opposing force.... This pattern is used for gripping a hammer, a pot handle, a drinking glass, or the handhold on a walker or crutch" (answer B, p. 766). Answer A is a form of prehension commonly referred to as tip prehension. Answer C, carrying a pail of bolts, requires a hook grasp. This requires the MCP joints to be placed in extension and the PIP and DIP joints to be flexed, and may not include the use of the thumb. Answer D is considered a spherical grasp pattern that requires the fourth and fifth digits to assume a more flexed position for enhanced cupping of the palm. See Reference: Pedretti. (2013). Lashgari, D. & Yasuda, L.: Orthotics.

126. (D) position the person in an upright posture, making sure head is flexed slightly and in midline. Making sure that the resident is correctly positioned is the first step in addressing eating problems. Improper posture can result in difficulties with swallowing. Depending on the particular problems of the individual, providing adaptive devices (answer A) may or may not be helpful, but nonetheless would not be the first step given without assessment of need. Observing for swallowing after each bite (answer B) and instructing caregivers as to proper setup (answer C) also would be important steps, but these would occur later in the intervention process. See Reference: Pedretti. (2013). Smith, J. & Jenks, K.N.: Eating and swallowing.

127. (D) Emphasize the importance of participation rather than the end product. Individuals with depression are aware when they are not performing at their usual level and recognize when they have not done a good job. It is important to offer "understanding and empathic responses and a validation of the client's feelings or thoughts" (p. 241) by acknowledging that he is not happy with the outcome, and at the same time encouraging him by recognizing his progress (answer D). He will recognize the implied praise (answers B and C) as false and may be too ashamed or embarrassed to give a poorly executed project as a gift (answer A). See Reference: Cara & MacRae. (2013). Cara, E.: Mood disorders.

128. (C) Accept her choice and support the decision to, at a minimum, avoid diet pills, laxatives, and/or diuretics. The harm reduction model is utilized with individuals who "may be unwilling to participate in treatment if the expectation is full recovery. Therefore a focus on harm reduction serves as a means of engaging the client and addressing the most dangerous behaviors" while promoting "weight gain and/or symptom interruption to minimize risk" (p. 134). Harm reduction concepts emphasize safety and include maintaining a minimum body mass index and avoiding diet pills, diuretics, laxatives (answer C) and other dangerous behaviors. Setting limits and coercing her into eating (answer A) would be inconsistent with the harm reduction model. Meal planning and preparation (answer B) and stress management (answer D) are all important occupational therapy interventions to focus on with this population. However, these answers do not specifically address the issue of safety, which is primary in the harm reduction model. See Reference: Brown & Stoffel. (2011). Lock, L.C. & Pepin, G.: Eating disorders.

129. (B) Tip the wheelchair backward and guide it down the ramp forward. "To push the client down a ramp, the caretaker should tilt the wheelchair backward by pushing his or her foot down on the anti-tippers to its balance position, which is a tilt of approximately 30 degrees. Then the caregiver should ease the wheelchair down the ramp in a forward direction, while maintaining the chair in its balance position. The caregiver should keep his or her knees slightly bent and the back straight" (answer B, p. 252). The individual sitting in the wheelchair also can help to control the wheels, if capable of doing so, by grasping the hand rims. It would be difficult for the person guiding a wheelchair backward down a ramp (answer A) to see where he or she is going. Only extremely strong individuals can propel themselves independently down a steep ramp (answer C). Using two people to move a wheelchair down a steep ramp could be awkward and dangerous (answer D). See Reference: Pedretti. (2013). Bolding, D., Adler, C., Tipton-Burton, M., Verran, A., & Lillie, S.M.: Mobility.

130. (B) seated sponge bathing. "The energy costs of an activity or occupation and the factors that influence energy costs can further guide the clinician in the safe progression of activity or participation in occupation. Oxygen consumption suggests how hard the heart and lungs are working and is indicative of the amount of energy needed to complete a task. Resting quietly in bed requires the lowest amount of oxygen per kilogram of body weight, roughly 3.5 mL of O_2/kg body weight. This can also be expressed as 1 basal metabolic equivalent (MET). As activity increases, more oxygen is needed to meet the demands of the task" (p. 1209). The MET value for sitting at the edge of the bed is 1 to 2, and the MET value for seated sponge bathing is 2 to 3 MET (indicating answer B is correct). The MET values for knitting (answer A) is similar to what the client is already doing (1 to 2 METs); engaging in sexual intercourse and taking a hot shower (answers C and D) range between 4 and 6 METs. Although it is unrealistic to expect the entry-level practitioner to memorize a MET table, several factors can help the therapist assess the demand of any given task. For example, upper extremity activity work produces a greater cardiovascular response than does lower extremity work. Because both peeling potatoes and propelling a wheelchair primarily use the upper extremities, one can deduce that the cardiac demand from those activities would be greater than walking very slowly. Taking a shower not only involves repeated UE use, but also adds the environmental factor of heat, which also contributes to the demands on the cardiovascular system. See Reference: Pedretti. (2013). Matthews, M.M.: Cardiac and pulmonary diseases.

131. (C) Use a calm voice and explain each step of the hair wash prior to doing it. Answer C is correct. To promote personal hygiene skills for children with autism, "behavioral methods are thought to be the most appropriate, but specific sensory strategies also may be helpful for some children" (p. 457). Even if the child does not yet understand language, each time hair is shampooed and dried, use a soothing voice to repeat what will happen next. The routine and rhythmic repetition of words can be calming. Answers A and B are inappropriate strategies, because washing the hair with only water or waiting until the child goes to the barber would not be efficient techniques to maintain proper hygiene in a young child. Answer D, the use of cool water, can be contraindicated. Water temperature should be warm, not hot, to increase relaxation. See Reference: Kuhanek & Watling. (2010). LaVesser, P. & Hilton, C.L.: Self-care skills for children with an autism spectrum disorder.

132. (D) Encourage the patient to speak with the rehabilitation psychologist. "If the OT is not the one to educate the client or the client's partner, the therapist should anticipate the need for information and have resources available for the client to acquire information.... OTs can provide information and referrals to clients who are concerned about sexual issues. Trained therapists can provide counseling. Issues of sexual function, sexual abuse, and values need to be considered in providing sex education and counseling" (p. 309). The OT should refer the individual to the psychologist (answer D), whose role is

to provide more extensive sexual or marital counseling, which appears to be what is required in this situation. OT practitioners often need to address functional issues related to sexuality when working with individuals who have been seriously injured or disabled and should be well versed and comfortable with the topic. Answer A may require counseling skills beyond the scope of the OT. The physiatrist (answer C), a physician specializing in rehabilitation, is responsible for attending to the medical needs of the individual and coordinating the rehabilitation process. Discussing the increased chances of divorce (answer B), although true, would not be helpful to this individual at this vulnerable time. See Reference: Pedretti. (2013). Tipton-Burton, M. & Umphred Burton, G.: Sexuality and physical dysfunction.

133. (A) Preparing a variety of foods using different cooking methods and recipes. Generalization is "the ability to apply a skill or strategy to an altogether new task in an environment that is different from the one in which the original training occurred" (p. 383). In order to achieve the ability to generalize newly learned skills, the training environment context should be varied. In order to achieve generalization of new strategies, both training tasks and environments should be varied (p. 393). Practicing a variety of tasks in a nonsystematic, but repetitive, way (variable practice) can enhance learning retention and generalization of skills because the novelty introduced into the task engages more cognitive effort. The practice methods identified in answers B, C, and D focus more on systematic or constant practice. This type of practice may result in better performance of different parts of the task, or of one task, but not in improved learning retention and generalization. See Reference: Trombly. (2008). Flinn, N.A. & Radomski, M.V.: Learning.

134. (C) Oversized T-shirts and elastic-top pants. For a child who experiences difficulty in self-dressing due to incoordination (as seen with athetoid cerebral palsy), clothing should be loose fitting with simple or no fasteners (p. 505). Loose clothing is preferred to tight-fitting garments (answers A and B). Garments with elasticized waist bands are more functional than those using zippers (answer B) or snaps and buttons (answer D). See Reference: Case-Smith & O'Brien. (2010). Shepherd, J.: Activities of daily living.

135. (D) Long, thin. Answer D, a long, thin nipple, is correct. "A variety of nipples are available to compensate for oral structural problems" (p. 468) and a long, thin nipple can encourage a recessed tongue forward during the feeding process (Table 15-5, p. 469). Answer A, the Habermann nipple, "was developed specifically for infants with cleft palate to deliver flow without requiring suction" (p. 468). Answer B, a nipple with a single hole, is most effective for children who perform better with a steady flow of liquid versus a burst of fluid as is typically provided via nipples with several holes (Table 15-5, p. 469). Answer C, a broad-based nipple, is most effective for children with a cleft lip because it tends to create suction (Table 15-5, p. 469). See Reference: Case-Smith & O'Brien. (2010). Schuberth, L.M., Amirault, L.M., & Case-Smith, J.: Feeding intervention.

136. (D) Breathlessness. A feeling of breathlessness, or dyspnea, "is a key feature of COPD. Damage to the lung results in flattening of the diaphragm due to hyperinflation. This flattening takes away the ability of the diaphragm to act effectively in assisting with expansion of the lungs during inspiration. To compensate for the lack of inspiratory pressure, patients with COPD tend to use their shoulder girdle muscles to expand their lungs, making it difficult to use those muscles in unsupported upper extremity activities" (p. 1307, answer D). Answer A, a deficit in postural control, would be correct if the client had been unable to maintain his balance while putting on the shirt. A deficit in muscle tone (answer B) would have been evident if the client had demonstrated spasticity while putting on the shirt. Inability to push his arms through the resistance created by the shirt sleeve would demonstrate a deficit in strength (answer C). See Reference: Trombly. (2008). Huntley, N.: Cardiac and pulmonary diseases.

137. (A) Discuss options and the consequences of each option. "The combination of the right equipment, behavior changes, and environmental modifications depend upon the individual's needs, resources, and personal preferences. Scheduled follow-ups are recommended to determine the need for new or further modifications as changes occur" (p. 1089, answer A). Then the following steps can be implemented to encourage acceptance of change: (1) identify options and the consequences of each option; (2) allow time for reflection and consideration of options (answer D); (3) practice with a "demo" device (answer C); (4) reassess the decision; (5) if acceptable, order the equipment; and (6) if rejected, document the steps taken and the reasons for rejection (answer B). See Reference: Trombly. (2008). Forwell, S.J., Copperman, L.F., & Hugos, L.: Neurogenerative diseases.

138. (B) Having the only red toothbrush. This individual appears to be performing at Allen's Cognitive Level 4.4 to 4.6. Individuals at this level "can display a heavy reliance on simple visual cues" (p. 63). The environmental adaptation strategy of using a red toothbrush (answer B), which stands out from the others, provides a strong visual cue. This is an envi-

ronmental adaptation and does not require new learning that may be beyond the individual's ability. Switching to an electric toothbrush (answer A) requires a new set of skills and this individual is likely to have difficulty with new learning. A built-up handle (answer C) is appropriate for individuals who have difficulty grasping the handle of a toothbrush. Having the individual's teeth brushed by a caregiver (answer D) is not desirable if the individual is able to do it himself. See Reference: Pollard, 2010 Pollard, D.: Appendix I: Functional cognition report forms for use by healthcare clinicians.

139. (B) Flex the child's hips and knees. Answer B is correct because flexing the hips and knees inhibits ankle plantarflexion (which makes the task very difficult) through the key point of the hip (p. 503). Answer A is incorrect, because hip and knee extension would contribute to, not inhibit, plantarflexion of the ankle. Answer C is incorrect, because shoulder extension would probably have more influence on hip and knee flexion than on ankle plantarflexion. Answer D is incorrect, primarily because the abnormal pattern at the ankle is usually influenced by inhibition from the key point of the hip. See Reference: Case-Smith & O'Brien. (2010). Shepherd, J: Activities of daily living.

140. (B) hemi-inattention. The correct answer is hemi-inattention (answer B), which is the inability to respond or orient to perceptions from one side of the body. This deficit also is apparent when an individual eats only half the food on his plate or shaves only half of his face. Hemi-inattention is contralateral to the side of a brain lesion; therefore, left hemi-inattention would result from right-sided brain damage. "Hemi-inattention is often confused with the presence of a left VFD (visual field deficit) in the client. Although both conditions may cause the client to miss visual information on the left side, they are distinctly different conditions and do not have the same effect on performance. When a left VFD occurs, the client attempts to compensate for the loss of vision by engaging visual attention. The client directs eye movements toward the blind left side in an attempt to gather visual information from that side. Because of the field deficit, however, the client may not move the eyes far enough to acquire the needed visual information from the left side and as a result may appear inattentive. In contrast, a client with hemi-inattention has lost the attentional mechanism in the CNS that drive the search for visual information on the left. No attempt will be made by the inattentive client to search for information on the left side of visual space, and no eye movement or head turns will be observed toward the left" (p. 615). A cataract (answer C) would cause a visual impairment with detail on both sides of a page. Bitemporal hemianopia (hemianopia also is referred to as hemianopsia), also known as "tunnel vision," occurs when the individual's peripheral vision is lost (answer D). The individual would still be able to cross midline with cataracts or bitemporal hemianopsia (answers C or D). A right neglect would not see the right side, and this type of patient would draw all the figures on the left side of the page. Visuospatial deficits are an important factor influencing functional independence outcomes. Visuospatial ability should be taken into account when establishing treatment goals as well as during discharge planning. See Reference: Pedretti. (2013). Warren, M.: Evaluation and treatment of visual deficits following brain injury.

141. (B) Associative. In groups at the associative (answer B) level, individuals are able to "begin to share and collaborate briefly when others approach; participate in some joint activities; participate in activities/games briefly for a few minutes; respond when the leader reinforces norms and encourages sharing" (p. 50). Individuals working in parallel groups (answer A) would not be sharing with others. Individuals at the cooperative group level (answer C) are more interested in engaging with others and maintaining participation for longer periods of time. Individuals at the mature group level (answer D) are able to participate independently. See Reference: Cole & Donohue. (2011). Cole, M.B.: Social participation basics.

142. (C) Tip. "In tip prehension, the IP joint of the thumb and the DIP and PIP joints of the finger are flexed to facilitate tip-to-tip prehension" (p. 765). This type of prehension is used to pick up objects such as a pin, nail, or coin. "It is difficult to substitute for tip prehension because it is rarely a static holding posture" (p. 765). Lateral prehension (answer A) is formed by positioning the pad of the thumb against the radial side of the finger. This prehension pattern is used for holding a pen, utensil, or key. Palmar prehension (answer B), also known as three-jaw chuck, is formed by positioning the thumb in opposition to the tips of the index and middle fingers, forming a pad-to-pad opposition. This form of prehension is commonly used to lift objects from a flat surface and to tie a shoelace. A spherical grasp (answer D) is typically used for holding a ball or other round objects. See Reference: Pedretti. (2013). Lashgari, D. & Yasuda, L.: Orthotics.

143. (C) Righting. Righting reactions are "designed to align the head with gravity (keep the head upright)" (p. 255). Answer A is incorrect, as the amphibian reaction occurs when the child is in prone position. Lifting the pelvis causes flexion of the arm and leg on the same side. This appears from 6 months and is maintained. Prehensile reactions refer to grasping patterns and reach, which differentiate humans from other primates. Equilibrium reactions develop after righting reactions and allow the child to maintain a standing and walking posture. See Reference: Case-Smith & O'Brien. (2010). O'Brien, J. & Williams, H.: Application of motor control/motor learning in practice.

144. (D) Meeting the vocational instructor weekly to discuss adaptations to work tasks. Occupational therapy consultation is a collaborative process designed to "identify and solve problems with engagement in occupations" (p. 1090). Answers A and B are activities typically completed by the vocational teacher. A vocational instructor should already be able to perform assessments (answer C). See Reference: Schell, Gillen, & Scaffa. (2014). Holmes, W.M. & Leonard, C.: Consultation.

145. (B) Identify the individual's abilities, needs, and goals. Identifying the individual's abilities, needs, and goals should occur before any other steps in the process in order to make a match between the individual's abilities, environmental demands, and the appropriate technology to carry out desired daily occupations. Answers A, C, and D are steps that would come later in the process. See Reference: Pedretti. (2013). Schultz-Krohn, W. & McHugh Pendleton, H.: Application of the occupational therapy practice framework to physical dysfunction.

146. (B) A lettuce, tomato, and cucumber salad. Grading "refers to systematically increasing the demands of an occupation to stimulate improved function or reducing the demands to respond to client difficulties in performance. When grading, the OT practitioner increases the demands of the task at hand to potentially reduce an underlying impairment or performance skill deficit. In other cases, the OT practitioner may downgrade the demands of an activity so that the task can be achieved despite a client's limitations" (p. 323). Upgrading the activity to a salad (answer B) involves using more steps and more ingredients, thereby increasing the level of complexity in both sequencing and problem-solving. More advanced meal preparation activities can be structured to increase in complexity in the following sequence: prepare a cold meal, prepare a hot one-dish meal (answer C), and prepare a hot multidish meal (answer D). Making a cheese sandwich (answer A) does not represent an upgrade of the activity. See Reference: Schell, Gillen, & Scaffa. (2014). Gillen, G.: Occupational therapy interventions for individuals.

147. (A) Each group member holds up a sign with his or her name on it, and the new mem-

ber reads the names of each. In errorless learning, "the person learns something by saying or doing it, rather than being told or shown by someone. In addition, the person is not given the opportunity to make a mistake," thereby minimizing the possibility of making mistakes. "The hypothesis is that the reduction or prevention of incorrect or inappropriate responses facilitates memory performance" (pp. 228–229). When the new member reads from signs (answer A), it increases the likelihood of accuracy and errorless learning. Imagery is a technique of creating associations between an individual's name and characteristics (answer B). Asking the new group member to say the names of one or two individuals who she remembers (answer C) would be the next step after demonstrating consistency in identifying those individuals. Having each group member state his or her name (answer D) is a good beginning activity but does not have a "doing" component requisite to the errorless learning approach. See Reference: Gillen. (2009). Managing memory deficits to optimize function.

148. (D) Provide wrist extension, MCP extension, and thumb extension. A low-level radial nerve injury results in decreased extension of the MP joints of the thumb and fingers. The purpose of this orthosis is to prevent the extensor tendons from overstretching as well as provide proper positioning of the hand for functional use. Answers A, B, and C are inappropriate functions for a dorsal dynamic orthosis. See Reference: Pedretti. (2013). Kasch, M.C. & Walsh, J.M.: Hand and upper extremity injuries.

149. (A) Coordinate with consistent timing of medications. "The most frequently used medical management strategy for PD (Parkinson's Disease) is prescription of a dopamine agonist to make up for the depletion of dopamine caused by destruction of the substantia nigra. Levodopa is the medication most commonly used for the treatment of PD.... A decrease in tremors and rigidity occurs during the 'on' period after the administration of Levodopa, but the client may also experience various dyskinesias, such as abnormal movements of the limbs. As the dosage of Levodopa wears off, the motor symptoms, specifically tremors and rigidity, associated with PD return. Timing of the medication and the periods of 'on-off' are important in planning the client's daily activities" (p. 942). An individual with Parkinson's disease should learn to effectively utilize the time period of reduced symptoms resulting from medication use to efficiently engage in ADLs. Medications taken regularly and consistently aid the establishment of routines for self-care (answer A). Performance of self-care activities before medications (answer B) and spread throughout the day (answer D) would not

make best use of the medication's positive effects. Answer C is incorrect because it discourages attempts for independent functioning. See Reference: Pedretti. (2013). Schultz-Krohn, W., Foti, D., & Glogoski, C.: Degenerative diseases of the central nervous system.

150. (C) Wide-barreled pencil. "Writing muscle tension and fatigue may be reduced for some children by using a wider-barreled pencil" (p. 573). Answers A, B, and D are all adaptations that can be used with a child who has JRA for various reasons; however, extended reaching and jar opening (answers A and B) are infrequently performed by children throughout the day in typical classroom settings. Because printing and handwriting are common tasks for children this age, it is important to reduce fatigue from hand weakness. The plate guard (answer D) is a useful device for those with incoordination or one-handedness, but is not particularly necessary when hand strength is decreased (adapting the utensil would be more reasonable). See Reference: Case-Smith & O'Brien. (2010). Schneck, C. & Amundson, S.L.: Prewriting and handwriting skills.

151. (B) Raise the toilet. The minimum doorway width that allows a standard wheelchair to pass through easily is 32 inches. A standard toilet is 15 inches, which is 3 inches lower than the standard wheelchair seat. Raising the toilet to 18 inches would make transfers easier for this individual. See Reference: Schell, Gillen, & Scaffa. (2014). Rigby, P., Trentham, B., & Letts, L.: Modifying performance contexts.

152. (B) Encourage the individual to take a relaxation break. Many addicts use drugs and alcohol as a way to fill leisure time and to manage stress or boredom. When this individual experienced frustration with the birdhouse project, he was unable to cope with the stress, became agitated, escaped the challenge, and sought out an addictive substance (the cigarette). The term *coping* is used to "describe the explicit actions taken by individuals as they encounter difficult conditions in their daily lives" (p. 313). Relaxation techniques (answer B) "can decrease the stress response and facilitate adaptive coping" (page 323). Providing a project with larger pieces (answer A) is an adaptation that would benefit individuals with coordination deficits. Clearly labeling the parts of the birdhouse (answer C) is an adaptation that would benefit individuals who have difficulty with visual perception. Moving to a less distracting environment (answer D) would benefit an individual with attention deficits. See Reference: Brown & Stoffel. (2011). Haertl, K. & Christiansen, C.: Coping skills.

153. (C) Preparing a frozen dinner. Preparing macaroni and cheese, a hot one-dish meal, is a multistep activity requiring the use of heat and following directions. Because the individual is unable to successfully perform at this level, the activity must be downgraded. Preparing a frozen dinner (answer C) involves the use of heat but requires fewer steps. Having the individual prepare a multicourse meal, such as chicken and mashed potatoes (answer A), would be upgrading an activity that is already too difficult. Cold meals and foods such as instant pudding and peanut butter and jelly sandwiches (answers B and D) would be downgrading the activity more than necessary. Once the OT has determined the area of difficulty, he or she "can choose to grade the activity down by providing scaffolding, changing the objects and properties, space demands, social demands, or sequence and timing...by changing some of these activity demands or providing assistance" (p. 161). The Rehabilitation Institute of Chicago identified five levels of complexity for meal preparation ranging from easiest (level one) to hardest (level five). Preparing macaroni and cheese, a hot one-dish meal, falls into the fourth level. Because the individual is unable to perform successfully at this level, the task must be downgraded to the next lowest level, i.e., level three, which includes preparation of hot beverages, soups, or frozen dinners. Having the individual prepare a multicourse meal, such as chicken and mashed potatoes (answer A), would be upgrading the activity to level five. Cold meals and foods such as instant pudding and peanut butter and jelly sandwiches (answers B and D) are at level two. Downgrading to this level would be appropriate if the individual had experienced significant difficulty, not minimal to moderate as demonstrated here. See Reference: Thomas. (2012). Grading and Adapting.

154. (D) Discuss parents' concerns and provide appropriate information and resources. Contemporary approaches in NICU environments embrace developmentally supportive care that acknowledges "parenting an infant in the NICU is stressful and difficult, and that both the infant and family must receive individualized support through the NICU hospitalization for optimal outcome" (p. 651). Answers A, B, and C are all strategies used in NICU intervention. However, answer D is clearly the optimal strategy for fostering parental observation and interpretation skills, building positional and handling skills, and responding to their infant's behaviors. Initial chart review and updating with nursing staff (answers A and B) are essential; however, they are the least optimal strategies to pursue while the family is present. Answer C, providing written materials, does not enable the OT to interact with the family, develop rapport, and hear about their immediate concerns. See Reference: Case-Smith & O'Brien. (2010). Hunter, J.G.: Neonatal intensive care unit.

155. (D) A buttonhook attached to a cuff that fits around the palm. Individuals with C6 to C7 quadriplegia/tetraplegia may have a tenodesis grasp or no grasp available to them. Therefore, a buttonhook attached to a cuff (answer D) or possibly a buttonhook with a built-up handle are the only appropriate choices. "Many assistive devices and equipment items can be useful to the person with SCI.... When appropriate, the universal cuff for holding eating utensils, toothbrushes, pens, and typing sticks is a simple and versatile device that offers increased independence" (p. 966). A buttonhook with a knob handle (answer B) or on a 5-inch dowel (answer C) is appropriate for an individual with a functional grasp but limited dexterity. A buttonhook with an extra-long, flexible handle benefits an individual with limited range of motion. See Reference: Pedretti. (2013). Adler, C.: Spinal cord injury.

156. (A) Constructional apraxia. "Constructional apraxia is a specific deficit in spatial-organization performance.... It can be seen functionally as difficulty with such activities as setting a table, making a sandwich, and making a dress and with any mechanical activity in which parts are to be combined into a whole" (p. 250, answer A). An individual with constructional apraxia may have full sensory awareness of the affected side of the body, but still may be unable to perform the assembly of one or more objects on to each other to carry out a verbal command or don clothing (answers B and C) in the proper sequence or position. Unilateral neglect (answer D) occurs as the individual neglects the affected side of the body and performs activities toward or with the unaffected side, for example, in the case of an individual combing only one side of his head or shaving one side of his face. See Reference: Trombly. (2008). Quintana, L.A.: Assessing abilities and capacities: Vision, visual perception and praxis.

157. (D) Block out areas of a page to expose material that is the immediate focus. Answer D is correct because this compensatory technique is a way of dealing with visual figure-ground or visual discrimination problems, "giving specific attention to the distinctive features of a visual stimulus through highlighting" (p. 380). The child can then focus on the important area of a task, such as reading. Answer A is incorrect because this is a technique used to orient a child with left-right visual tracking problems. Answer B is incorrect because it is a technique used to deal with visual attention problems. Answer C is incorrect because it is a technique used to help children deal with visual memory problems. See Reference: Hinojosa & Kramer, (2009). Schneck, C.: A frame of reference for visual perception.

158. (B) Decreased edema and prevention of tendon adhesions. "Gentle muscle contraction, as seen with ROM, acts as a vasopneumatic pump to encourage return of the excess fluids to the heart, prevent the adhesion of surrounding tissues, and minimizing resulting discomfort in the acute state of healing. OTs encourage this process by means of teaching range of motion programs, such as tendon gliding exercises for edema [answer B] accumulating in the hand.... Tendon gliding exercises specifically are completed at the intensity of five repetitions twice daily at regular intervals, until the edema has diminished" (p. 43). Answers A, C, and D are all potential outcomes as a result of implementing a tendon gliding program after the edema and potential for tendon adhesions are prevented. See Reference: Meriano & Latella. (2008). Proulx-Sepelak, D.: Foundational skills for functional activities.

159. (B) Offer even-tempered acceptance, reflection, and assurance that they will get better. "When working with someone who is depressed, it is essential to relate with understanding and empathy.... [O]ne should provide...understanding and empathetic responses and a validation of the client's feeling or thoughts...and assurance that the person will get better although he or she may not know or feel it now" (p. 241). Answer B is a good example of an empathetic response that validates the individuals' feelings. In contrast, a cheerful approach (answer A) can be perceived as denying the significance of the person's feelings. Silence (answer C) also may be perceived as unaccepting. Having the individual be responsible for structuring and leading the group (answer D) is incorrect because initiating and maintaining discussions is often difficult for depressed individuals. See Reference: Cara & MacRae. (2013). Cara, E.: Mood disorders.

160. (A) Reassess the physical environment and location of AT. "Ergonomic work arrangements allow users to work in neutral, relaxed positions that consider energy conservation, which is important to maximize productivity for all users while protecting health and minimizing the risk of injury" (p. 596). Answer B addresses other relevant factors in computer use, but none that would directly affect fatigue, whereas answers C and D do not coincide with the student's independent use of the computer. See Reference: Case-Smith & O'Brien. (2010). Schoonover, J., Argabrite Grove, R.E., & Swinth, Y.: Influencing participation through assistive technology.

161. (C) Utilize a leg-bag for the trip. Using a leg-bag for the trip (answer C) is the best option. A leg-bag can be hidden under most pants or trousers. A "urine collection bag must not be placed above the level of the bladder for longer than a few minutes" (p. 144); therefore, placing it in the lap (answer D) or hanging it on the back of the wheelchair (answer B) are not good options. A condom catheter (answer A) still requires some type of bag in which to collect the urine, so it does not solve the problem. See Reference: Pedretti. (2013). George, A.H.: Infection control and safety issues in the clinic.

162. (A) As an adjunct to intervention to promote child's function. Answer A is correct, as studies (listed on pp. 316–317) have demonstrated that following a period of restraint of the less involved arm and hand, gains in the frequency of use, accuracy, and strength of the involved arm and hand were maintained. "Constraint-induced movement therapy...seems to be a potential adjunct to other interventions for children with asymmetric motor involvement due to CNS dysfunction" (p. 315). Answers B and D are incorrect, as studies of CIMT do not suggest these results. Answer C is incorrect as it describes a characteristic of CIMT and not an outcome. See Reference: Case-Smith & O'Brien. (2010). Exner, C.: Evaluation and intervention to develop hand skills.

163. (B) Begin writing periods with students completing "chair push-ups" and elastic band stretches. "Postural and arm preparation activities are an important component of a comprehensive handwriting program.... In the classroom...they may perform heavy work such as an arm push up in a school chair" (p. 568). Answer A is not an optimal strategy, as students will do these activities only when in physical education class and the "preparation" is not connected to routine handwriting periods. Answers C and D promote visual-motor integration, through tracing activities also challenging pencil grasp and accuracy of drawn lines. Neither of these two strategies is an intervention to influence arm and hand muscle strength and motor control. See Reference: Case-Smith & O'Brien. (2010). Schneck, C. & Amundson, S.L.: Prewriting and handwriting skills.

164. (C) Position the stander at 75 to 80 degrees from the floor. Answer C is correct because by adjusting the prone stander nearest to vertical (the least effect of gravity on the head or posture), the child will be able to work on head righting. "The child who cannot maintain a righted head in a full prone lying position may be successful in a prone stander at 75 degrees upright" (p. 546). Answer A is incorrect because while working on the floor in prone, the head and neck are doing the most work against gravity. The demand for the child to right his head against gravity when at a 45-degree angle (answer B) are still greater than when the stander is raised to 75 degrees. Answer D is incorrect because the head and neck work the least against gravity in the vertical upright position. See Reference: Hinojosa & Kramer. (2009). Colangelo, C.A. & Shea, M.: A biomechanical frame of reference for positioning children for functioning.

165. (C) "Client stated she was too tired to continue." One of the main symptoms of major depressive disorder is decreased energy; therefore, the response of "I'm too tired" indicates fatigue or it may be reflective of the individual's level of motivation. Regardless, the only response that is appropriate as a subjective entry is "Client stated she was too tired to continue" (answer C). The subjective portion of the note contains "subjective information obtained from the client...that cannot be verified or measured during the treatment session" (p. 63). Clinical judgments, such as the client's potential for progress (answer B) or factors contributing to impaired performance (answers A and D) belong in the assessment part of the SOAP note. See Reference: Gateley & Borcherding. (2012). Writing the "S"—subjective.

166. (B) Confront the individual's behavior and ask, "Are you aware that your frequent interruptions prevent others from having a chance to contribute?" The individual has not responded to the more subtle and indirect cues provided by the therapist. The OT must be able to "provide clients with structure, direction, and feedback in a way that they can understand it.... An important aspect of providing clients with structure and direction involves providing them feedback" (p. 168). In this case, the OT needs to take a more directive approach. Providing tactile cues (answer A), redirection (answer B), and restructuring the task (answer D) are examples of indirect feedback, which has not worked in the past. Considering that the more conservative attempts have not been effective, a more direct approach, such as confronting the behavior, would be the best approach for the OT to take at this time. See Reference: Taylor. (2008). Therapeutic communication.

167. (C) Painting. Because the patient shows no preference, the OT should first recommend the safest activity. "Individuals with peripheral neuropathy...need to use extra care not to stick themselves with the needles" (p. 139), so needlepoint would not be the first choice. Splinters would be a risk factor with woodworking (answer B) and paper cuts would be a risk factor with scrapbooking (answer A). That leaves painting (answer C) as the best option. See Reference: Tubbs & Drake. (2012). Needlework.

168. (C) Folding laundry. "Therapists should consider overarching themes when deciding which interventions to use to address a client's inability to re-sume meaningful roles and successfully participate in chosen occupations.... Approaches that focus on the use of functional activities as the therapeutic change agent (e.g., task oriented approaches) show promise from both a research and a clinical perspective" (pp. 855–856). Folding laundry (answer C) challenges balance and upper extremity function in ways that are more functional than stacking cones or throwing a ball. Rather than seeking contrived activities (answers A, B, and D) that challenge single skill deficits, the focus of home care is to find ways for the patient to actually perform the daily activities that are presenting the challenges. Because this patient is the mother of four, it is presumed that her occupational role includes homemaking activities. See Reference: Pedretti. (2013). Gillen, G.: Cerebrovascular accident/stroke.

169. (B) Pants with an elastic waistband. Elastic waistbands that are not too tight and stretchy materials are suggested adaptation strategies for easier dressing (p. 505). Also, pants with an elastic waistband is the option with the least need for adaptations. Answers A, B, and C typically make dressing and undressing easier, but because of this particular child's incoordination and weakness, elastic waistbands are the preferred method to introduce in order to promote independence with this particular dressing skill. Adaptations to clothing should be recommended for people who need to compensate for a skill that will likely not improve. Given the child's recent head injury, the likelihood of recovering lost motor skills is good. See Reference: Case-Smith & O'Brien. (2010). Shepherd, J.: Activities of daily living.

170. (A) A transfer bench with a handheld shower. Answer A is the most appropriate choice, because an individual with paraplegia would most likely be able to transfer himself out of the wheelchair and onto a transfer bench. Because the child will not have use of his legs, a handheld shower would permit the child to wash without having to adjust the faucet overhead. Answer B, a hydraulic lift, would be indicated for an individual who is obese or for someone who has limited function of both the upper and lower extremities. Answer C also would be used for an individual with limited function because the child can be rolled onto the tub prior to its inflation. Answer D, a wheeled shower chair, would be a choice made for washing in a shower, not a tub. The chair can simply be rolled into a stall. See Reference: Case-Smith & O'Brien. (2010). Shepherd, J: Activities of daily living.

171. (B) Obtain a raised toilet seat. The individual will most likely continue to require a raised toilet seat for several months in order to avoid flexing the hip past the designated range. A handheld shower (answer D) is not always necessary; however, a shower chair with adjustable legs and grab bars could be helpful. High-contrast tape (answer C) may help to make ascending and descending stairs safer for individuals with limitations in vision. Moving items from low cabinets to higher locations may help this individual comply more readily with the necessary hip precautions, but moving objects from high to lower cabinets (answer A) would not. See Reference: Pedreitti, 2013. Lawson, S.C. & Murphy, L.F.: Hip fractures and lower extremity joint replacement.

172. (D) Assist clients in the selection of simple, short-term tasks. "Parallel groups are the lowest level, made up of clients doing individual tasks side by side.... Little interaction is required, and the OT leader defines the task and provides clients with the necessary assistance and emotional support" (p. 141). At this level, the OT must be available to provide support, encouragement, and assistance when indicated (answer D). Parallel group members typically work on individual tasks within the group. Therefore, it would not be expected that the OT would encourage experimentation (answer A), which would require the client to be working at the project group level. Project groups focus on clients working with other group members while encouraging trust. The OT participates as an active member when the group is at the mature level, at which point individuals take on the roles necessary to achieve a balance between meeting the group task, and the emotional needs of the group. Because the OT must act as an authority figure in the parallel group in order to set limits, encourage interaction, and assist the patient in feeling safe, answer B is incorrect. See Reference: Cole. (2012). Psychodynamic approaches.

173. (D) A raised-bed garden. The individual with back pain must avoid activities that stress the lumbar spine, such as prolonged bending/flexing of the spine. A raised-bed garden would allow gardening without bending. A wheelbarrow with elongated handles (answer B) would be more difficult to control while pushing than a wheelbarrow with normal handles, and therefore would place undue stress on the low back. A 12-inch-high seat with tool holders (answer C) could benefit an individual with low endurance, but working on the ground from that position would be very difficult for an individual with back pain. Answer A, ergonomically correct hand tools, would assist individuals requiring joint protection of the hands and upper extremities as opposed to those with back pain. See Reference: Pedretti. (2013). Grangaard, L.: Low back pain.

174. (D) Role-playing with dolls. Answer D, role-playing with dolls, is the most appropriate choice as it provides opportunity for playfulness through pretend play, during which "the child begins to create situations, [and] objects take on new purpose" (p. 417). Role-playing is focused primarily on the activity at hand, rather than on the end product, such as in answer A (playing a game of "Go Fish") and answer B (playing a game of checkers). Answer C, jumping rope, might frustrate the child secondary to her difficulty with motor tasks. The end goal of an occupational therapy treatment for this child would be to increase the child's play skills with the expectation that the child will begin to interact more comfortably within the home, school, and peer environments. See Reference: Parham & Fazio. (2007). Lane, S. & Mistrett, S.: Facilitating play in early intervention.

175. (C) Minimizing scar hypertrophy through compression garments and proper skin care. "Ideally, clients should be fitted with custom-made compression garments no later than 3 weeks after wound healing; otherwise, wearing of interim garments is continued until custom garments can be applied. Custom-made compression garments are constructed to provide gradient pressure.... They should be worn 23 hours a day and be removed only for bathing, massage, skin care, or sexual activity.... Compression therapy should be applied to burned areas for approximately 12 to 18 months or until scar maturation is complete" (p. 1136). Minimizing scar hypertrophy through compression garments and proper skin care is imperative upon wound closure (answer C). Answer A, preventing scar formation via static use of orthosis, is typically performed during the surgical or postoperative phase of treatment. Controlling edema (answer B) and promoting self-care skills (answer D) are not goals directly related to scar management and are more commonly initiated during acute care intervention. See Reference: Pedretti. (2013). Reeves, S.U. & Deshaies, L.: Burns and burn rehabilitation.

176. (C) Provide a screen to reduce peripheral visual stimuli. Although all the answers given describe techniques that could assist the student, the use of a screen (answer C) is most appropriate in a mainstream classroom. The other methods or adaptations (answers A, B, and D) could have a negative impact on the other children's ability to learn. See Reference: Case-Smith & O'Brien. (2010). Schneck, C.: Visual perception.

177. (B) Based on his refusal, do not treat the individual and document the interaction in the chart. As stated in principle 3 of the Code of Ethics, the occupational therapy practitioner will "respect the recipient of service's right to refuse [answer B] occupational therapy services temporarily or permanently without negative consequences" (p. 5). Treating the individual against his wishes (answers A and C) go against this ethical principle. Treating the individual without recording the appropriate charges would be cheating the facility. According to the principle of veracity of the AOTA Code of Ethics, "Occupational therapy practitioners shall record and report in an accurate and timely manner all information related to professional activities" (p. 9), so charging for time spent reviewing the chart is not acceptable. See Reference: AOTA Code of Ethics. (2010).

178. (D) Participation in all classroom activities and routines with agreed upon adaptations. As school-based OT is designed to enable the student to participate and learn in the curriculum, services are no longer provided when this criterion is met. Services are discontinued "when the student has acquired the needed skills and uses them during school, when needed adaptations and supports are in place, or when services have failed to produce the desired outcomes despite numerous approaches and lengthy attempts" (p. 735). Answers A and B would most likely indicate to the OT that changes/adjustments/alternate approaches are necessary to assist the student in attaining identified objectives. Answer C, transitioning from middle to high school, is not a reason to end OT services if the student continues to demonstrate a need for OT services within the school setting. See Reference: Case-Smith, Rogers, & Johnson. (2001). Bazyk, S. & Case-Smith, J.: School-based occupational therapy.

179. (D) A patient with the diagnosis of CVA and left neglect caught his left arm in the wheel of the wheelchair, resulting in a cut and bruise. "Most institutions have specific policies and procedures to follow. In general, the therapist should...notify the supervisor of the incident and file the incident report with the appropriate person within the organization" (p. 151). An incident report should be completed whenever a situation occurs that is harmful to the patient or practitioner. This includes, but is not limited to, falls, burns, cuts, and contact with hazardous materials. Although the information in answers A, B, and C is worthy of report in the appropriate form of documentation, only answer D would result in an incident report. See Reference: Pedretti. (2013). Hewitt George, A.: Infection control and safety issues in the clinic.

180. (C) The client independently selected one of six craft designs presented. The notation of the client's response to treatment that contains the most objective information is answer C. "The objective section consists of factual or professional information that is confirmed or validated by the therapist. Baseline data and/or progress on goals, observations, and client performance may be included" (p. 25). The no-

tations that address the client's wants and hostility (answers A and B) are interpretations of behavior versus directly observable responses. The use of the word *appropriate* (answer D) reflects the OT practitioner's judgment. See Reference: Meriano & Latella. (2008). Meriano, C. & Latelle, D.: Introduction.

181. (A) Non-experimental. Surveys are considered to be non-experimental, answer A. "Non-experimental designs primarily rely on statistical manipulation of data rather than mechanical manipulation and sequencing. By definition, non-experimental designs are those in which none of the three criteria for true experimentation exists in the structure of sample selection, exposure to an experimental condition, and data collection. These designs are most useful when testing a concept or construct or set of relationships among constructs that naturally occur.... Survey designs are primarily used to measure characteristics of a population. Through survey designs, it is possible to describe population parameters as well as to predict relationships among these characteristics" (p. 114). Answers B, quasi-experimental, C, pre-experimental, and D, a time series tool, are all considered forms of experimental design. See Reference: DePoy & Gitlin. (2011). Experimental-type designs.

182. (B) The child demonstrated tongue thrust with food presented in five of 10 trials. Answer B is correct, as it reports the therapist's "objective observations and measurements" (p. 471). Tongue thrust is an objective, well-defined term. The other answers are subjective. Answer A infers the child's emotional reaction. Answer C implies or judges the child's behavior. Answer D interprets data based on insufficient evidence. See Reference: Schell, Gillen, & Scaffa. (2014). Sames, K.: Documentation in practice.

183. (D) Sheltered workshop. "Sheltered Workshops are noncompetitive employment settings intended to provide many of the positive benefits of a work atmosphere for individuals with disabilities" (p. 692) and would best meet this individual's needs for a protected environment. Supported employment (answer B) and working with the job coach (answer C) in a fast-food restaurant, for example, are both examples of competitive and integrated work environments. Clubhouse models (answer A) offer a range of employment options but are typically used in psychiatric rehabilitation. See Reference: Schell, Gillen, & Scaffa. (2014). King, P.M. & Olson, D.L.: Work.

184. (D) Evaluate participants' performance strengths and weaknesses. Answer D is correct. The first step in any intervention is almost always evaluation. The next step in this process, based on a developmental model because of the age and backgrounds of the clients, is developing trust and exploration (answer A). This is followed by skill development (answer B). Once basic skills are in place, greater emphasis is placed on work quantity and quality (answer C) (p. 194). See Reference: Case-Smith & O'Brien. (2010). Stewart, K.B.: Purposes, processes, and methods of evaluation.

185. (D) autonomy By reporting concerns about the individual that could result in the loss of his driver's license, the OT would be directly impacting his autonomy, or self-determination (answer D). "The principle of autonomy and confidentiality expresses the concept that practitioners have a duty to treat the client according to the client's desires." Respect for autonomy ...acknowledges a "person's right to hold views, to make choices, and to take actions based on personal values and beliefs" and the "right to make a determination regarding care decisions that directly impact the life of the service recipient should reside with that individual." (AOTA Code of Ethics, 2013). Social justice (answer A) requires that "Occupational therapy personnel shall provide services in a fair and equitable manner." Veracity (answer B), according to the AOTA Code of Ethics, requires that "Occupational therapy personnel shall provide comprehensive, accurate, and objective information when representing the profession." The principle of Fidelity in the AOTA Code of Ethics (answer C) states that "Occupational therapy personnel shall treat colleagues and other professionals with respect, fairness, discretion, and integrity." See Reference: AOTA Code of Ethics

186. (D) Comply with the parent's request and allow the OT student to observe the treatment session. OTs should always respect the recipients of their services. According to the Occupational Therapy Code of Ethics (2010), under Principle 3C, "occupational therapy personnel shall: Respect the recipient of service's right to refuse occupational therapy services temporarily or permanently without negative consequence" (p. S21). Attempts to persuade the parent to allow the OT student to lead the session (answers A and B) conflict with this principle. Canceling the session (answer C) is punitive and withholds services from the child. See Reference: American Occupational Therapy Association, Inc. (2010). Occupational Therapy Code of Ethics and Standards. Am J Occup Ther, 2010 Nov-Dec; 64: Supplement: S17-26.

187. (D) Transdisciplinary. Answer D, transdisciplinary team, is correct. One team member provides the direct intervention and other team members function in collaborative consultant roles so "the family benefits from the expertise of many professionals but interacts with only one" (p. 459). Answer

A is incorrect because a unidisciplinary team is not really a team; as the term implies, there is only one member. Answer B is incorrect as in the multidisciplinary approach, "each professional is responsible for identifying and carrying out one's own discipline-related evaluation and intervention" (p. 457). Answer C also is incorrect, because the interdisciplinary team is "composed of members representing and using knowledge and skills of their respective discipline, the team members identify goals and plan intervention collaboratively" (p. 458). See Reference: Schell, Gillen, & Scaffa. (2014). Falk-Kessler, J.: Professionalism, communication, and teamwork.

188. (D) Benefit or cost center analysis. "An important function of most managers is the planning and controlling of a departmental budget. Budgets are typically planned for a calendar year or a fiscal year.... The process of planning and managing a budget requires that a manager have a comprehensive understanding of the goals and objectives of the larger organization so that he or she can establish priorities for funding that support this mission over time.... Budgets also include revenue and expenses.... Subsets of revenues and expenses are commonly referred to as cost centers" (p. 1025). Outcomes measurements (answer A) are taken at the completion of service intervention and are used to evaluate the effectiveness of the intervention. Utilization reviews (answer B) assess the care that is provided to ensure that services were appropriate and not overutilized or underutilized. Program evaluation (answer C) is a method used to determine how well the program's goals have been achieved. See Reference: Schell, Gillen, & Scaffa. (2014). Braveman, B: Management of occupational therapy services.

189. (B) 3-inch screw-top jar. Answer B is correct. Because the goal was written as a functional behavioral objective, the OT should collect information about the functional progress that the child has made in this specific performance area. Assessing progress by measuring range of motion with a goniometer (answer A), the strength of grip using a dynamometer (answer C), or degree of coordination using a fine motor scale assessment (answer D) may provide useful information of individual performance components addressed; however, none of these will provide sufficient information to measure progress of a functionally written goal. See Reference: Case-Smith & O'Brien. (2010). Bazyk, S. & Case-Smith, J.: School-based occupational therapy.

190. (C) Respect, beneficence, and justice. "The ethical issues of conducting research have only recently been a focus of national concern. In 1974, the National Research Act created a commission to delineate the ethical issues and guidelines for the involvement of humans in behavioral and biomedical research in the United States.... The resulting Belmont Commission issued a report in 1979 that outlined three basic ethical principles to guide all research activity in order to protect human subjects.... The second principle in the Belmont Report describes three areas that must be addressed: respect for persons, beneficence, and justice" (p. 152). HIPAA guidelines, answer A, and annual review, answer B, do not relate to the Belmont Report, whereas answer D, the Nuremberg Code, was part of the impetus for the development of the Belmont Commission. See Reference: DePoy & Gitlin. (2011). Protecting the boundaries.

191. (A) Pain management techniques. Work-hardening programs focus on returning individuals to work in physically appropriate settings, as quickly as is feasible, through reconditioning. As part of that program, pain management techniques (answer A) are included to assist the person with managing and coping with pain during work-related activities. A work-hardening program would teach proper body mechanics to prevent further injury rather than focus on energy conservation (answer C), which is emphasized with individuals who need to minimize or avoid fatigue. Vocational counseling (answer D) helps individuals enhance their vocational potential and addresses skills necessary for job seeking and job acquisition. Although balancing work and leisure (answer B) is important for maintaining overall health, it is not the emphasis of a work-hardening program. See Reference: Pedretti. (2013). Haruko Ha, D., Page, J.J., & Wietlisbach, C.M.: Work evaluation and work programs.

192. (B) a presentation to local physicians with flyers and business cards. Answer B, a presentation to physicians, is correct because this is an example of marketing to a potential referral source(s) who refer based on Medicare requirements. "The private practitioner has prepared for the establishment of their business by preparing marketing materials which may include: business cards, flyers, educational lectures and outreach communication" (p. 5). Answers A, C, and D are all examples of internal (answer D) and external marketing strategies (answers A and C), that may not directly target Medicare recipients. See Reference: http://www.aota.org//media/Corporate/Files/Advocacy/Reimb/Pay/Private/OTPPP%20%201-08%20finaloptimized.ashx p. 5.

193. (A) G8988—Self-care. The two G-codes that are most appropriate in this situation are G8988—Self-care and G8979–Mobility. Given that the patient is also getting physical therapy, and only one G-

code can be used at a time, the most appropriate answer is G898—Self-care (answer A). The G-code G8978—Mobility (answer B) would most likely be used by physical therapy in this situation. G8985—Moving, handling and carrying objects (answer C) was not an area that was specifically identified. Because two G-codes cannot be used at the same time, G8979—Mobility and G8988—Self-care (answer D) would not be an option. See Reference: http://www.cms.gov/Regulations-and-Guidance/Guidance/Transmittals/Downloads/R165BP.pdf

194. (D) is no longer homebound. "You must be homebound and a doctor must certify that you are homebound" (Centers for Medicare and Medicaid, p. 5). After the individual is able to leave the residence, the individual cannot continue to receive home care services (answer A) and would be referred to outpatient services. Without knowing the individual's specific goals, it is not possible to say whether she has achieved them (answers B and C). See Reference: Schell, Gillen, & Scaffa. (2014). Lohman, H.: Payment for services in the United States.

195. (A) whether occupational therapy services support participation in the education program. Related services are defined as services needed to help students benefit from their education program. School-based OT services "support the student's participation in the curriculum, access to the school environment, and participation in extracurricular activities" (p. 663). Intervention to develop functional skills (answer B) and independence in ADL (answer C) are addressed in school programs only when they impact the student's participation and ability to benefit from their education program. Accessibility of the learning environment (answer D) is an important concern, but it would be covered by consultation with the school or teacher, not through direct service provision. See Reference: Schell, Gillen, & Scaffa. (2014). Swinth, Y.L.: Education.

196. (B) The OTA updates the OT on the progress a patient has made in the past week, and both provide information to update the goals. A collaborative relationship between an OT and an OTA supports sharing of information and the use of each professional's skills. In this type of relationship, communication is two-way, and both individuals work as a team to the benefit of the patient. Answers A and D demonstrate one-way communication in which the OT tells the OTA what to do. In answer C, the OT takes information from the progress note, but does not receive input or recommendations from the OTA for the patient's discharge summary. See Reference: American Journal of Occupational Therapy,

November/December 2009, Vol. 63, 797-803. doi: 10.5014/ajot.63.6.797 AJOT document.

197. (C) Interpreting results of assessments for the purposes of treatment planning. "An occupational therapist initiates and directs the screening, evaluation, and reevaluation process and analyzes and interprets the data in accordance with federal and state law, other regulatory and payer requirements, and AOTA documents" (p. 4). The functions noted in answers A, B, and D may all be performed by the OTA in a long-term care facility. See Reference: AOTA Standards of Practice. (2010). http://www.aota.org//media/Corporate/Files/Practice/OTAs/ScopeandStandards/Standards%20of%20Practice%20for%20Occupational%20Therapy%20FINAL.ashx (downloaded 7/20/13).

198. (B) Understand how Medicaid coverage varies from state to state. Medicaid "is a cooperative venture funded jointly by the federal and state Governments to assist states in furnishing medical assistance to eligible needy individuals...and [varies] considerably by state [answer B].... Thus, a person who is eligible for Medicaid in one state might not be eligible in another" (p. 1041). Many healthcare plans use preauthorization (answer A) as a cost-containment measure. The frequency of reevaluation (answer C) may be determined by the patient's third-party payer, but Medicaid does not mandate monthly reevaluation. Because Medicaid programs are managed by individual states, billing would be directed to the state, not federal, government (answer D). See Reference: Schell, Gillen, & Scaffa. (2014). Hammel, J. et al: Disability rights and advocacy.

199. (A) Convenience. Convenience sampling, answer A, is "also referred to as accidental sampling, volunteer sampling, and opportunistic sampling.... Convenience sampling involves enrollment of available subjects or elements as they enter the study until the desired sample size is reached. The investigator establishes inclusion and exclusion criteria and selects those individuals who fit these factors and volunteer

to participate in the study in the case of human subjects and that meet the criteria in the case of nonhuman elements" (p. 169). See Reference: DePoy & Gitlin. (2011). Boundary setting in experimental-type designs.

200. (C) Help place food on the spoon for a patient learning how to use a universal cuff in the patient's room at lunchtime, while the OT supervisor runs a lunch group in the dining room. "An aide, as used in occupational therapy practice, is an individual who provides supportive services to the occupational therapist and the occupational therapy assistant. Aides do not provide skilled occupational-therapy services. An aide is trained by an occupational therapist or an occupational therapy assistant to perform specifically delegated tasks. The occupational therapist is responsible for the overall use and actions of the aide. An aide first must demonstrate competency to be able to perform the assigned, delegated client and nonclient tasks, (AOTA, Guidelines for Supervision, p. 177). An aide may be delegated client-related tasks when (a) the outcome of the task being delegated is predictable; (b) the client's situation and the environment are stable and will not require that judgment, interpretations, or adaptations be made by the aide; (c) the client has demonstrated some previous performance ability in executing the task; and (d) the task routine and process have been clearly established. The aide also must be trained and demonstrate service competency while carrying out certain tasks as well as be aware of signs and symptoms that would indicate the assistance of an OT or OTA. When these conditions are met, answers A, B, and D are all acceptable. Answer C states that the patient is "learning" to use a universal cuff. This would indicate that changes may still be in progress that could require the judgment and skill of an OT practitioner. See Reference: http://www.aota.org//media/Corporate/Files/Practice/OTAs/Supervision/Guidelines%20for%20Supervision%20Roles%20and%20Responsibilities.ashx Guidelines for supervision, roles and responsibilities during the delivery of occupational therapy services.

Simulation Examination 4

Directions: Circle the correct answer to the following questions. When you have completed this examination, check your answers against the answer key that follows. As you will see, an explanation is given for each answer along with a reference for further study. The book author is listed as well as the chapter author. See the bibliography for complete references. Study the areas in which your comprehension was low.

PEDIATRICS

1. During the interview with the parents of a 3-year-old child with mild cerebral palsy, the OT learns that the child is regularly fed by his grandmother and does not have any independent feeding skills. Before setting self-feeding goals, what should the OT explore?

A. Degree of abnormal muscle tone in the child's upper extremities.
B. Possibility of developmental delay.
C. Cultural context and family interaction patterns.
D. Need for adapted equipment.

2. A child with significantly low muscle tone caused by Duchenne muscular dystrophy is losing trunk control when sitting. The OT assesses the child's range of motion, strength, and endurance, which indicates that the OT is MOST likely relying upon which frame of reference?

A. Neurodevelopmental treatment.
B. Sensory integration.
C. Biomechanical.
D. Visual perceptual.

3. A young child with hypertonicity is unable to bring his hands to midline to reach for a toy while in supine and sitting positions. What is the BEST position to use to reduce the effects of abnormal patterns and facilitate midline grasp?

A. Supported standing.
B. Prone.
C. Side-lying.
D. Quadruped.

4. An OT receives a referral for an infant in the NICU whose mother has a history of drug use during pregnancy. What is the FIRST action the therapist should take?

A. Determine the mother's current drug use, medical status, parental involvement, and support systems.
B. Recommend a social work referral, provide support and community program information, and refer to the Department of Human Services.
C. Modify the environment to protect the infant from excessive and/or inappropriate sensory stimulation prior to direct intervention.
D. Assess infant's motor and behavioral skills and begin gentle handling to promote positive sensory experiences.

5. An OT is selecting activities for a child's treatment plan to achieve an IEP goal concerning the student's completion of written expression during independent seatwork in the language arts curriculum. To BEST support the student's engagement and provide optimal therapeutic value the OT should:

A. have the student complete tracing activities in progressively smaller physical areas to refine pencil control, increase visual-motor accuracy, and promote writing endurance.
B. interview the student to learn how seatwork is most challenging and then engage student in skill-building activities to increase self-efficacy in that specific component.
C. embed self in the classroom during language arts seatwork periods to assess performance and trial multiple strategies as student participates in the assigned work.
D. use teacher evaluation data to define student's specific areas of need and implement activities that target practice in the teacher's highest priority area.

6. An OT is exploring assistive technology options to help a student with autism produce written assignments in the classroom. The team is concerned that because of the student's rigid and perseverative behaviors, additional computer use in the classroom will intensify maladaptive behavior and promote his isolation from peers. What is the BEST option for this child?

- A. Do not implement increased computer usage in the classroom at this time.
- B. Emphasize handwriting over this marking period and determine the student's progress.
- C. Include specific strategies in the plan to incorporate variable use and avoid isolation.
- D. Allow student to use the computer only in a group setting with other students.

7. Impulse control difficulties limit a 12-year-old boy with conduct disorder in the classroom. Which is the MOST effectively written functional goal for his IEP?

- A. By end of marking period, student will participate in classroom activities for 1 hour without disruptive outbursts for 4 of 5 days.
- B. By end of the marking period, student will attend to an activity for 30 minutes, demonstrating improved impulse control.
- C. Student will show a 50% reduction in the frequency of disruptive outbursts by end of the marking period.
- D. When presented with a new activity, the student will follow directions without protest, four out of five times, within 6 months.

8. Following the inclusion of occupational therapy in a student's IEP, what is the PRIORITY for the school-based OT?

- A. Develop IEP goals related to the child's fine motor performance to handle classroom tools and learning materials.
- B. Meet with classroom teacher to review methods for collecting progress-monitoring data to track student's performance.
- C. Readminister test used in initial evaluation to update scores for the educational record.
- D. Facilitate child's performance in student roles expected in the school setting.

9. A child with athetoid cerebral palsy is working in OT to develop self-feeding skills. When the child attempts to pick up food, it is inadvertently pushed off the plate. Which adaptation should the OT provide to solve this problem?

- A. A swivel spoon.
- B. A nonslip mat.
- C. A mobile arm support.
- D. A scoop dish.

10. An OT in the school system is developing transition activities for a group of 16- to 18-year-old students with developmental disabilities. Which activities are BEST to address goals related to transition?

- A. Role-play ordering food in the classroom.
- B. Go out for lunch at a fast-food restaurant.
- C. Order a takeout lunch by phone.
- D. Select lunch items from a picture menu in the classroom.

11. A therapist is discussing discharge plans with the parents of a 7-year-old child with sensory defensiveness. What is the MOST appropriate strategy to introduce proprioceptive input to heighten the child's arousal?

- A. Walking barefoot on textured surfaces.
- B. Slow, repetitive rocking over a large therapy ball.
- C. Playing in a large box full of Styrofoam pellets.
- D. Playing tug-of-war with rope.

12. Through the school-based evaluation process, the OT may consider many possibilities for intervention; however, the determination that occupational therapy will be included in the student's IEP is made at which point in the IEP process?

- A. After the OT reviews and interprets all evaluation data.
- B. During the interview with the classroom teacher who referred the child for evaluation.
- C. At the IEP meeting once the occupational therapy evaluation results are summarized to team members.
- D. After the student's goals and objectives are determined for the IEP.

13. An OT is planning treatment activities to use for a child with postural instability. What would be the BEST preparatory activities to recommend?

    A. Weight shifting and weight-bearing activities.

    B. Activities that provide tactile and proprioceptive input.

    C. Activities while the child is prone over a wedge.

    D. Activities that increase the time child is upright against gravity.

14. An OT needs to assess the performance skills in a 10-year-old child with autism. Which observation will provide the MOST information?

    A. Child's use of sandpaper, glue, and paint while constructing a birdhouse.

    B. Occurrence of self-stimulation behaviors during classroom circle.

    C. Child's ability to place a backpack in a designated cubby when entering the classroom.

    D. Teacher's appraisal of the child's capacity in role of "learner" in the classroom.

15. An OT observes a child with a learning disability use an unusually tight grip when writing with a pencil. The child also frequently breaks the pencil point by applying too much pressure on the paper. What is the MOST likely cause of these observations?

    A. Inadequate sensory processing related to the vestibular system.

    B. Limited motor planning.

    C. Inadequate sensory processing related to the kinesthetic system.

    D. Difficulty with visual system processing.

16. Which would the OT recommend for a 12-year-old child with mild visual impairments who desires independent use of the home telephone?

    A. A speaker phone.

    B. A hands-free phone.

    C. A phone with extra-large buttons.

    D. A phone with a receiver holder.

17. Using a "top-down" approach for a middle school student, where should the school-based occupational therapy process begin?

    A. School-related performance skills.

    B. The student's participation in curricular and extracurricular activities.

    C. Client-factors related to class participation.

    D. An understanding of the head-toe and proximal-distal pattern of development.

18. An OT is working with an 8-year-old child who has mild spastic cerebral palsy. The evaluation has shown that the child has poor in-hand manipulation skills. What would MOST likely improve the development of this skill?

    A. Grasping blocks to build a building.

    B. Placing pegs from one pegboard to another.

    C. Carrying books in a bag with a handle.

    D. Removing a nut from a bolt.

19. An OT is evaluating developmental stages in a 10-month-old baby who is beginning to "cruise" while holding on to furniture. How would the OT MOST likely describe the child's development?

    A. Compensatory.

    B. Advanced.

    C. Typical.

    D. Delayed.

20. An OT is working with a school-age child to improve her power grasp technique. Which activities would the OT MOST likely encourage the child perform to practice this grasp?

    A. Pegboard activities over increasingly longer time periods.

    B. Brushing her own hair in the morning and evening.

    C. Carrying a lightweight book bag in her hands, rather than on back.

    D. Throwing a weighted ball at a target on the wall.

21. In using an assessment that is "norm-referenced" for children, what assumption can the OT make about the test?

    A. It measures typical behavior of children.

    B. It compares performance with a normative sample.

    C. It is valid and reliable.

    D. It was standardized on groups of typically developing children.

22. An OT working in an outpatient setting is considering the use of Ayres Sensory Integration™ for a child with a learning disability. Which intervention is MOST consistent with this approach?

A. Student is included in classroom-based group that includes a program of varied sensory stimulation activities.

B. Student uses a small, weighted blanket on his lap during seat work periods in the classroom.

C. OT encourages child to engage in a playful environment with ramps, scooters, ladders, balls, manipulatives, and vibrating toys.

D. OT develops a planned sensory diet that includes "Sensory Stories" to promote student's participation in the classroom activities and routines.

23. A school-age child with multiple disabilities is beginning to develop some controlled movement in the upper extremities. When would it be MOST appropriate to introduce switch-operated assistive technology?

A. Once the child develops the ability to sit upright for 10 minutes.

B. After the child can reach and point with accuracy.

C. When the child demonstrates any reliable, controlled movement.

D. Once the child develops isolated finger control to push buttons.

24. An OT is working with a 3-year-old child who has spastic diplegia. What mobility device would be MOST appropriate to use in assisting this child to explore space?

A. Body-length prone scooter.

B. Aeroplane mobility device.

C. Tricycle.

D. Power wheelchair.

25. An infant is beginning to sit and lean forward onto his arms. The OT considers recommendations to the family to increase opportunities for the infant to practice this developing postural control and balance reactions during their everyday routines. Which is the MOST likely suggestion given to this family?

A. During trips to the mall, the family should carry the infant in an upright position, holding the child's lower torso enabling the child to practice balance while looking at the variety of stimuli in this environment.

B. Each day as she watches the morning news, mother should continue to practice the trunk control and balance activities modeled by the OT during home visits.

C. Extended family members who spend time with the child should attend the OT's home visit to learn ways the parent embeds new strategies that support child's development into their daily routines.

D. Family should use cushions to support the child in seated play on the living room floor, with toys present, while parent watches nightly news or folds laundry.

26. An OT in the NICU is instructing the parents to bottle feed their infant. To facilitate suck-swallow-breathe coordination, the OT would instruct the parents to hold the baby comfortably in the breast-feeding position and do what next?

A. Stroke the infant's cheek before feeding her a bottle.

B. Gently touch the infant's lips before introducing the bottle.

C. Tip the bottle back to allow the infant to include a breath in her suck-swallow pattern.

D. Gently rub the infant's gums and cheek simultaneously before feeding the baby her bottle.

27. What is the BEST position in which the OT can place an 8-month-old child to provide the opportunity to further develop reaching skills for play?

A. Supine.

B. Prone.

C. Side-lying.

D. Sitting.

28. A teenager with fine motor incoordination reports difficulty with self-care. Which option would this individual find MOST beneficial?

    A. Wash mitt.
    B. Spray deodorant.
    C. Toothpaste with a flip-open cap.
    D. Toothbrush with a built-up handle.

29. Which BEST represents a school-based consultative relationship between the OT and school teacher?

    A. The teacher identifies a child's needs so the OT can follow up with appropriate intervention.
    B. The OT provides an in-service program to the teachers in the school.
    C. OT reports student's progress to other team members at IEP meetings.
    D. OT implements services that support the teacher's classroom goals.

30. An OTA with previous school-based occupational therapy experience has joined the school district staff. The supervising OT is developing the OTA's workload. Which is the MOST likely action taken by the OT?

    A. Evaluations the OTA completed in her previous setting are identified, and students needing these evaluations completed are assigned to the OTA's caseload.
    B. OTA will not complete any evaluations until the probationary period in employment is complete.
    C. OTA will observe the OT completing each evaluation once, then the OTA will administer the measure for the next student identified by the OT.
    D. The OTA demonstrated administering assessments completed in previous setting, OT reviewed OTA's scoring, and then determined which ones the OTA could complete in this setting.

31. After a variety of interventions have not led to the improvement a parent anticipated in her 4-year-old's social participation, she asks the OT for information about the benefit of vitamins, special diets, and other alternative approaches for children with autism. What is the BEST response for the OT to give this parent?

    A. Advise the parent that these are not researched-based interventions, so the family should not pursue them.
    B. Encourage the mother to be patient and allow her son to participate in the current therapy program for a longer time.
    C. Suggest the parent contact her insurance company to learn about their policies on reimbursement for these types of treatments.
    D. Offer to bring summaries on the research into various complementary and alternative approaches for children with ASD and review them during the next home visit.

32. A second-grade student with muscular dystrophy operates a manual wheelchair, but his mobility is slow because of muscle weakness. When should the OT consider a power wheelchair?

    A. In junior high school when child switches classrooms several times daily.
    B. When child's speed over long distances becomes less than that of a walking person.
    C. After the home can be made accessible.
    D. After it becomes impossible to propel a manual wheelchair.

33. Which is MOST likely to provide relevant evaluation information about how a child with motor delays completes self-care activities?

    A. Standardized tests of dressing skills.
    B. Review of the medical record.
    C. A developmental screening test.
    D. Observation of child during self-care activities.

34. In assessing the dressing skills of a 5-year-old child, the OT observes that the child is able to put on a jacket, zip the zipper, and tie a knot in the draw string but needs verbal cuing to tie a bow. At what level would the OT MOST likely describe the child's dressing skills?

    A. Age-appropriate.
    B. Delayed.
    C. Advanced.
    D. Limited.

35. A goal for a child with a neuromuscular disorder is to develop postural reactions for increased participation in play. Which activity BEST addresses this goal?

   A. Introduce pulley exercises to increase upper extremity strength.
   B. Engage the child in reaching activities while seated on the floor.
   C. Encourage the child to engage in play dough activities while in the prone position.
   D. Engage the child practice finger painting while in a supported seated position.

36. The parents of a 12-month-old with a significant motor dysfunction due to cerebral palsy asked the OT when a means of assisted mobility should be introduced. What is the earliest age the OT should suggest to the parents?

   A. 18 months.
   B. 2 years.
   C. 3 years.
   D. 4 years.

37. An OT observes a child with autism spectrum disorder flapping his right hand in front of his eyes repeatedly. This behavior MOST likely serves which purpose?

   A. Helps focus vision at close range.
   B. Relieves pain in his right hand.
   C. Relieves paresthesia in his fingers.
   D. Helps child maintain his state of arousal.

38. A child with a learning disability has significant problems with visual memory that limit performance during test activities. How can the OT enhance visual memory?

   A. Provide memory tasks in mass practice trials.
   B. Decrease demands for visual attention just prior to memory tasks to prime visual memory abilities.
   C. Help student identify simple rhymes to remember steps to complete homework independently.
   D. Repeat visual memory activities so student can anticipate next steps.

39. Part of an OT's documentation reads, "Continue social skills training program and encourage child to attend one new after-school club activity within the next week." Which section of a SOAP note is the MOST appropriate to place this statement?

   A. Subjective.
   B. Objective.
   C. Assessment.
   D. Plan.

40. As part of an initial evaluation in an outpatient setting, the OT is developing an occupational profile on an 18-month-old with Erb's palsy. Which approach BEST represents the OT's use of narrative clinical reasoning skills?

   A. Perform interviews with the parents regarding their daily routines, social life, and child-rearing practices.
   B. Rely on information gathered from the collaboration between the OT and the family.
   C. Determine the child's performance level through an activity analysis task and occupational performance checklist.
   D. Focus energy on the available social and financial resources of the family to target goals for participation in community-based activities.

41. During the process of planning an intervention program, the therapist relies on data gathered through narrative reasoning. What information do these data provide to the OT?

   A. Student's knowledge of the classroom activities and routines.
   B. Teacher's report of how the student has adjusted in this new classroom.
   C. Estimate of the student's fine motor skills compared with those of peers.
   D. History of therapy services the student has received.

42. Which BEST represents a typically developing 12- to 15-month-old child's functional mobility?

   A. The child uses a wide base of support and takes small, inconsistent steps.
   B. The child uses a wide base of support and can navigate uneven ground.
   C. The child uses a narrow base of support and low arm guard position.
   D. The child uses a narrow base of support, can walk well, and can run for short distances.

43. Which approach should the OT implement to best support learning and development for a child with autism spectrum disorder?

    A. Incorporate customized social stories as a part of daily recess to promote the child's social skills development.

    B. Use a family-centered approach to learn about parent concerns and priorities and provide interventions that help them increase parenting skills and promote their child's learning.

    C. Help the family adapt the home environment to include strategies that support the child's individual sensory preferences.

    D. Emphasize therapist/child intervention sessions that provide ample opportunities for child to explore multisensory play.

44. When preparing an evaluation summary for a child with juvenile rheumatoid arthritis, what is the MOST important information to share with the child's schoolteacher?

    A. A summary of the child's cognitive and visual perceptual skills.

    B. Adaptive equipment/ADL needs in the classroom.

    C. Information on the child's range-of-motion status.

    D. Recommended home exercise program.

45. When performing a "naturalistic observation" of dressing skills with a young child with developmental delay in an outpatient setting, what should the OT do FIRST?

    A. Provide oversized clothing to ensure success.

    B. Have the child dress and undress in a distraction-free corner of the clinic.

    C. Give assistance as needed to minimize frustration.

    D. Observe the child entering the clinic and taking off his coat and shoes.

46. An OT is instructing a family how to observe for stress in their preterm infant in the NICU. What are the MOST important autonomic responses to watch?

    A. Frantic movements in upper extremities and shaking.

    B. Limpness in upper and lower extremities and crying.

    C. Twitches, or jerky movements while infant is asleep.

    D. Hiccups and skin color change to flushed.

47. A child with cerebral palsy and visual impairment is learning to use a computer for classroom work and is frustrated because it takes a long time for her to type a sentence. What is the BEST solution for this problem?

    A. A larger monitor.

    B. Voice recognition word processing software.

    C. Word prediction software.

    D. Masking some of the keys on the keyboard.

48. A child has mastered brushing her teeth while the OT gave verbal and physical cues. To progress with the process of reducing the intrusiveness of cues, what is the OT's NEXT step?

    A. Verbal cues only.

    B. Verbal and general gestural cues only.

    C. Physical cues only.

    D. Gestures and physical cues.

49. A 17-year-old individual who wears a hip brace is measured for a wheelchair. What are the correct seat dimensions for the OT to recommend?

    A. 2 inches wider than the widest point across the child's hips with the brace on.

    B. 2 inches wider than the widest point across the child's hips.

    C. 2 inches more than the distance from the back of the bent knee to the buttocks.

    D. The same as the distance from the back of the bent knee to the buttocks.

50. The OT is selecting activities for a school-age child with postural control limitations. Which activity would BEST promote postural control?

    A. Sliding down a playground slide.

    B. Playing simple "Simon Says."

    C. Swimming laps.

    D. Playing on a trampoline.

51. The OT working with an infant observes the presence of the first stage of voluntary grasp. How would the OT describe the grasp pattern exhibited in documentation?

    A. Radial palmar grasp.

    B. Pincer grasp.

    C. Ulnar palmar grasp.

    D. Raking grasp.

52. An OT witnesses a seizure in a child with hydrocephalus. What is the MOST relevant information to document?

    A. Child's positioning during the seizure.

    B. Objective signs and duration of the seizure.

    C. Responsiveness during the seizure.

    D. Facial expression during and after the seizure.

53. When adapting a toilet for use by a 6-year-old child with limited postural control, what should the OT PRIMARILY pay attention to?

  A. Whether the toilet paper can be reached without a major weight shift.
  B. Whether the flush handle is easy to manipulate.
  C. Whether the child's feet reach the floor.
  D. Whether a nonskid mat is available on the floor to prevent slipping.

54. A 6-year-old student is confusing the direction in which letters of the alphabet are oriented. What is the BEST way for the OT to advise the teacher?

  A. It is suggestive of a problem and warrants further evaluation of visual perceptual skills.
  B. There is a need to develop visual memory skills to improve spatial recognition.
  C. A formal vision screening is indicated.
  D. Research suggests that position in space development is complete at 7 to 9 years of age.

55. The OT plans to use a top-down approach for evaluating a child's self-feeding performance skills. How will the assessment MOST likely begin?

  A. Assessing seating and positioning needs.
  B. Observing the child eating during a meal.
  C. Identifying assistive devices.
  D. Isolating performance component limitations.

56. A child's long-term goal is to increase participation in classroom learning activities that require fine motor skill. The assessment has revealed a deficit in tactile discrimination, specifically stereognosis. What is the MOST relevant short-term goal?

  A. Child will correctly identify five out of five fingers touched when given tactile stimulus.
  B. Child will correctly identify five out of five shapes drawn on the dorsum of her hand.
  C. Child will correctly identify five out of five matching textures.
  D. Child will correctly identify, by feel only, five out of five common objects.

57. An OT is working with a child whose ability to perform schoolwork in a busy second-grade classroom is affected by his limited visual attention. What is an adaptation of the sensory environment that would MOST improve attention during a visual task?

  A. Work with soft music playing near his desk.
  B. Place child's seat work against a patterned background.
  C. Use headphones during seat work.
  D. Attach a small reading lamp to his desk.

58. A young child has been wearing a left upper extremity prosthesis for 3 weeks. What is the MOST important activity recommendation for the OT to give to the child's preschool teacher?

  A. Offer toys that the child can manipulate with one hand so play is successful.
  B. Stress bilateral arm/hand use, incorporating both arms to hold and stabilize objects.
  C. Help the child play by stabilizing and holding toys for him as he plays.
  D. Involve the child in activities that do not require manipulation.

59. When developing a self-care program for a 3-year-old child with significant visual impairment, what would the OT MOST likely do?

  A. Create a reliable route to the bathroom, encouraging the child to familiarize herself with the smells and sounds of the bathroom.
  B. Have the child practice various obstacle courses created in the family's living room to improve body image/awareness.
  C. Practice fine motor skills with a light-up peg activity board.
  D. Connect the family to other families with children who have visual impairments.

60. The parents of an adolescent with a mental health disorder are meeting with the OT in an outpatient center to plan areas for evaluation. What will the OT MOST likely want to include as part of the evaluation?

  A. Assessment of the child's visual motor integration related to schoolwork performance.
  B. Assessment to measure child's cognitive and visual perceptual skills.
  C. Interview about challenges and successes within the family's current daily activities and routines.
  D. Involve other members of the school team for the purpose of carryover.

61. When evaluating an adolescent with an attention deficit hyperactivity disorder (ADHD), the OT will be PARTICULARLY observant for which behaviors?

  A. Excessive talking and inability to remain seated and wait for his turn.
  B. Frequent references to oneself as "the authority" and "the smartest" in the group.
  C. Use of profanities and displays of aggressive behavior.
  D. Expressions of anxiety about working on a project and fear of failure.

62. The OT is working to develop play behavior in a child with low muscle tone who has difficulty engaging in activities against gravity. What is MOST likely position for the OT to use with this the child?

    A. Long sitting along a wall.

    B. Side-lying on a mat.

    C. Supine on a large wedge.

    D. Prone over a bolster.

63. A 7-year-old boy with hemiplegia has difficulty putting on his socks each morning before school. What should the OT recommend?

    A. Encourage the child to wear tight-fitting socks.

    B. Teach the child to sit in a chair with a back support, lift the affected leg and use socks with a wide opening.

    C. Encourage the child to request assistance from his mother when putting on socks.

    D. Teach the child to sit in a chair and lift and place the unaffected foot up on a small stool, and use socks with a wide opening.

MENTAL HEALTH/COGNITION

64. An OT is training an OTA to administer a standardized assessment. Which one of the following is the best method to evaluate the OTA's service competency with that assessment tool?

    A. Observe a competent OT's performance of the standardized test.

    B. Observe a competent OT practice and then teach another how to administer the test.

    C. Follow procedures exactly as outlined in the test manuals.

    D. Obtain the same results as another OT does who has demonstrated service competency.

65. An individual with a panic disorder feels so overwhelmed he cannot get himself from his room to OT group each morning. Which of the following strategies will be MOST helpful?

    A. Reduce distractions and keep the lights low.

    B. Provide a stimulating environment with real-life opportunities.

    C. Give him a tour of the OT department and a schedule of activities.

    D. Leave doors open and avoid being alone with the individual.

66. An OT is working with an adult diagnosed with dementia who is experiencing moderately severe cognitive decline and who was admitted to the hospital after accidentally setting a kitchen fire. What are the MOST appropriate follow-up services to identify relative to this patient's meal-planning needs after discharge?

    A. OT services to teach the patient to cook safely.

    B. Volunteer companion services to supervise cooking at home.

    C. Transportation services to bring the person to a community meal site.

    D. Home-delivered meal services.

67. The goal of a work program for homeless youths is to develop job skills that will improve housing status. The OT plans to evaluate each participant. Based on the transtheoretical model, which area of assessment/evaluation should the OT begin with?

    A. Environmental.

    B. Social skills.

    C. Work skills.

    D. Readiness for change.

68. A client with chronic pain is working with an OT through a workers' compensation program. Despite collaborative development of goals and strategies to begin volunteer activities, the individual has not yet identified a location at which to volunteer. Concerns about losing workers' compensation benefits because of volunteering have been raised. Using a motivational interviewing approach, what is the BEST action for the OT to take?

    A. Reply that the client is ready and needs to make a decision.

    B. Collaborate to find a location and the phone number.

    C. Reassure the client that the workers' compensation benefits will remain intact.

    D. Identify a volunteer opportunity for the client and schedule an appointment.

69. An individual being interviewed by an OT experienced repeated sexual abuse by a parent as a child. The individual states that parent's actions were due to the stress of being fired from a job and that everyone finds different ways to manage stress. In the evaluation report, the OT should identify this as the use of what defense mechanism?

    A. Identification.

    B. Projection.

    C. Denial.

    D. Intellectualization.

70. An OT student has been assigned the task of creating a reality orientation board for a dementia unit. What are the key elements to include?

    A. Illustrated step-by-step instructions for that day's activity.

    B. Pictures of family members now and when they were younger.

    C. The time, date, next meal, and the weather.

    D. A list of the individual's medications and times they should be taken.

71. An extremely withdrawn individual has developed the ability to tolerate interaction with one other group member while making greeting cards using rubber stamps. Which of the following steps should be taken NEXT in order to develop this individual's ability to interact with others?

    A. Involve the individual in a three-member task group.

    B. Progress the individual from rubber stamping to stenciling.

    C. Instruct the individual in how to make stamps from various materials.

    D. Encourage the individual to choose stamps and colors.

72. Task-specific training is being used to train an individual with severe cognitive limitations to put on a T-shirt. How will this training be MOST effective?

    A. In the individual's home.

    B. In the OT department.

    C. At least twice a week.

    D. When the client is feeling cooperative.

73. An individual admitted for alcohol abuse is preparing for discharge and has made it clear that he does not plan to completely abstain from alcohol. What type of community-based self-help program would be MOST appropriate for this patient?

    A. A harm reduction program.

    B. Alcoholics Anonymous.

    C. Narcotics Anonymous.

    D. A health promotion program.

74. An individual with a traumatic brain injury is impulsive during self-feeding, which is exemplified by placing too much food in the mouth at one time. What method would MOST effectively develop safer eating habits?

    A. Cut the food into smaller pieces prior to serving.

    B. Count to 10 between bites of food.

    C. Set down the utensil until the mouth is cleared.

    D. Serve the food in separate containers on the meal tray.

75. An OT is planning a program for men with co-occurring disorders who are currently residing in a supported housing environment. The needs assessment should focus on issues common to individuals for which of the following conditions?

    A. Depression and substance abuse.

    B. Mental retardation and sensory processing disorders.

    C. Diabetes and hypertension.

    D. Post-traumatic stress disorder and amputation.

76. An OT is running a sensorimotor group in an adult day program for individuals with chronic mental health conditions. Using Ross's Five-Stage Group Approach, which would be the MOST appropriate activity to follow the introduction and orientation?

    A. Task activity such as making a fruit salad.

    B. Line-dancing involving movement in three planes.

    C. Group planning for the next session.

    D. Group members taking turns introducing themselves.

77. An individual with an anxiety disorder has been placed on new anti-anxiety medication. While monitoring the individual over the next few days, the OT practitioner should be particularly observant for which of the following side effects?

    A. Akathisia.

    B. Decreased arousal and drowsiness.

    C. Extrapyramidal syndrome.

    D. Tardive dyskinesia.

78. An OT is working with three individuals in a cooking group who demonstrate difficulty attending to tasks, frequently ask to leave the room, and do not interact with each other. Based on the developmental group frame of reference, which of the following is the MOST appropriate goal for this group for each group member?

A. Experiment with trying one different group role.

B. Share materials and tools with at least one other group member.

C. Express two positive feelings about oneself within the group session.

D. Share space while working on a task without disrupting others for 15 minutes.

79. The OT is working with an individual diagnosed with Alzheimer disease. Evaluation revealed profound memory loss, severe intellectual deterioration, incontinence, and nearly complete loss of basic ADL performance. The family is concerned about the agitation the individual demonstrates when getting undressed in the evening. What is the MOST appropriate intervention for the OT to implement?

A. Modifying the bathroom to ensure safety with toilet and tub transfers.

B. Training the caregiver in the use of memory strategies such as labeling.

C. Working with the caregivers to help them utilize routines that will facilitate caregiving.

D. Instructing the caregiver to use visual and verbal cues to enable the individual to be as independent as possible.

80. A patient with a spinal cord injury is on a rehab unit and constantly flirts with the OT. What is the MOST appropriate way for the OT to respond?

A. Firmly reject the patient's advances and stop treatment.

B. Acknowledge the patient's actions and mildly flirt back in order to promote the patient's self-esteem.

C. Request that the supervising OT discuss the effects of SCI and sexual functioning with the patient.

D. Set personal boundaries appropriate to the therapist-patient relationship.

81. An individual with severe depression is withdrawn and exhibiting a low energy level. Which of the following interventions would be most effective in supporting participation at this time?

A. Selecting a leisure activity of interest and identifying materials needed.

B. Performing a simple task.

C. Practicing meditation.

D. Writing suggestions for coping with daily life stresses.

82. An OT working in a state-owned outpatient facility for adults with intellectual disabilities receives a referral for an individual recently admitted to the facility. While observing the individual's performance on the job line in the sheltered workshop, the OT notice the individual appears bored, hits his legs with his fists, and talks loudly. Which type of environment would BEST meet this individual's needs?

A. A quiet workroom with minimal noise and lowered blinds to reduce lighting.

B. A job that offers structure and repetition.

C. Rotation between several job stations, with an alarm to alert the individual when it is time to rotate.

D. A workroom with upbeat music and a variety of jobs from which to choose.

83. An OT in a residential community mental health setting is developing a psychoeducational program to promote healthier eating habits among the residents. To accomplish the group's goals using this approach, what is the OT be MOST likely to do?

A. Have each client make a healthy food collage.

B. Have the group plan and shop for a meal.

C. Designate 1 day a week for the residents to be responsible for cooking dinner.

D. Show a video about nutrition and keep a meal diary for a week.

84. In the comfortable but crowded OT clinic of a mental health partial hospitalization program, a client is having difficulty concentrating on problem-solving tasks. Which of the following environmental strategies would be MOST likely to enhance the client's ability to perform the problem-solving tasks in this clinic setting?

A. Play pleasant background music.

B. Decrease the intensity of lighting in the clinic.

C. Allow the person to perform tasks in a quiet, separate area.

D. Adjust the temperature and ventilation in the clinic.

85. An OT has been hired to consult in a residential setting that provides housing and support for individuals with histories of substance abuse. Children under the age of 2 may reside with their parents, who have a maximum length of stay of 9 months. After administering the Parenting Well Strength and Goals assessment, the OT found that commonly identified areas of need included setting limits, having positive interactions, finding fun things to do, expressing anger without hurting anyone, and identifying their children's strengths. How can the OT most appropriately address this concern?

- A. Evaluate each parent and design individualized interventions to promote parenting and play skills.
- B. Provide educational materials about the impact of parental substance abuse on children.
- C. Provide a course to the day-care staff about age-appropriate expectations and play activities.
- D. Design a program focusing on developing parenting skills, beginning with a module on age-appropriate expectations.

86. During the course of treatment, an individual diagnosed with depression tells the OT that he leads a very isolated lifestyle and often feels alone and afraid. What is the BEST therapeutic response for the OT to make?

- A. Reassure the client that "we can be friends" or that "you will be his friend."
- B. Tell the client, "I know how you feel."
- C. Encourage the client to socialize more often.
- D. Acknowledge his feeling of isolation.

87. A young adult is hospitalized with anorexia nervosa. The OT wants to collect data on the individual's life history, patterns of daily living, interests, values, and needs. By what means would the OT best obtain this information?

- A. Overall physical assessment.
- B. Occupational profile.
- C. Activity configuration.
- D. Psychoeducational session.

88. During a group activity in a mental health setting, one client, Joe, grabs a tool from another client, Sam. The OT employs a modeling approach to encourage appropriate behavior. Which of the following best illustrates a modeling approach?

- A. Get Joe's attention, then return the tool to Sam and ask him whether you may use the tool when he has finished with it.
- B. Remind Joe about the way he had asked Sam to pass the sugar for his coffee that morning and praise him for it.
- C. Ask Joe to identify another method he might have used to obtain the tool.
- D. Tell Joe that you can see how frustrating it is to have to wait his turn for the tool.

89. An OT has been asked to design a series of leisure skill development sessions for individuals in recovery from substance abuse. What activities should be included in the FIRST session?

- A. Introduce healthy alternatives for leisure activities.
- B. Identify leisure skill strengths and weaknesses.
- C. Encourage problem-solving.
- D. Provide strategies for healthy social interaction.

90. A roofing contractor was diagnosed with the extrapyramidal disorder Parkinson's disease. When the OT is educating the client about hypokinesia, what symptoms would be described?

- A. Hyperextension or hyperflexion of the wrist and digits.
- B. Slow movements.
- C. Arrhythmic, or wormlike movements of the distal extremities.
- D. Purposeless, jerky movements.

91. An OT asks an individual in a manic state what he would like to do in craft group. The individual answers, "I'm a really good carpenter so I'm going to build my kids a club house." What is the OT's BEST response?

- A. Support him in this choice.
- B. Tell him he doesn't have the necessary attention span at this time.
- C. Redirect him toward an activity that doesn't require sharp tools.
- D. Suggest trying a small birdhouse first.

92. An individual who lives in a group home and has a history of sexual abuse has identified relaxation through physical activity as a method she would like to use to manage anxiety. Which activity would be MOST appropriate for the OT to introduce?
- A. Sewing and handcrafts.
- B. Yoga, initially in her own room.
- C. Progressive relaxation exercises in a group format.
- D. Aerobics class.

93. An OT interviewing an individual diagnosed with a TBI about his ADL performance realizes that the client is confabulating. What is the BEST way for the OT to gather the needed information?
- A. Complete the interview using closed-ended questions.
- B. Stop the interview and complete it the next day.
- C. Interview a reliable informant instead of the individual.
- D. Administer a written questionnaire using a checklist format.

94. An OT working in a psychosocial rehabilitation program has been asked to design a leisure-skills group for individuals functioning at the egocentric-cooperative group level. It is mid-December, and the OT wants to utilize a holiday theme. Which would the MOST appropriate activity be for this group?
- A. Provide a list of holiday songs for a sing-along.
- B. Have the group create a list of their favorite holiday songs and set a date for a performance.
- C. Organize a holiday cookie swap in which each group member brings a dozen cookies to contribute.
- D. Set up a reminiscence group in which participants express their memories of past holidays.

95. A young adult on the autistic spectrum has obtained a job at a coffee shop. Social skills are good, as evidenced by getting along well with the boss and coworkers, but the client has difficulty noticing when orders are ready, when areas need to be tidied up, and when the coffee machine needs to be refilled. What is the MOST appropriate recommendation to address potential sensory issues?
- A. Provide noise-canceling headphones.
- B. Move to a quieter work area.
- C. Rotate frequently from one station to another.
- D. Provide a job coach.

96. During a meal planning group, an individual with a brain injury is frequently observed looking out the window instead of engaging in the planning task. Which one of the following strategies will have the most effective and immediate impact on the individual's participation in the meal planning activity?
- A. Teach the individual how to use self-instruction statements.
- B. Instruct the client in the use of orienting procedures.
- C. Have the individual use time pressure management strategies.
- D. Position the individual with their back to the window.

97. As discharge time approaches for an individual hospitalized for mental illness, the OT is approached by the individual's parents who express their desire to help their adult child. What is the BEST action for the OT to take?
- A. Explain that HIPAA does not allow discussion of the client's situation with family members.
- B. Explain that recovery occurs best when family members are not involved.
- C. Emphasize the importance of putting their adult child's needs first.
- D. Provide them with information about the National Alliance on Mental Illness (NAMI).

98. An OT practitioner is working with a client experiencing anxiety after being in a physically and mentally abusive relationship. The treatment facility utilizes a psychodynamic-object relations approach. Which of the following interventions would be MOST consistent with this type of approach?
- A. Mediation and yoga poses.
- B. Journal and diary writing.
- C. Personal hygiene and grooming classes.
- D. Aerobics and fitness program.

99. An individual has been referred to OT for prevocational assessment upon admission to a community mental health day program. When considering likelihood of success in the workplace, what are the MOST important areas to assess?
- A. Time management, ability to accept feedback, following instructions.
- B. Attention, memory, and visual motor performance.
- C. Dressing, grooming, and hygiene skills.
- D. The anticipated work environment and level of supervision.

100. An elderly man is caring for his elderly wife who has dementia. He becomes frustrated when she repeatedly asks for her mother and then becomes upset when he tells her that her mother is not there. Which strategy should the OT recommend to the husband to help manage this situation?

- A. Use reality orientation by explaining that her mother has been dead for a long time.
- B. Set limits by firmly telling her to stop asking for her mother.
- C. Use therapeutic "fibbing" by telling his wife that her mother will be coming shortly.
- D. Help him to identify the feelings she is having but is unable to express verbally.

101. An OT public relations campaign is being instituted in your state. It was suggested by the OT state representative that a committee be formed in order to educate potential OT clients at the local level. Which of the following would be the BEST strategy for targeting this market?

- A. Write articles about occupational therapy for local newspapers.
- B. Hold an open house in your department and invite members of the hospital community.
- C. Provide an in-service workshop for nurses working for local home health companies.
- D. Conduct a workshop in your area of expertise at your local or state occupational therapy conference.

102. An OT is working with an adult who is 10 years post-brain injury, has severe attention and memory deficits, and has poor self-awareness. The client's goal is to develop basic job skills for working in a packaging plant. What is the BEST approach for teaching how to package three pieces into a plastic bag?

- A. Rote repetition of packaging task substeps with gradually fading cues.
- B. Preparatory activities to develop sequencing skills.
- C. Activities designed to improve memory and attention.
- D. Use of instructional cards to use as a reminder of how to perform the packaging task.

103. During evaluation, the OT responds using paraphrasing to an individual who recently lost a spouse in a car accident. Why is the OT MOST likely implementing this technique?

- A. Refocus or redirect the individual's comments.
- B. Show acceptance and understanding regarding the individual's situation.
- C. Persuade the individual to make a choice.
- D. Encourage the individual to provide additional information.

104. An OT is working with an older adult who has been admitted for depression with concerns about upcoming retirement. The individual has progressed from the precontemplation stage to the action stage. Which is the BEST action stage activity for this individual?

- A. Record the pros and cons of retiring.
- B. List five concerns about retiring.
- C. Choose one goal to address in the next session.
- D. Identify potential community groups of interest to join.

105. An individual in an OT group has a history of monopolizing the group without giving others an opportunity to participate in the group process. What is the MOST effective approach for working on the individual's social conduct and group skills during a discussion about planning a community outing?

- A. Appeal to the group to give the individual feedback about how his behavior affects them.
- B. Have the individual assign tasks to various group members.
- C. Have the individual observe the group while saying nothing.
- D. Pair the individual with another group member to investigate expenses for the outing.

106. The OT is working with a patient who needs to be independent in medication management prior to discharge. What is the MOST effective strategy for the OT to teach the patient to remember if medication has been taken?

- A. Establish a routine of taking medications the same time every day.
- B. Keep the medications in a special, labeled location.
- C. Use a diary to record each dosage after it is taken.
- D. Arrange for a caregiver to remind the patient when medications should be taken.

107. An OT is preparing to complete an initial evaluation on an individual diagnosed with obsessive-compulsive disorder. Which strategy for modifying the environment is likely to be MOST effective while interviewing this individual?

    A. Minimize environmental distractions.

    B. Utilize open-ended questions.

    C. Instruct the individual to take her time and not rush.

    D. Limit the time available to answer each question, interrupting when possible.

108. A school-based occupational therapist has been asked to develop a suicide prevention program for teens. What would be the BEST program goal for this age group?

    A. Create a volunteer program in a readily accessible environment.

    B. Identify peer leaders who can model and train their peers to identify adults they can trust.

    C. Collaborate with school faculty to develop a filmmaking course for school credit.

    D. Create an after-school tutoring program to develop self-esteem.

109. An OT is running a social skills group and the activity involves planning a trip to the aquarium. The OT starts with a warm-up activity. Next, the OT introduces the goal for the session, which is determining what time they would need to get the bus from their building in the morning in order to arrive at the aquarium by 10:00 a.m. What would be the NEXT step for the OT to take?

    A. Provide feedback to group members who are not respecting the opinions of other group members.

    B. Assign homework involving working with a partner to determine when to get the bus back to the center.

    C. Ask the group members whether anyone has ever been to an aquarium, and see how many fish they can name.

    D. Point out where on the schedule to find times for buses leaving the center in the morning.

110. At a weekly meeting of a responsive social skills group, one individual states he has a job interview the next day and is concerned about how much to reveal about his personal history. What is the NEXT step the OT should take in the problem-solving process?

    A. Involve the group in generating possible solutions for the problem.

    B. Select the best solution or combination of solutions.

    C. Instruct the group in how to role-play for this client's situation.

    D. Identify the pros and cons of each possible solution.

111. An OT has been asked to design a social skills group for individuals functioning at the project group level. What is the MOST appropriate activity to include?

    A. A game of Social Bingo.

    B. An exercise group.

    C. Planning a birthday party.

    D. Attending a church service.

112. An OT is working on money management skills with an individual with cognitive deficits following a stroke. Which of the following components would be LEAST amenable to an errorless learning approach?

    A. Identifying coins.

    B. Making change.

    C. Writing a check.

    D. Creating a budget.

113. Members of an OT group at a psychosocial rehabilitation program who have physical disabilities in addition to mental illness began expressing anger about the lack of accessibility in the building where the day program is housed. Which of the following offers the action that will MOST empower the group members?

    A. Employ an OT practitioner to assess the facility for ADA compliance.

    B. Incorporate advocacy skill training into the group format.

    C. Bring a lawsuit against the facility for violating the ADA.

    D. Involve the clients in a stress management group.

114. An OT is developing a stress reduction and management program for an individual recently diagnosed with multiple sclerosis. One stressor that the individual has identified is that her teenage children are resistive to helping with chores that were previously her responsibility (e.g., cleaning the bathrooms, taking out the trash). Which coping strategy could the OT recommend that would be MOST effective in dealing with this stressor?

    A. Assertive communication skills.

    B. Time management techniques.

    C. Deep breathing and muscle relaxation.

    D. Laughter.

115. An OT has been hired to design and implement a lifestyle redesign program for recently retired older adults. With which activity should the OT begin each module?

    A. Occupational self-analysis.

    B. Transportation.

    C. Safety.

    D. Social relationships.

116. An individual exhibits limited awareness of functional limitations resulting from his recent brain injury, attempts to perform transfers unsafely without assistance, and says that he doesn't see the need for therapy. What is the best way for the OT to promote awareness and insight for this patient?

    A. Have the individual explain why he believes he is not impaired.

    B. Provide a checklist of skills that must be present to perform various activities and review it with the patient.

    C. Have the individual predict his performance before an activity, then have him self-evaluate the performance.

    D. Disregard the individual's perceptions and proceed with therapy.

117. An OT has been asked to develop a skills training program for individuals with cognitive limitations who will be working on a dairy farm. What is the first step in designing an intervention that will effectively address the needs of this population?

    A. Interview consumers to identify solutions to the problems using open-ended questions.

    B. Create a skills training curriculum based on identified problems and solutions.

    C. Develop a list of problems and solutions based on the literature.

    D. Using consumer input, create a list of potential problems.

118. An OT has been asked to design a group to promote self-efficacy for women in a domestic violence shelter. The task part of the activity involves the women giving each other facials and manicures. How should the OT follow up the activity for these women, who are functioning at a cooperative group level?

    A. Identify the steps for planning a fashion show.

    B. Have the participants take "glamour shots" of each other.

    C. Institute a participant-led discussion of how the activity made them feel and identification of reasons they deserve to feel so good.

    D. Solicit program feedback from the group members and encourage them to plan how to implement this type of group again.

119. During a group session for individuals in an inpatient facility, one of the members repeatedly interrupts others, grabs tools and supplies, and states that "the group is a waste of time." What is the BEST approach for the OT?

    A. Encourage other group members to express their frustration with the individual using "I statements."

    B. Tell the individual she may not return to the group until she is able to treat others with dignity and respect.

    C. Ignore the behavior during the group and speak to her about it afterward.

    D. Explain to her that this type of behavior is unacceptable.

120. An OT consulting in a supervised living environment is teaching the residential staff strategies to help minimize the effect of hallucinations for residents with schizophrenia. What is the MOST effective strategy for the OT to teach staff?

    A. Avoid disturbing persons while they are experiencing the hallucinations.

    B. Move individuals experiencing hallucinations to areas where they can be isolated

    C. Provide meaningful activities that will divert attention from the symptoms.

    D. Move the individuals experiencing hallucinations to more stimulating environments.

121. During lunch, an OT observes one individual who grabs the ketchup away from her neighbor, chews with her mouth open, and does not make eye contact with those around her while others seem to be trying to avoid her. The behaviors exhibited by this individual MOST likely indicate a deficit in which of the following?

- A. Social interaction skills.
- B. Physicality in communication.
- C. Self-control.
- D. Coping skills.

122. An agency placing individuals with mental health conditions in a municipal jobs program has hired an OT to make recommendations for reasonable accommodations. Which of the following areas would be MOST essential to assess in order to make these recommendations?

- A. Work environment, structure of work tasks, rules, and supervision.
- B. Architectural barriers within the work site.
- C. Work aptitudes and interests of the persons to be placed in the work program.
- D. Capacity of the individuals to perform specified work tasks.

123. An OT consulting with a drop-in shelter for homeless women is developing a leisure activity group. The OT has observed high levels of anxiety and distrust in the residents. One of the goals of the group activity is to foster a sense of competence and mastery over the environment. Which of the following activities BEST addresses this goal?

- A. Participating in a small group collage activity.
- B. Making leather lacing change purses from kits.
- C. Going to see a movie at a local theater.
- D. Presenting a resident talent show.

124. After administering an interest checklist, the OT practitioner documents that an individual has identified a few vague, solitary leisure interests. Based on this information, what is the BEST activity to use in the next session focusing on healthy use of leisure time?

- A. A leisure inventory assessment.
- B. An activity exploring leisure opportunities and problems.
- C. An activity that encourages the individual to sign up for social activities.
- D. A calendar of community leisure activities for the next few weeks.

PHYSICAL DISABILITIES

125. The OT is working with an injured bus driver who is planning on returning to work soon. The bus driver works evenings and needs to sleep during the day. The client reports not sleeping well since the accident and asks the OT for suggestions. Which environmental adaptations are MOST important for the OT to recommend?

- A. Use room-darkening curtains and lower the temperature.
- B. Use a fan to drown out noise and raise the temperature.
- C. Have a glass of wine before bed and participate in a quiet activity.
- D. Recommend evaluation for a CPAP machine.

126. An individual with joint changes that moderately limit finger flexion would be MOST comfortable using utensils with:

- A. regular handles.
- B. weighted handles.
- C. a universal cuff attachment.
- D. built-up handles.

127. An individual sustained a right upper extremity soft tissue injury and is currently experiencing swelling of the hand and joint stiffness. Which of the following should be implemented FIRST in the acute phase of edema management?

- A. Cold modalities, elevation, and active assist and/or passive range of motion.
- B. Electrical stimulation and dynamic use of orthosis.
- C. Resistive exercises, weight-bearing, and lifting.
- D. Joint mobilization, serial casting, and dynamic use of orthosis.

128. When fabricating an orthotic device for an individual with rheumatoid arthritis, which type of splint or orthoses is MOST appropriate for the purpose of resting the joints, decreasing pain, and preventing contractures?

- A. MP joint orthosis.
- B. Wrist stabilization.
- C. Ulnar drift positioning.
- D. Resting hand orthosis.

129. The OT is working with a client with a spinal cord injury. Which level of injury would benefit MOST from using a wrist-driven flexor hinge orthosis during a prehension activity?

    A. C1

    B. C3

    C. C6

    D. T1

130. In order to promote tenodesis when performing PROM, how should the OT position the wrist?

    A. Neutral to promote finger flexion and extension.

    B. Flexion to promote finger flexion and extension.

    C. Extension to promote finger flexion, and flexion to facilitate finger extension.

    D. Flexion to encourage finger flexion, and extension to promote finger extension.

131. An individual who is several days post-sustaining a myocardial infarction experiences nausea during a bathing evaluation. Which of the following is the FIRST action the OT should take?

    A. Stop the activity.

    B. Document the symptoms.

    C. Instruct the individual to sit and then continue the activity.

    D. Ask the individual whether he can continue the activity.

132. After fabricating an antispasticity splint/orthotic device, the MOST important thing for the OT to determine is that:

    A. the fingers are flexed.

    B. the thumb is in an opposable position.

    C. the patient is wearing the splint/orthotic device at all times.

    D. pressure marks or redness from the splint/orthotic device disappear within 20 minutes.

133. An OT is treating an individual who demonstrates progressive weakness and atrophy of the thenar muscles and numbness and tingling in the thumb and the index and middle fingers. The client also complains of difficulty while grasping a coffee cup. The individual is not experiencing proximal upper extremity limitations; therefore, the OT will MOST likely suspect problems with which of the following?

    A. Ulnar nerve.

    B. Median nerve.

    C. Radial nerve.

    D. Brachial plexus

134. An OT is preparing a presentation for a business with a high incidence of workers diagnosed with cumulative trauma disorders. What are the MOST significant risk factors associated with cumulative trauma disorder?

    A. Repetition, high force, and awkward joint postures.

    B. Progressive resistive exercise, joint mobilization, and weight-bearing.

    C. Inflammation, swelling, and pain.

    D. Fatigue, muscle cramps, and paresthesias.

135. An individual with COPD has identified a long-term goal of being able to shop independently for groceries. Which statement is the BEST short-term goal for this individual?

    A. Individual will purchase 10 items at the supermarket with supervision.

    B. Individual will cook a one-dish meal with items purchased at the supermarket.

    C. Individual will identify food items needed for developing a shopping list.

    D. Individual will learn energy-conservation techniques that apply to grocery shopping.

136. An OT is assisting an individual with mild hemiparesis in transferring from the wheelchair to a mat table using a stand-pivot transfer technique. After locking the brakes, what is the FIRST verbal cue the OT gives to the individual?

    A. Stand up.

    B. Scoot forward to the edge of the wheelchair seat.

    C. Unlock the wheelchair brakes.

    D. Position the wheelchair so that it directly faces the mat table.

137. An individual with low endurance complains of becoming too fatigued during sexual activity to enjoy it. The BEST strategy for the OT practitioner to recommend is for the individual to:

    A. time sex for the end of the day.

    B. take the top, prone position.

    C. assume the bottom, supine position.

    D. experiment with a variety of positions.

138. An individual with Parkinson's disease is at risk for aspiration. When instructing the primary caregiver in proper positioning during feeding, the OT practitioner should recommend:

A. feeding the individual in bed in a supine position.

B. seating the individual upright on a firm surface with the chin slightly tucked.

C. positioning the individual in a semireclined position in a reclining chair.

D. providing food to the individual in bed in a side-lying position.

139. An individual who uses a wheelchair is being discharged from a rehabilitation facility to home. In determining accessibility of the interior home environment, what areas should be of the GREATEST concern to the OT?

A. Location of telephones and appliances.

B. Arrangement of furniture in bedrooms.

C. Steps, width of doorways, and threshold heights.

D. Presence of clutter in the environment.

140. The OT is working with a young woman with motor-control deficits following a TBI and feels the client would benefit from deep proprioceptive input. Which craft activity would BEST provide the needed type of input?

A. Mixing papier-mâché dough by hand.

B. Rolling clay into a 1/4-inch slab using a rolling pin.

C. Gluing mosaic tiles on to a premade form.

D. Stringing glass and silver beads on to a leather cord.

141. An OT is instructing an individual how to perform stand-to-sit transfers after a total hip replacement (posterior lateral approach). Prior to sitting down from a standing position, the therapist should instruct the individual to:

A. extend the operated leg forward, reach back for the armrests, then slowly sit.

B. extend the nonoperated leg forward, reach back for the armrests, and slowly sit.

C. extend the operated leg forward, hold the walker securely, and slowly sit.

D. extend the nonoperated leg forward, reach back for the armrest with one hand while holding the walker securely with the other, and slowly sit.

142. Which of the following BEST meets the criteria for an individual to be a candidate for a mobile arm support?

A. Diagnosis of quadriplegia.

B. Lateral trunk stability.

C. Fair plus elbow flexion.

D. At least 90 degrees of passive shoulder flexion and abduction.

143. A long-term goal for an individual following a hip arthroplasty is independence in lower extremity dressing with adaptive equipment. The MOST relevant short-term goal for the OT practitioner to work on would be for the individual to:

A. increase standing tolerance to 10 minutes.

B. increase hip flexion to 90 degrees.

C. demonstrate adherence to prescribed hip precautions.

D. apply energy-conservation techniques during dressing activities.

144. An OT provides a leather-working activity to an individual with complete C8 tetraplegia to increase current grip strength. Which component of this activity would be MOST effective in promoting this goal?

A. Holding the hammer.

B. Grasping the stamping tools.

C. Squeezing the sponge to wet the leather.

D. Lacing the leather with a needle.

145. The OT is instructing an individual with COPD in energy conservation techniques. Which of the following should the OT recommend in order to limit the amount of energy expended during bathing?

A. Using a reacher to retrieve and place items.

B. Showering on a tub bench while incorporating rest breaks.

C. Using a bath mitt while bathing.

D. Encouraging the use of proper body mechanics.

146. An individual is beginning to demonstrate return in the right upper extremity following a CVA, but has mildly impaired sensation in the right hand, which results in the inability to identify objects. Which would be the BEST method to help improve stereognosis?

A. The OT practitioner verbally describes how an object looks prior to touching it.

B. The individual looks at the object before touching it.

C. The individual works with "putty" to strengthen her hand.

D. The individual attempts to find coins in a pocket while occluding vision.

147. A patient who had a CVA has difficulty using his left upper extremity for reaching activities because of fluctuating muscle tone. According to the Neurodevelopmental Treatment approach, one of the MOST effective ways to teach a person to normalize high muscle tone in affected extremities prior to functional activities is by:

A. placing a weighted cuff on the extremity.

B. weight-bearing through the upper extremity in sitting or standing.

C. using the unaffected arm for all reaching activities.

D. forced use of the affected extremity.

148. The OT is working on feeding skills with an individual with amyotrophic lateral sclerosis who is in the late stages of the disease process. Which of the following is the MOST appropriate intervention for this individual?

A. Provide a rocker knife, plate guard, and non-skid mat.

B. Implement a pureed diet and allow adequate time for eating.

C. Emphasize upper extremity strengthening.

D. Minimize the use of adaptive equipment.

149. An individual who works as a nurse reports difficulty squeezing the bulb of the sphygmomanometer when taking blood pressure readings and difficulty opening pill bottles. Which of the following instruments would be MOST appropriate for assessing this individual?

A. Goniometer.

B. Aesthesiometer.

C. Volumeter.

D. Dynamometer.

150. An individual with ALS swims three times a week to maximize strength and endurance. Initially able to swim for only 10 minutes, the individual is now able to swim 20 minutes without becoming fatigued. What is the NEXT step to take to increase endurance?

A. Continue the program of swimming 20 minutes, three times a week.

B. Decrease swimming frequency to two times a week.

C. Increase swimming time to 25 minutes or to tolerance.

D. Provide adaptive equipment that will enable the individual to swim using less energy.

151. An OT has been working with an individual who sustained a deep laceration of the median and ulnar nerves, resulting in complete sensory loss. Upon reevaluation, what sensation would the OT expect to see return FIRST?

A. Vibration and pain.

B. Temperature and pain.

C. Light touch and proprioception.

D. Tactile localization and proprioception.

152. An OT is teaching an individual who recently sustained an above-elbow amputation how to tie shoelaces with one hand. Which of the following methods would the OT practitioner MOST likely implement to facilitate success with shoe tying?

A. Problem-solving.

B. Retraining.

C. Altering the task.

D. Compensation.

153. A multidisciplinary team is conducting a needs assessment to develop a falls prevention program for the frail hospital population. The MOST likely section of the needs assessment for the OT practitioner to perform would be:

A. analysis of statistical data on the number of falls occurring each year.

B. environmental hazard analysis and falls risk during performance of ADL.

C. evaluation of gait and mobility device use of those at high risk for falls.

D. assessment of medication impact on fall incidence.

154. An individual recovering from a peripheral nerve injury demonstrates weakness in thumb opposition. Which of the following instruments most effectively evaluates strength in the affected area?

A. Aesthesiometer.

B. Pinch gauge.

C. Dynamometer.

D. Volumeter.

155. Evaluation results for a person with arthritis will MOST accurately reflect true functional abilities if scheduled to take place at what time of day?

A. Early morning (8 a.m. to 10 a.m.).

B. Afternoon and evening.

C. Late morning (10 a.m. to 11 a.m.).

D. Early morning and again at another time of day.

156. An OT who needs to transfer a morbidly obese man is not confident that it can be managed by one person. The BEST action for the practitioner to take is to:

A. use proper body mechanics.

B. request that a PT perform the transfer.

C. ask another person for assistance.

D. refrain from transferring the patient.

157. When assessing an individual who is suspected of having carpal tunnel syndrome, the OT tests for Tinel sign by gently tapping the median nerve at what level?

A. Elbow.

B. Midforearm.

C. Palmar crease.

D. Volar wrist.

158. An individual's weight has changed during the course of hospitalization, and there is now a space of 2.5 inches between the individual's hips and the sides of the wheelchair. Which is the BEST recommendation regarding proper wheelchair fit?

A. Obtain a wider wheelchair because this one is now too narrow.

B. Encourage the individual to lose weight.

C. Pad the sides of the wheelchair to improve the fit.

D. Obtain a narrower wheelchair because this one is now too wide.

159. An individual in stage I of amyotrophic lateral sclerosis who is currently ambulatory, is independent in ADLs, and complains of overall weakness has been referred for OT in an outpatient setting. Which of the following interventions is MOST appropriate for this individual?

A. Moderate exercise in uninvolved muscles and active range-of-motion exercise.

B. Progressive resistive exercises of involved muscles and active range-of-motion exercises.

C. Use of orthosis and identification of adaptive equipment needs.

D. Passive range-of-motion exercises and use of orthosis.

160. An individual is being discharged from inpatient rehabilitation following a CVA. The individual requires minimal assistance in ADLs, is independent in transfers, demonstrates continuing improvement in RUE function, and plans on eventually returning to work. What would the recommendations for continued OT services MOST likely be for the individual?

A. Home health.

B. Outpatient.

C. A work-hardening program.

D. Discontinuation of services.

161. An OT practitioner is ordering a wheelchair for an individual with progressive MS who complains of chronic overall weakness. The MOST important consideration the practitioner can make is the adaptability of the wheelchair in anticipation of:

A. gradual gains in strength.

B. growth of the individual.

C. fluctuating weakness and/or further decline.

D. improved wheelchair mobility.

162. An individual with rheumatoid arthritis complains of joint pain and inflammation. The individual reports continuing with the home program despite the pain and demonstrates a series of briskly executed active range-of-motion movements. After evaluation, the OT should instruct the individual to:

A. continue performing the program as demonstrated.

B. perform gentle active range of motion with weights as tolerated.

C. eliminate all range-of-motion exercises for a week.

D. perform only gentle active range of motion.

163. The OT is assessing sensory awareness in an individual who had a right CVA. From observation, the OT notices the client using visual compensation to complete ADL tasks. Which of the following techniques is MOST appropriate?

A. Establish a rapport, then test the affected side, followed by the unaffected side.

B. Demonstrate the procedure on the unaffected extremity, then occlude the individual's vision and test the affected side.

C. Occlude the individual's vision, demonstrate the procedure on the affected extremity, then unocclude vision and test both sides.

D. Interview the individual and assess only the areas that the client reported to be impaired.

164. Which of the following devices is required for an individual with C7 to C8 quadriplegia when performing oral hygiene activities?

A. Mobile arm support with utensil holder.
B. Universal cuff.
C. Toothbrush with built-up handle.
D. Wrist support with utensil holder.

165. The goal for a patient who has had a traumatic brain injury is to be able to put on a shirt independently. The MOST effective way for the OT practitioner to structure dressing training for maximum learning retention and generalization of this skill is:

A. teaching and practicing each segment of the dressing procedure during consecutive treatment sessions.
B. practicing the whole task of putting on a shirt in a setting similar to the real environment.
C. providing dressing simulation activities (button boards, etc.).
D. allowing the client to view a videotape on how to put on a shirt and providing written directions for completing steps for dressing.

166. An individual with complete C7 tetraplegia demonstrates fair plus (3+) strength in the wrist extensors. Which of the following interventions would the OT practitioner introduce to MOST effectively increase strength in the wrist extensors?

A. A craft activity using increasingly heavy hand tools.
B. Mildly resistive activities that are halted as soon as the individual begins to fatigue.
C. Electric stimulation to the wrist extensors.
D. Mild resistance during AROM to the wrist.

167. An individual with amyotrophic lateral sclerosis has asked how to maintain strength in weak (fair plus) wrist extensors. Which is the MOST appropriate intervention for the OT to recommend?

A. Wearing a cock-up wrist support.
B. Playing hook and loop checkers to tolerance.
C. Performing active range of motion of the wrist daily without resistance.
D. Completing wrist extension exercises several times a day against maximal resistance.

168. When evaluating an individual with dysphagia for MOTOR problems associated with swallowing, the OT practitioner should look for:

A. coughing or choking.
B. disorientation or confusion.
C. pain while swallowing.
D. decreased smell and taste.

169. In order to screen an individual referred for a work-hardening program, the OT practitioner needs to locate background information about the individual's work history. The BEST method for obtaining detailed information about the individual's job requirements is to:

A. interview the individual.
B. examine the results of a job-demand analysis.
C. look up the individual's job in the *Dictionary of Occupational Titles*.
D. request information from the referring physician.

170. An individual in overall good health has expressed the overarching goal to remain "as functional and independent as possible" after recently being diagnosed with osteoarthritis of the upper and lower extremities. Using a client-centered approach to prevent further complications, what is the OT practitioner MOST likely to recommend to this client?

A. Lifting weights three times a week for 1 hour.
B. Listening to relaxation tapes three times a week before bedtime.
C. Vocational retraining.
D. Low-impact aerobics three times a week for 1 hour.

171. An OT is treating an individual who has been refusing to wear his splint/orthotic device, and now reports it is lost. Prior to fabricating another splint/orthotic device, the therapist should FIRST:

A. give the individual 48 hours to locate the splint/orthotic device, then fabricate a new one if the first cannot be found.
B. determine whether there are any motivational or cultural issues interfering with splint/orthotic device wear compliance.
C. ask the individual to find the splint/orthotic device and demand that he begin wearing it or you will call his physician.
D. discharge the individual because he has no interest in regaining function.

172. An OT is instructing an individual with arthritis how to maintain functional range of motion while performing household activities. Which of the following activities will MOST effectively accomplish this goal?

A. Use short strokes with the vacuum cleaner.
B. Keep elbow flexed when ironing.
C. Place lightweight objects on low shelves.
D. Use a dust mitt to keep fingers fully extended.

173. An individual who had total hip arthroplasty (posterior lateral approach) is working on independence in lower extremity dressing. Which of the following instructions is MOST important to convey to this individual regarding safety?

A. Sit during dressing activities.
B. Avoid internal rotation and adduction of the involved hip.
C. Use a long-handled shoehorn and dressing stick.
D. Wear shoes with elastic laces.

174. The MOST appropriate goal for an individual who sustained a C7 to C8 spinal cord injury is to be able to perform wheelchair-to-commode transfers at which of the following levels?

A. Independent with a transfer board.
B. Minimal to moderate assistance with a transfer board.
C. Dependent in all transfers.
D. Assisted, using a stand-pivot transfer.

175. An OT working in an outpatient setting has completed ROM measurements on an individual who had hand surgery. After bandaging the open wounds, what should the OT do with the stainless steel goniometer?

A. Place it in a plastic bag and label it with the individual's name.
B. Sterilize it before using it again.
C. Store it with the used equipment, and sterilize it at the end of the day.
D. Wash it with hot, soapy water before using it again.

176. An OT with expertise in hand rehabilitation is assessing an OTA's service competency in hand function assessment. At what point is service competency established?

A. When the OTA consistently obtains the same results as the OT.
B. After the OTA passes the NBCOT examination.
C. When the OTA has obtained a specified number of continuing education credits in in-hand rehabilitation.
D. After the OTA has practiced for a minimum number of years in in-hand rehabilitation, as specified by state licensure.

177. An OT practitioner is selecting foods for a treatment session with a client who has decreased oral motor control and difficulty chewing. In general, which of type of foods would be MOST appropriate to introduce?

A. Pureed foods such as pudding or applesauce.
B. Mechanical soft-textured foods such as ground tuna.
C. Soft foods, such as banana or macaroni and cheese.
D. Thin flavored liquids, such as juice.

178. An individual with a diagnosis of lung cancer is admitted to a rehab unit following a lobectomy. The OT should design and implement a treatment plan that focuses on:

A. palliative care.
B. prevention and changing habits.
C. restoration of function.
D. symptom management.

179. When assessing the sense of proprioception at an individual's joint, the OT would hold the lateral aspect of the elbow, wrist, or digit, and then move the body part into flexion or extension. The response of the client would then be to:

A. identify where the pain is.
B. demonstrate the stretch reflex.
C. demonstrate full active range of motion.
D. indicate whether the body part is being moved up or down.

180. An OT providing accessibility consultation services to a local library finds a reference room with a doorway that has a threshold height of 2 inches, making wheelchair access difficult. Which of the following recommendations would be MOST appropriate?

A. Hang signage to increase awareness of the threshold.
B. Provide a throw rug that covers the threshold.
C. Remove the threshold altogether.
D. Install a ramp over the threshold.

181. An OT is assessing hand function in an individual with arthritis. While making a peanut butter sandwich, the individual is unable to remove the lid from a peanut butter jar but is able to stand at the counter, spread peanut butter on the bread with a knife, and replace the lid. These observations would MOST likely reflect a deficit in which of the following?

A. Range of motion.
B. Coordination.
C. Endurance.
D. Strength.

182. The OT investigator is attempting to gain insight into family beliefs related to children who experience blindness. The OT would like to explore attitudes, values, communication preferences, and overall expectations of the parents in relation to the children who experience blindness. Which of the following would be the MOST likely naturalistic design that would capture the desired information?

    A. Participatory action research.
    B. Grounded theory.
    C. Phenomenology.
    D. Ethnography.

183. A male patient with an indwelling catheter asks the OT practitioner for advice concerning sexual activity. Which of the following responses is MOST appropriate?

    A. Refer the patient to his physician.
    B. Discuss precautions necessary for sex.
    C. Teach the individual how to remove and replace the device.
    D. Explain that it is dangerous and to avoid having sex.

184. An individual demonstrates flaccidity in the left upper extremity following a CVA. While performing PROM to the affected arm, the OT notes marked pitting edema of the left hand. What should the OT do next to decrease the edema?

    A. Elevate the affected extremity.
    B. Fabricate a resting splint/orthotic device for the affected extremity.
    C. Provide mild resistive exercises.
    D. Have the individual attempt to squeeze a ball.

185. An OT is working with an individual who complains of hypersensitive fingers following a crush injury to the hand. Which of the following methods would be MOST appropriate for achieving desensitization?

    A. Textured material, rubbing, tapping, and prolonged contact.
    B. Massage, functional electrical stimulation, and a progressive desensitization program.
    C. Pressure, percussion, vibration, icing, and edema massage.
    D. Visual compensation and functional use of the extremity.

186. An individual with an upper extremity fracture has asked how to maintain arm strength until the cast is removed. What activities would BEST accomplish this goal?

    A. Isometric muscle contractions.
    B. Isotonic muscle contractions.
    C. Progressive resistance movements
    D. Passive movement.

187. An OT is developing a prevention program for a local company with many workers who have developed tendonitis, nerve compression syndromes, and myofascial pain. A primary focus of the prevention program should be to:

    A. educate company workers about osteoarthritic conditions.
    B. develop a pamphlet on peripheral vascular disease.
    C. produce a flyer identifying risk factors for cumulative trauma disorders.
    D. offer screening for neuroma-related conditions.

188. An individual uses a mouth stick when working with a computer. Which of the following devices will prevent the mouth stick from accidentally striking other keys?

    A. A moisture guard.
    B. A key guard.
    C. An autorepeat defeat.
    D. One-finger-access software.

189. An individual with hand weakness has difficulty holding a fork. Using a biomechanical frame of reference, the OT practitioner should:

    A. elicit functional grasp using reflex-inhibiting postures.
    B. stimulate the hand flexors using quick stretch to promote a functional grasp.
    C. have the individual repeatedly squeeze with the hand against increasing amounts of resistance.
    D. build up utensil handles.

190. The OT is working with a client who takes cardiac medications because of abnormal cardiac rhythms and chest pain. Which of the following medications is typically utilized to treat these symptoms?

    A. Diuretics.
    B. Statins.
    C. Beta blockers.
    D. Antiplatelet agents.

191. An individual has been referred to OT following an upper extremity injury resulting in partial paralysis. Which of the following assessments would be MOST important for an OT practitioner guided by a biomechanical frame of reference?

    A. Adaptive equipment needs.

    B. Tone, reflex development, automatic reactions.

    C. Strength, range of motion, coordination.

    D. Habits, values, roles.

192. During an interview following a total hip replacement, it is CRITICAL that the OT practitioner determine the individual's:

    A. marital status.

    B. cognitive status.

    C. leisure interests.

    D. work responsibilities.

193. When evaluating light touch of the primary somatic system, the OT will MOST likely use:

    A. a tuning fork on the skin.

    B. alternating pressure of both ends of a safety pin.

    C. warm and cold water tubes placed on the skin.

    D. a cotton swab to apply light touch to a small area of the skin.

SERVICE MANAGEMENT AND PROFESSIONAL PRACTICE

194. An OT evaluating a child notices a bruise on the child's shoulder that looks like an adult's handprint and fingerprints. Which is the MOST critical step for the OT to take?

    A. Discuss this with the family member who picks up the child.

    B. Observe for additional injuries.

    C. Make a report to appropriate authorities.

    D. Avoid becoming involved in personal family matters.

195. An OT observes another OT exit a patient's room laughing loudly, clearly intoxicated, and with alcohol on her breath. After having discussed his concerns privately with the OT and witnessing this for the third time, the OT believes the individual is a danger to patients in the facility and should be prevented from practicing. In order to achieve that outcome, to whom should the OT report the colleague?

    A. NBCOT.

    B. State licensure board.

    C. AOTA Ethics Commission.

    D. Facility administrator.

196. When ordering a wheelchair for an individual who has Medicare, Part B, the OT must be sure to document that the wheelchair:

    A. increases functional independence.

    B. is medically necessary.

    C. maintains patient function.

    D. reduces deformity.

197. During the OT treatment session, a child begins a grand-mal seizure. What is the MOST important action for the OT to take during the seizure?

    A. Check breathing and administer mouth-to-mouth resuscitation if necessary.

    B. Attempt to restrain the child's movements to prevent injury and place something in the mouth.

    C. Ease the child to a lying position, remove or pad nearby objects, and loosen clothing.

    D. Observe the child, document behavior, and record the duration.

198. An OT/OTA team begins to provide occupational therapy services through a certified home health agency. What is the MOST critical component for establishing a successful collaborative relationship in this treatment setting?

    A. Determining reimbursement when completing joint visits.

    B. Establishing a system for the OT to countersign the OTA's documentation.

    C. Creating effective communication via weekly staff meetings, voice mail, and faxes.

    D. Developing a handout to educate clients regarding how the team will provide services.

199. A home health OT has received a referral for an individual with Medicare coverage. Which one of the following actions must occur before the therapist can initiate evaluation or treatment?

- A. Identify the deficits that impair functional abilities.
- B. Establish short- and long-term goals.
- C. Obtain a physician's plan of care identifying services to be provided.
- D. Collect the individual's history of the current illness.

200. The OT is working with an individual insured through Medicare Part B. Which of the following activities can the OT delegate to an aide?

- A. Assisting with routine dressing, after training and competency have been demonstrated.
- B. Introducing a new piece of adaptive equipment with a feeding activity.
- C. Completing a billable ADL training session with distant supervision.
- D. Selecting an appropriate tub bench from a variety of options in a catalog.

Answers for Simulation Examination 4

1. (C) Cultural context and family interaction patterns. Answer C is correct. Cultural expectations may determine behavior standards and the expression of family roles. "In some cultures, children are fed by a caregiver throughout the preschool years" (p. 47). Answers A, B, and D may be valid issues as well, but should be addressed after the OT has familiarized himself or herself with the cultural and familial context of the feeding process. See Reference: Case-Smith & O'Brien. (2010). Schuberth, L.M., Amirault, L.M., & Case-Smith, J.: Feeding intervention.

2. (C) Biomechanical. "The biomechanical frame of reference for positioning children for functioning is applied when a person cannot maintain posture through appropriate automatic muscle activity because of neuromuscular or musculoskeletal dysfunction" (p. 489). This child's physical status has changed with decreasing postural control. Adaptive support devices need to be considered, and a biomechanical frame of reference provides this approach. Answer A is incorrect because the neurodevelopmental treatment frame of reference is concerned with improving posture and movement, and supportive equipment is prescribed for that purpose. Answer B is incorrect as sensory integration concerns interactions between the sensory systems to provide information that contributes to complex behaviors. Answer D is incorrect because the visual perceptual frame of reference is concerned with receiving and understanding visual stimuli and is used to guide intervention for visual perceptual problems, not postural dysfunction. See Reference: Hinojosa & Kramer. (2009). Colangelo, C.A. & Shea, M.: A biomechanical frame of reference for positioning children for functioning.

3. (C) Side-lying. The side-lying position (answer C) is correct. This position reduces the influence of tonic labyrinthine reflexes, extensor tone, and gravity, all of which make protraction of the shoulders and forward reach difficult (p. 527). Answer A is incorrect because the standing position will not reduce extensor tone. Moreover, it encourages shoulder retraction and makes forward reaching of both arms to midline more difficult. Answer B is incorrect because in the prone position the upper extremities are involved in weight-bearing. However, this position may help facilitate forward reach by developing shoulder protraction. Answer D is incorrect because in the quadruped position, the upper extremities are involved in weight-bearing. However, if the position is attainable, shoulder protraction and forward reach may be facilitated. See Reference: Hinojosa & Kramer. (2009). Colangelo, C.A. & Shea, M.: A biomechanical frame of reference for positioning children for functioning.

4. (C) Modify the environment to protect the infant from excessive and/or inappropriate sensory stimulation prior to direct intervention. Answer C best represents developmentally supportive practices that view "protecting the newborn from excessive and inappropriate sensory input is often a more urgent priority than direct interventions or interactions with the infant" (p. 652). Answers A and B are important in determining appropriate treatment plans for the infant and family and eventual educational and disposition recommendations; they are team-managed activities that are not the priority focus for the OT. Answer D is incorrect, as early direct handling of the infant is not compatible with contemporary developmentally supportive practices. See Reference: Case-Smith & O'Brien. (2010). Hunter, J.G.: Neonatal intensive care unit.

5. (C) embed self in the classroom during language arts seatwork periods to assess performance and trial multiple strategies as student participates in the assigned work. "Whole activities with multiple steps and a meaningful goal (versus repetition of activity components) elicits the child's full engagement and participation...Functional magnetic resonance imaging (fMRI) studies indicate that more areas of the brain are activated when individuals engage in meaningful whole tasks versus parts of the tasks.... Children use multiple systems and organize their performance around that goal" (p. 5). Answers A, B and D are incorrect, as "(r)epeating a single component.... has minimal therapeutic value" (p. 5). See Reference: Case-Smith & O'Brien (2010).

6. (C) Include specific strategies in the plan to incorporate variable use and avoid isolation. Answer C, strategies to vary computer use and avoid unwarranted behaviors, is correct. "Individuals with ASD may develop habits, routines, or inflexible behaviors when presented with the consistent repetition of computer-based activities" (p. 557). Computer platforms and software programs offer features that enable variability by altering auditory (visual rather than sound alerts) and visual characteristics (contrast, font size/color) of word-processing tasks. The OT can recommend activities and environments to promote the student's participation in school activities and routines. Progress monitoring is important so that the team can assess the benefits of this strategy to increase the student's assignment production. Without a trial and evaluation of the increased computer use, answers A and B are inappropriate. "Because the OT should carefully plan the technology activities to meet the unique needs of the individual" (p. 559), answer D, which does not address any specific individualization, is incorrect. See Reference: Kuhanek & Watling. (2010). Hartmann, K.: Technology tools and strategies.

7. (A) By end of marking period, student will participate in classroom activities for 1 hour without disruptive outbursts for 4 of 5 days. Answer A is correct, as it relates the performance to be developed to a child's environment or life tasks, therefore, making it more meaningful. Functional goals target "actions and skills that students typically do or need to develop" (p. 725) for successful participation in the curriculum. Answers B, C, and D are measurable, but not functional goals because they do not address the context in which the skill is applied. Answer C describes a reduction in negative behavior and focuses the team on measuring that negative behavior, rather than the preferred, functional performance. See Reference: Case-Smith & O'Brien. (2010). Bazyk, S. & Case-Smith, J.: School-based occupational therapy.

8. (D) Facilitate child's performance in student roles expected in the school setting. Facilitating performance in student roles (answer D) is correct. "Going to school and being at school require children to adopt multiple roles that enable them to survive, 'fit in,' and enjoy a significant part of their lives that lasts for more than a decade.... [O]ccupational therapists must ensure that children can fully engage in their new roles" (p. 84). Answer A is incorrect as OTs work together with other team members to generate the student's IEP goals. Further, goals should reflect functional outcomes related to the child's participation in the curriculum, rather than increases in isolated performance skill areas. OTs and teacher do collaborate to develop progress monitoring strategies (answer B); however, this occurs after the OT has designed specific intervention approaches to enhance the student's role performance when desired outcomes are defined. Answer C is incorrect as many tests are not appropriate to measure change. For those tools that do measure change, it is too soon to readminister the tools that contributed to this student's recent evaluation. See Reference: Lane & Bundy. (2012). Chapparo, C. & Lowe, S.: School: Participating in more than just the classroom.

9. (D) A scoop dish. A scoop dish (answer D) is correct as its high rim provides a surface against which to push the food. The child would have less difficulty with controlling movement of food because the sides of the scoop dish would provide a shape that aids scooping of food onto the spoon. A swivel spoon (answer A) helps primarily when supination is limited. A nonslip mat (answer B) helps stabilize the plate itself, and a mobile arm support (answer C) positions the arm to help weak shoulder and elbow muscles to position the hand. See Reference: Case-Smith & O'Brien. (2010). Schuberth, L.M., Amirault, L.M., & Case-Smith, J.: Feeding intervention.

10. (B) Go out for lunch at a fast-food restaurant. Answer B, go out for lunch at fast-food restaurant, is correct because a key principle in intervention for effective transition includes using natural environments and cues, and increasing community-based instruction as the student gets older (p. 820). Classroom-based activities and simulated activities (answers A, C, and D) do not provide as many opportunities for the student to practice the community member role in activities that actually take place in the community. See Reference: Case-Smith & O'Brien. (2010). Spencer, K.: Transition services: From school to adult life.

11. (D) Playing tug-of-war with rope. Playing tug-of-war (answer D) is correct. This activity affords alternating pushing and pulling and tasks such as this "that are constantly changing in their proprioceptive demands facilitate increased arousal" (p. 161). The combination of two types of sensory input, proprioception (pulling) and tactile stimulation (touching the rope fibers), "develop[s] self-regulation, sensory awareness, and awareness of movement in space" (p. 161). Answers A and C are incorrect because they emphasize additional tactile input. Answer B is incorrect because it emphasizes slow vestibular input. See Reference: Hinojosa & Kramer. (2009). Schaaf, R.C., Schoen, S.A., Smith Roley, S., Lane, S.J., Koomar, J., & May-Benson, T.A.: A frame of reference for sensory integration.

12. (D) After the student's goals and objectives are determined for the IEP. After IEP goals and objectives (answer D) are correct, the team is able to discuss "which professional(s) should address particular goals..., when they will be addressed..., and where they will be addressed.... Each of these decisions is made on the basis of the student's need, not the personal preferences of professionals" (p. 666). Answers A, B, and C refer to points in the evaluation and IEP processes that occur prior to establishment of the student's goals and objectives, so they are each incorrect. See Reference: Schell, Gillen, & Scaffa. (2014). Swinth, Y.L.: Education.

13. (A) Weight shifting and weight-bearing activities. Answer A is correct as weight shifting and weight-bearing are used to activate motor control. "All postural movements, whether gross or subtle, occur with a shift of weight.... Weight bearing assists in the developing cocontraction of stabilizing muscles around a joint with the intention of enhancing proximal stability" (p. 225). Answers B, C, and D are incorrect because the weight shift and movement are not clear. See Reference: Hinojosa & Kramer. (2009). Barthel, K.A.: A frame of reference for neuro-developmental treatment.

14. (A) Child's use of sandpaper, glue, and paint while constructing a birdhouse. Answer A is correct. Assessing whether the child can use tools in accordance with their intended purpose while constructing a bird house provides opportunity to observe goal-directed "discrete purposeful actions [that] can be discerned.... Performance skills are links in a larger chain of actions, which...become the whole chain—the task performance" (p. 249). Answers B, C, and D are most representative of performance patterns, such as engaging in self-stimulation behaviors, daily routines, and role performance. "Performance

patterns are those habits, routines, rituals, and roles that support or hinder occupational performance" (p. 344). See Reference: Schell, Gillen, & Scaffa. (2014). Fisher, A.G. & Griswold, L.A.: Performance skills: Implementing performance analyses to evaluate quality of occupational performance.

15. (C) Inadequate sensory processing related to the kinesthetic system. Answer C, inadequate sensory processing related to kinesthetic system, is correct. "Good kinesthetic information enhances speed, reduces the need to visually monitor the hand during writing, and influences the amount of pressure applied to the writing implement" (p. 557). Answer A, vestibular system, is not the correct answer because, although it is difficult to completely separate one sensory system from another, the vestibular system primarily affects balance and general motor coordination. Answer B, limited motor planning, is not the correct answer because this refers to the ability to conceive of, plan, and carry out unfamiliar motor tasks. Answer D, the visual system, is incorrect because although the visual system does monitor motor control such as pencil grip and pressure, the use of a pencil requires unconscious awareness of body position and pressure at times when the task is not monitored visually. See Reference: Case-Smith & O'Brien. (2010). Schneck, C. & Amundson, S.L.: Prewriting & handwriting skills.

16. (C) A phone with extra-large buttons. Answer C is correct. Phone companies offer adapted phone systems for children and adults who have various limitations. Some phones have extra-large buttons for those with incoordination or visual impairments. A phone with extra-large buttons would most likely be the best solution for the child with mild visual impairments who desires to use the phone without assistance. Answers A, B, and D would assist individuals who are unable to hold the phone independently due to incoordination, weakness, or loss of function in the hand or upper extremity. See Reference: Case-Smith & O'Brien. (2010). Russel, E. & Nagaishi, P.S.: Service for children with visual or hearing impairments.

17. (B) The student's participation in curricular and extracurricular activities. Student participation (answer B) is correct, as "(p)ractice models and theories that begin with consideration of occupational performance, roles, habits, time use, interests, or routines lend themselves readily to a top-down approach.... Practice models that attempt to explain the underlying causes of functional deficits are consistent with a bottom-up approach" (p. 326). Answers A and C represent a bottom-up approach. Answer D refers to traditional motor development theories and is an incorrect response. See Reference: Lane & Bundy. (2012). Brown, T.: Assessment, measurement, and evaluation.

18. (D) Removing a nut from a bolt. Answer D is correct. Unscrewing a nut requires the in-hand manipulation skill called simple rotation. This "involves the turning or rolling of an object held at the finger pads approximately 90° or less" (p. 285). Answers A, B, and C are incorrect because they describe activities with no in-hand manipulation skill and the hand essentially keeps the object in a certain position as it is grasped, released, or carried. See Reference: Case-Smith & O'Brien. (2010). Exner, C.: Evaluation and intervention to develop hand skills.

19. (C) Typical. Answer C, typical development, is correct because children between the ages of 10 and 12 months may take first steps and walk with one hand held or behind a push toy (p. 65). Children 10 to 12 months old typically begin to cruise (walking sideways while holding on to furniture), thus making answers A, B, and D incorrect. See Reference: Case-Smith & O'Brien. (2010). Case-Smith, J.: Development of childhood occupations.

20. (B) Brushing her own hair in the morning and evening. Answer B is correct, as a power grasp is "used to control tools or other objects. Oblique object placement in the hand, flexion of the ulnar fingers, less flexion with the radial fingers, and thumb extension and adduction facilitate precision handling with this grasp (e.g., for brushing hair)" (p. 280). Answer A, pegboard activities, would most likely be introduced to facilitate the pincer grasp or tip pinch, whereas answer C, carrying a briefcase, such as a child's art case, would encourage the hook grasp position. Finally, the activity of ball throwing would most likely be introduced to encourage a spherical grasp position. See Reference: Case-Smith & O'Brien. (2010). Exner, C.: Evaluation and intervention to develop hand skills.

21. (B) It compares performance with a normative sample. Answer B is correct; "norm-referenced" tests have been given to a large number of persons in a specific population that is called "the normative sample, and norms, or average scores, are derived from this sample" (p. 221). When a child is tested with a norm-referenced test, scores earned are compared with those of the normative sample, providing information on how the child performed compared with the average performance of the normative sample. Answers A and D are incorrect, because although norm-referenced tests for children generally are de-

veloped with samples of individuals without developmental delays or adverse health conditions, "some tests include smaller subsamples of clinical populations as a means of determining whether the test discriminates between children whose development is proceeding normally and those who have known developmental delays" (p. 222). Answer C also is incorrect as "norm-referencing" does not ensure that the test is valid and reliable. Evidence for these characteristics is provided in the test manual. Further, validity and reliability are "never definitively determined, and ongoing evaluation of validity and reliability is necessary" (p. 227). See Reference: Case-Smith & O'Brien. (2010). Richardson, P.K.: Use of standardized tests in pediatric practice.

22. (C) OT encourages child to engage in a playful environment with ramps, scooters, ladders, balls, manipulatives, and vibrating toys. Answer C is correct. Ayres Sensory Integration™ is a distinct and highly individualized intervention method with child-directed activities, implemented by a therapist who has advanced training and understanding in the area of neuroscience. The ASI fidelity measure describes a safe environment with "affordances...that invite interactions with the environment including space to move and jump and crash and items that stimulate creativity and engagement,...[and] sensory opportunities that feature varied and appropriate vestibular, tactile and proprioceptive sensations" (p. 841). Answer A is incorrect because the child's program is not being "individualized," but is included in a group program. The weighted blanket (answer B) is an intervention that uses sensation as a modality for a specific therapeutic purpose (p. 847). A sensory diet (answer D) is a "sensory menu of individualized, structured activities and/or modalities used as part of one's daily routines to meet the individual's values, needs, and occupational performance goals" (p. 848). See Reference: Schell, Gillen, & Scaffa. (2014). Lane, S.J., Smith Roley, S., & Champagne, T.: Sensory integration and processing: Theory and applications to occupational performance.

23. (C) When the child demonstrates any reliable, controlled movement. As long as the child can produce any reliable, controlled movement, switches can be adapted to meet positioning and mobility needs (p. 597). Accurate reach and pointing (answer B) or isolated finger control (answer D) are not necessary to use simple pressure switches. An upright sitting position (answer A) would not be required if the child needed to be positioned in a reclining or side-lying position. See Reference: Case-Smith & O'Brien. (2010). Schoonover, J., Argabrite Grove., & Swinth, Y.: Influencing participation through assistive technology.

24. (A) Body-length prone scooter. Children with spastic diplegia have abnormal tone affecting all four extremities, but with primary movement limitations in the lower extremities. Therefore, answer A, a body-length prone scooter, is correct. This child may use his upper extremities to propel himself through space while his lower extremities are positioned on the scooter surface (p. 626). The aeroplane mobility device (answer B) is designed for children with good lower extremity function who need support in the upper body (p. 627). A tricycle (answer C) requires good lower extremity control, including reciprocal movement (p. 626). A power wheelchair (answer D) is designed for individuals with limited upper and lower extremity function (p. 633). See Reference: Case-Smith & O'Brien. (2010). Wright-Ott, C.: Mobility.

25. (D) Family should use cushions to support the child in seated play on the living room floor, with toys present, while parent watches nightly news or folds laundry. Answer D is correct because it reflects the use of "natural environments" (p. 53) as a context for intervention and embedding therapeutic intervention into the family's everyday activities and routines. Answer A is incorrect as it provides only a limited opportunity for the child to practice supported postural responses while held by the parent. When a person models/demonstrates behavior for others (answer B and C), there is no assurance that the intended learners (parent or extended family member) understand and can replicate the situation, or even if that opportunity fits within their routine. A better option would have been for the parent or extended family member to demonstrate how they would help the child practice trunk control and then problem-solve with the OT about how and when this can fit into their everyday routines. See Reference: Lane & Bundy. (2012). Morrison, C.D.: Early intervention.

26. (C) Tip the bottle back to allow the infant to include a breath in her suck-swallow pattern. Answer C is correct. "Suck-swallow-breathe coordination can be facilitated by providing secure positional support, reducing stimuli, using a slow-flow nipple, and pacing to allow breathing pauses" (p. 673). Tipping the bottle back stops the flow of milk and forces a swallow break so the infant can take a breath. Answer A, touching the infant's cheek before feeding, would most likely facilitate the rooting reflex. Answer B, gently touching the infant's lips before introducing the bottle, does not help the infant swallow once liquid is in the mouth. Answer D, rubbing the infant's lips and cheeks simulta-

neously, would most likely frustrate the infant because several different reflexes are being encouraged at the same time (e.g., the rooting reflex and phasic-bite reflex). See Reference: Case-Smith & O'Brien. (2010). Schuberth, L.M., Amirault, L.M., & Case-Smith, J.: Feeding intervention.

27. (D) Sitting. Answer D is correct because an upright sitting position provides the child with the opportunity to develop a variety of functional skills while promoting proximal activation of trunk, neck, and pelvis to facilitate a play response with the child's arms: "[a]nterior/posterior and lateral stability of neck and trunk;...[a]rms liberated; shoulder position independent of trunk—shoulder girdle provides stable base for arm movements" (p. 529) as the child looks for toys and reaches toward the opposite side of the body. Answers A and B are incorrect because head and neck stability have most likely developed primarily in the prone and side-lying position, before the child attains a seated position. Answer D is incorrect as arm reaching out into space is limited by the floor surface on which the child lies. See Reference: Hinojosa & Kramer. (2009). Colangelo, C.A. & Shea, M.: A biomechanical frame of reference for positioning children for functioning.

28. (C) Toothpaste with a flip-open cap. A tube of toothpaste with a flip-open cap (answer C) is correct. This child could manage a toothpaste cap that flips open much more easily than a cap that must be removed completely from the tube. Also, toothpaste tubes with flip-open caps are larger in diameter, which make them easier to manage. A wash mitt (answer A) and a toothbrush with a built-up handle (answer D) are good options for those with weak grasp. Spray deodorant (answer B) has a small button to push, which would be difficult to operate for someone with incoordination. (p. 490) See Reference: Case-Smith & O'Brien. (2010). Shepherd, J.: Activities of daily living.

29. (B) The OT provides an in-service program to the teachers in the school. Answer B is correct. "The purpose of consultation is to identify and solve problems with engagement in occupations, prevent future problems, or achieve identified goals (p. 1090). Answers A, C, and D do not reflect the mutual relationships and ongoing collaborative process that are characteristic of the consultation approach. See Reference: Schell, Gillen, & Scaffa. (2014). Holmes, W.M. & Leonard, C.: Consultation.

30. (D) The OTA demonstrated administering assessments completed in previous setting, OT reviewed OTA's scoring, and then determined

which ones the OTA could complete in this setting. Answer D is correct as it requires the OTA demonstrate proper administration and scoring of evaluations. The OT is responsible to confirm the OTA's competency for any procedures delegated to the OTA. "The OT will observe the OTA...and note whether the OTA can perform the identified skills and tasks" (p. 1084). The OTA's demonstration and review of scoring is one method for the OT to confirm the OTA's competence. Answer A is incorrect, as it omits the necessary step for the OT to confirm the OTA's competence prior to delegating test administration to the OTA. Answer B is incorrect, as it restricts the OTA from carrying out tasks for which he or she is likely competent, and also is an inefficient way to manage the workload in the school setting. Answer C is incorrect, as it may not be necessary for the OTA to observe evaluations that have been administered in the past, and, more important, it also omits the necessary step for the OT to confirm the OTA's competence prior to delegating test administration to the OTA. See Reference: Schell, Gillen, & Scaffa. (2014). Youngstrom, M.J.: Supervision.

31. (D) Offer to bring summaries on the research into various complementary and alternative approaches for children with ASD and review them during the next home visit. Answer D reflects a collaborative and well-informed approach that is correct. Occupational therapists should be "open-minded and support the family as they make decisions. Armed with information and a family-centered approach to therapeutic interactions, the OT has an important role in assisting the parents of children with an ASD" (p. 614). Answers A, B, and C refer the parent to other resources and do not respond to the parent's need for information and support. See Reference: Kuhanek & Watling. (2010). Kuhanek, H.M. & Gross, M.: Complementary and alternative interventions.

32. (B) When child's speed over long distances becomes less than that of a walking person. Answer B is correct. The OT should consider a power wheelchair to increase independence if the child "cannot propel a wheelchair long distances at the same speed and efficiency as demonstrated by the average walking person" (p. 633). Because the child will be experiencing progressive muscle weakness, energy conservation is of primary importance. Answers A and C address valid environmental considerations to be made after determining the general need for a powered chair. Waiting until the child becomes unable to propel the wheelchair (answer D), would make the transition more difficult and prevent the child from getting around independently in the

meantime. See Reference: Case-Smith & O'Brien. (2010). Wright-Ott, C.: Mobility.

33. (D) Observation of child during self-care activities. Answer D is correct. "Interview, inventories, and structured and naturalistic observations are evaluation methods typically used to measure ADL performance in occupational therapy" (p. 479). Observation of children in familiar settings and routines also helps the OT learn about how the child is expected to perform. Parent interviews can identify the priorities of the child's caregiver. Answers A, B, and C provide necessary information about performance components, development, and other parameters, but are not as effective in helping the evaluator learn about the child's self-care functioning. See Reference: Case-Smith & O'Brien. (2010). Shepherd, J.: Activities of daily living.

34. (A) Age-appropriate. Answer A is correct as the child is performing a dressing activity that is age-appropriate for a 5-year-old child. A typical child at this age can dress unsupervised and is able to tie and untie knots, but generally does not know how to tie a bow independently (p. 501). See Reference: Case-Smith & O'Brien. (2010). Shepherd, J.: Activities of daily living.

35. (B) Engage the child in reaching activities while seated on the floor. Answer B is correct. "All postural movements...occur with a shift of weight...[and] occur in degrees of amplitude and in various planes (e.g., anterior-posterior, laterally, and diagonally)" (p. 225). The OT can grade the weight shift demands through the location of objects as the child reaches. The reaching activity will cause the child to change his or her center of gravity during the reaching phase, which will require a further postural response to compensate for the change of position. Answers A, C, and D are not necessarily related to postural reaction development, but instead to strengthening, decreasing tactile defensiveness, and visual perception. See Reference: Hinojosa & Krame. (2009). Barthel, KA: A frame of reference for neurodevelopmental treatment.

36. (A) 18 months. Answer A is correct. Research "continues to substantiate the fact that children as young as 18 months can achieve independent skills in powered mobility" (p. 623). See Reference: Case-Smith & O'Brien. (2010). Wright-Ott, C.: Mobility.

37. (D) Helps child maintain his state of arousal. Answer D is correct. These repetitive acts are believed to "help the individual maintain a state of homeostasis, calmness, or arousal" (p. 103). A child with autism may have the ability to focus at close range (answer A). Answers B and C, pain and paresthesia, are incorrect. See Reference: Kuhanek & Watling. (2010). Audet, L.R.: Core features of autism spectrum disorders: Impairment in communication and socialization, and restrictive acts.

38. (C) Help student identify simple rhymes to remember steps to complete homework independently. Answer C is correct. The OT embedded a recommended memory strategy into the child's daily routines to help him organize his work and "to enhance the retrievability through the use of language cues such as songs, rhythms, and acronyms" (p. 380). Answer A is incorrect as the mass practice is not optimal for generalization into functional tasks. Answer B is incorrect as visual attention is a prerequisite to visual memory (p. 380). Answer D is incorrect because serial or varied repetition enhances visual memory. See Reference: Hinojosa & Kramer. (2009). Schneck, C.: A frame of reference for visual perception.

39. (D) Plan. The Plan section of a SOAP note (answer D) is correct. This section includes statements related to continuing intervention; the frequency and duration of the treatment; suggestions for additional activities or treatment techniques; the need for further evaluations; and, when needed, recommendations for new goals (p.148). The subjective portion of a SOAP note (answer A) refers to an individual's or caregiver's comments about the intervention or their condition (p. 143). The objective portion of the SOAP note (answer B) focuses on measurable and/or observable data obtained by the OT through specific evaluations, observations, or use of therapeutic activities (p. 144). The assessment part of a SOAP note (answer C) refers to the effectiveness of the treatment and any changes needed, the status of the goals, and any justification for continuing OT intervention (p. 147) See Reference: Sames. (2010). Sames, S.: SOAP and other methods of documenting ongoing intervention.

40. (A) Perform interviews with the parents regarding their daily routines, social life, and child-rearing practices. Answer is correct, as this method enables the therapist to "understand the meaning of this experience from the client's perspective" (p. 390). Understanding the client's life story (family's priorities, concerns, lifestyle, medical history, etc.) helps the therapist focus on what is important to the family. Answer B is most representative of the interactive facet of clinical reasoning (p. 391). Answer C is used by the OT to define specific "client diagnosis-related problems" when engaging in the procedural component of clinical reasoning (p. 390). Answer D is a task most related to the pragmatic or practical side of clinical reasoning (p. 391). See Refer-

ence: Schell, Gillen, & Scaffa. (2014). Boyt Schell, B.A.: Professional reasoning in practice.

41. (B) Teacher's report of how the student has adjusted in this new classroom. Answer B is correct, as narrative reasoning is a "strategy for understanding the meaning of the experience from the child's, family's, and other care provider's perspectives" (p. 28). The teacher's report about the student's adjustment generates information about the importance this person attributes to different aspects of the student's performance and these data inform the intervention plan. Answer A provides information about the student's awareness of activities during the school day, yet it does not explain the meaning of these events. An age-level score (answer C) and history of previous therapy (answer D) represent factual information, likely from a test administration and the child's record, respectively. See Reference: Dunn. (2011). Dunn, W.: Clinical reasoning for best practice services for children and families.

42. (A) The child uses a wide base of support and takes small, inconsistent steps. Answer A is correct. At 12 to 15 months of age, most infants are early in their walking development. During this time their "efforts toward unsupported forward movement are often seen in short, erratic steps, a wide-based gait and arms held in high guard" (p. 68). Answers B, C, and D are typical for an older toddler. See Reference: Case-Smith & O'Brien. (2010). Case-Smith, J.: Development of childhood occupations.

43. (B) Use a family-centered approach to learn about parent concerns and priorities and provide interventions that help them increase parenting skills and promote their child's learning. The correct response is answer B. Contemporary models of practice recognize the importance of the child's family as a consumer of pediatric occupational therapy. "It is critical for parents to be informed about their children, [and research has identified 'information'] as the most commonly expressed need for parents of young children with disabilities.... The goal of parent education is to promote the development and competence of the child by enhancing parents' knowledge about child rearing, parenting, or relationship skills.... The skill development component of parent education may involve concepts such as learning about strategies and techniques for playing and communicating with their young child at home...or learning specific behavioral techniques" (p. 495). See Reference: Lane & Bundy. (2012). Rodger, S. & Ziviani, S.: Autism spectrum disorders.

44. (B) Adaptive equipment/ADL needs in the classroom. Answer B is correct; the most essential information the teacher needs from the OT is how to provide adaptations for the child in the classroom, along with information on the client's ADL status and how juvenile rheumatoid arthritis (JRA) symptoms may affect the child's ability to participate in school activities. "The OT in the school setting focuses his or her evaluation on what is needed for the student to engage and participate in meaningful and purposeful school occupations" (p. 658). Information about the child's developmental skills and attributes (answers A and C) are of lesser importance, and may be unimportant for the teacher to support this student's learning. Answer D, home program information, is most useful to the child's family. See Reference: Schell, Gillen, & Scaffa. (2014). Swinth, Y.L.: Education.

45. (D) Observe the child entering the clinic and taking off his coat and shoes. Answer D is correct and represents a naturalistic observation, in which the therapist "gathers information in the typical or natural setting in which the activity occurs" (p. 482). Reliable information can be gained by observing the child as he or she typically completes the activity; this is especially true of children with developmental delay, who may have difficulty generalizing learning from one situation to another. Answer B may not provide a sample of the child's true skill level. Answers A and C describe situations in which assistance is provided, therefore not allowing the child to demonstrate his skill in independent dressing. See Reference: Case-Smith & O'Brien. (2010). Shepherd, J.: Activities of daily living.

46. (D) Hiccups and skin color change to flushed. Answer D is correct as hiccups and flushed skin are autonomic nervous system signs reflecting physiological instability/stress. Answers A and B are changes in motor behavior that reflect stress. Answer C, twitches and jerky movement while asleep, are not autonomic responses. Rather, they reflect disorganization in the infant's sleep state (p. 662). See Reference: Case-Smith & O'Brien. (2010). Hunter, J.G.: Neonatal intensive care unit.

47. (B) Voice recognition word processing software. Answer B is correct. In voice recognition systems, the "computer recognizes and translates voice sounds into text" (p. 607). A larger monitor (answer A) may be useful to help her see details on the screen; however, this student has both visual and motor impairments so typing on the keyboard is challenging for her. After several letters are typed, word prediction software (answer C) anticipates the word desired and increases the speed of input by decreasing the number of keystrokes required. This may help her complete this task, yet not provide an optimal solution. Masking inappropriate keys (answer D) reduces the number of letter options, and can limit

the variety of words this student is able to type. See Reference: Case-Smith & O'Brien. (2010). Schoonover, J., Argabrite Grove, R.E., & Swinth, Y.: Influencing participation through assistive technology.

48. (B) Verbal and general gestural cues only. Answer B, the combination of verbal and gestural cues, is correct (p. 265). Physical cues (answers C and D) are the most intrusive. Verbal cues only (answer A) is the least intrusive method. See Reference: Case-Smith & O'Brien. (2010). O'Brien, J. & Williams, H.: Application of motor control/motor learning in practice.

49. (A) 2 inches wider than the widest point across the child's hips with the brace on. Measuring the child with the brace on and adding 2 inches (answer A) allows the child to easily get in and out of the chair while preventing pressure to the child's sides (p. 500). Answer B measures only the hips and would not allow enough room for the child to sit or move easily in the chair while wearing the brace. Answers C and D are both incorrect measurements for seat length, because both would have the seat too deep for the individual's leg length. The correct length of the seat should be 2 inches shorter than the distance from the back of the bent knee to the back of the buttocks. See Reference: Radomski & Trombly. (2008). Dudgeon, B.J. & Dietz, J.C.: Wheelchair selection.

50. (D) Playing on a trampoline. Answer D, playing on a trampoline, is correct. Postural control refers to the ability to maintain balance during functional movements and depends on both posture and balance (p. 252). Activities that require a child to respond by changing body position to maintain balance encourage the use of postural reactions. Trampoline activity requires a child continuously change body position to adapt to changes in gravity while jumping. Answer A, sliding down a sliding board, stimulates vestibular processing and does not require the postural adjustments as needed for the trampoline. Imitating gestures when playing simple "Simon Says" (answer B) facilitates perceptual processing and does not provide dynamic movement that challenges postural control. Swimming (answer C) is a good activity to improve a child's endurance. The water supports the child and reduces the need for postural adjustments and balance. See Reference: Case-Smith & O'Brien. (2010). O'Brien, J. & Williams, H.: Application of motor control/motor learning in practice.

51. (C) Ulnar palmar grasp. Answer C is correct as the progression of grasp development is "ulnar grasp to palmar grasp to radial grasp" (p. 282). The infant first grasps on the ulnar side of the hand against the palm, then with all four fingers against the palm (palmar grasp), and finally the grasp moves to the radial side of the hand (radial grasp) at around 6 months of age. "Crude raking of a tiny object is present by about 7 months of age.... Between 9 and 12 months of age, refinement occurs in the ability to use thumb and finger pad control for tiny and small objects" (p. 283). See Reference: Case-Smith & O'Brien. (2010). Exner, C.: Evaluation and intervention to develop hand skills.

52. (B) Objective signs and duration of the seizure. Staff members are often asked to monitor the child for seizure activity (p. 162) to assess the efficacy of anticonvulsive medication or during periods of gradual withdrawal. Type and duration of seizures should be documented carefully. Observations about the child's position (answer A), responsiveness (answer C), and facial expression (answer D) are important observations, but not as significant as documenting the objective signs and duration of the seizure. See Reference: Case-Smith & O'Brien. (2010). Rogers, S.L.: Common conditions that influence children's participation.

53. (C) Whether the child's feet reach the floor. Answer C is correct. A relaxed position during toilet use is essential for success in elimination training. The seat should be low enough so the child's feet can be used to help with postural stability. In addition, a seat design featuring a wide base, back support, and placement at a height that enables the child to place the feet firmly on the ground or on foot supports will give the child a sense of comfort and security (p. 500). Answers A, B, and D describe other useful considerations that should be addressed after the issue of support has been resolved. See Reference: Case-Smith & O'Brien. (2010). Shepherd, J.: Activities of daily living.

54. (D) Research suggests that position in space development is complete at 7 to 9 years of age. Answer D is correct. "The ability to discriminate between mirror- or reverse-image numbers and letters, such as b and d, and p and q, does not mature in some children until around 7 years of age" (p. 380). Answer A is incorrect, as 6-year-old children are typically developing their understanding of position in space concept. In view of this, a focus on developing visual memory is not warranted. There is insufficient information available to justify a referral for vision screening beyond what is typically provided as children enter school. See Reference: Case-Smith & O'Brien. (2010). Schneck, C.: Visual perception.

55. (B) Observing the child eating during a meal. Answer B, observation of the child eating during a regular meal, is correct, as a "top-down approach considers the contexts in which the child performs valued occupations" (p. 482). In this evaluation, the OT considers the influence of the environment, identifies the steps of the task, and observes the child's capacities and needs. Answers A, C, and D center on client limitations and do not include other areas of the top-down evaluation approach. See Reference: Case-Smith & O'Brien. (2010). Shepherd, J.: Activities of daily living.

56. (D) Child will correctly identify, by feel only, five out of five common objects. Answer D is correct, as stereognosis is the "ability to identify objects through proprioception, cognition, and the sense of touch" (p. 213). Answer A demonstrates localization of tactile stimuli, answer B demonstrates graphesthesia, the "ability to identify numbers or letters traced on the skin" (p. 715), and answer C is an example of the tactile discrimination of textures. See Reference: Radomski & Trombly. (2008). Bentzel, K.: Assessing abilities and capacities: Sensations; Bentzel, K.: Optimizing sensory abilities and capacities.

57. (C) Use headphones during seat work. Answer C, using headphones, is correct, as this helps to filter out/reduce some of the auditory input from other activities and students in the classroom. "Reducing competing sensory input in both the auditory and visual modalities can be helpful for some students with poor visual attention" (p. 392). Increasing competing input (answers A, B, and D) may reduce the ability to attend to visual stimuli. See Reference: Case-Smith & O'Brien. (2010). Schneck, C.: Visual perception.

58. (B) Stress bilateral arm/hand use, incorporating both arms to hold and stabilize objects. Answer B is correct. "A person with a unilateral amputation can be expected to use the prosthesis primarily for sustained holding or for stabilization and to use it more slowly compared to the unaffected extremity" (p. 1282). Two-handed activities for play and school incorporate the prosthesis into the child's body image and help to develop bilateral skills. Activities that avoid the use of the prosthesis, as in answers A, C, and D, do not help the child to integrate the prosthesis into normal patterns of use. See Reference: Radomski & Trombly. (2008). Stubblefield, K. & Armstrong, A.: Amputations and prosthetics.

59. (A) Create a reliable route to the bathroom, encouraging the child to familiarize herself with the smells and sounds of the bathroom. Answer A is correct. A primary goal for the OT working with children with visual impairments is to "support participation in the contexts in which they function on a daily basis" (p. 758). By creating a reliable route to the bathroom, encouraging the child to focus on tactile and olfactory cues (answer A), the OT can establish compensatory techniques for the visual deficit. Having the child practice with obstacle courses (answer B) would be appropriate for the development of movement in space and body image/awareness, but does not directly support participation in self-care activities. Answer C, practicing fine motor skills, would be more closely related to the development of hand manipulation skills. Introducing the child to other children with similar impairments would be an appropriate socialization activity for the child, but is not directly related to participation in daily activities. See Reference: Case-Smith & O'Brien. (2010). Russel, E. & Nagaishi, P.S.: Service for children with visual or hearing impairments.

60. (C) Interview about challenges and successes within the family's current daily activities and routines. Answer C is correct, because "(w)hen a child has a mental illness, the typical roles and family occupations of all of the family members are challenged" (p. 518). Occupational therapists have skills to work with persons across the life span, they understand the impact of occupation on health and quality of life, and they are expert in designing daily activities and routines to support occupational performance. Answers A and B are incorrect, as there is no evidence in this question to drive specific evaluation in either of these areas. Answer D is incorrect as parents choose resources to help them parent their children with or without disabilities, and without further indication that contact with the child's school will help parents achieve their goal(s), this action is inappropriate. See Reference: Lane & Bundy. (2012). Cronin, A.: Emotional and behavioral disorders.

61. (A) Excessive talking and inability to remain seated and wait for his turn. The behaviors described in answer A correctly exemplify the excessive fidgeting and restlessness, inattention, and impulsiveness that is characteristic of ADHD (p. 529). Although some of the symptoms of overactivity and impulsiveness can be classified as part of a mood disorder of the manic type, such as the behaviors described in answer B, these behaviors are typically linked with symptoms of grandiosity and inflated self-esteem. The use of profanity and hitting another student (answer C) exhibit interference with the basic rights of other children or societal rules and is most related to conduct disorders, whereas answer D is typical of a child with an anxiety disorder in which the student shows signs of uneasiness, apprehension, or dread associated with the anticipation of danger. See Reference: Lane & Bundy. (2012). Chapparo, C. & Lane, S.: School: Learning disabilities & intellectual disabilities.

62. (B) Side-lying on a mat. Answer B, side-lying on a mat, is correct. In this position, the child has an

"excellent opportunity to try out skilled arm and hand movements on the upside arm. This horizontal position demands less trunk control than sitting.... [There are no] weight-bearing demands on the shoulder of the arm that is not reaching...nor does the infant have to work against gravity to use his or her hand in front of his or her face, as in the supine position" (p. 497). Answer A, long-sitting, answer C, supine positioning, and answer D, prone positioning, all require the child to work against gravity, and would most likely be too difficult for the child to maintain while engaging in play activities secondary to low tone. See Reference: Hinojosa & Kramer. (2009). Colangelo, C.A. & Shea, M.: A Biomechanical frame of reference for positioning children for functioning.

63. (B) Teach the child to sit in a chair with a back support, lift the affected leg onto a stool, and use socks with a wide opening. For a child with hemiplegia or limited balance, sitting with back support may be the best starting position for putting on and removing socks. The child lifts the affected leg onto a box or step to bring the foot closer to the unaffected hand...a wide sock opening can prevent frustration during the most difficult part of putting on socks (p. 505t). Answer A, encourage the child to wear tight-fitting socks, would make it more difficult for the child to put on and take off his socks. Answer C, encouraging the child to request assistance from his mother, and answer D, placing the unaffected foot on a small stool, would not assist in dressing skills independence for this child. See Reference: Case-Smith & O'Brien. (2010). Shepherd, J.: Activities of daily living.

64. (D) Obtain the same results as another OT does who has demonstrated service competency. "Service competency is the process of teaching, training, and evaluating in which the occupational therapist determines that the occupational therapy assistant performs tasks in the same way that the occupational therapist would and achieves the same outcomes [answer D]" (p. 1084). This does not mean "that the OTA will perform the task in exactly the same manner as the OT would, only that the outcomes will be similar" (p. 1085). Demonstrating service competency often requires more than one trial in order to refine techniques to obtain the same results. Answers A, B, and C are methods for developing service competency, but do not provide the opportunity for the OT practitioners to compare and contrast their techniques and measurements in order to obtain the same results. See Reference: Schell, Gillen, & Scaffa. (2014). Youngstrom, M.J.: Supervision.

65. (C) Give him a tour of the OT department and a schedule of activities. "The CBT (cognitive-behavioral therapy) approach to panic disorder involves having the individual approach situations that cause anxiety and reduce the catastrophizing associated with the event" (p. 176). Taking a tour of the OT department (answer C) is an example of a behavioral experiment, a typical CBT strategy, designed to let clients test thoughts, behaviors, and beliefs and to enable them to predict outcomes, allowing them to evaluate the results and use this feedback to revise or create new perspectives. Reducing distractions and keeping lights low (answer A) may be useful environmental adaptations for individuals with mania or hyperactivity. Providing a stimulating environment and real-life activities (answer B) is recommended for individuals experiencing delusions. OT practitioners should leave doors open and avoid being alone (answer D) with individuals who are hostile or violent. See Reference: Brown & Stoffel. (2011). Davis, J.: Anxiety disorders.

66. (D) Home-delivered meal services. Answer A, continued OT services to teach the patient to use the kitchen safely, is incorrect because individuals diagnosed with dementia tend to decline over time, and interventions aimed at improvement are unrealistic. Volunteer companions (answer B) provide companionship to elders at home but not skilled supervision of activities. Transporting to a community site for meals (answer C) on a daily basis could be inconvenient, overly challenging, and taxing for an elder with moderately severe dementia. Answer D, in-home meal delivery services such as Meals on Wheels, would be the best and safest option for providing consistent access to food in the home. See Reference: Cara & MacRae. (2013). MacRae, A. & Smith, J.: Mental health of the older adult.

67. (D) Readiness for change. "Readiness assessment (answer D) is an important first step in any rehabilitation assessment process, and...must come before conducting functional and resource assessments" (p. 701). The transtheoretical model describes the stages of readiness for change and recognizes that a level of readiness to change is a prerequisite to change occurring. Evaluation of the environment (answer A), social skills (answer B), and work skills (answer C) would all come later. See Reference: Brown & Stoffel. (2011). Pitts, D.B.: Work as occupation.

68. (B) Collaborate to find a location and the phone number. "Motivational interviewing is designed for people who are not ready to change or are ambivalent about changing. The fundamental approaches of motivational interviewing are collaboration, evocation, and autonomy" (p. 340). This individual is clearly ambivalent about changing his level of activity. Working with him to identify a volunteer

opportunity in which he would be interested (answer B) is a good example of this collaborative approach, in contrast to telling him that he is ready (answer A), which is a confrontational approach and can lead to defensiveness. Making decisions for the client by identifying where he should volunteer (answer D) does not represent a collaborative approach. Because the OT cannot determine how long the individual's benefits will continue, assuring him that he will not lose them (answer C) would be inappropriate. See Reference: Brown & Stoffel. (2011). Brown, C.: Motivation.

69. (D) Intellectualization. By employing the defense mechanism of intellectualization (answer D), the patient protects herself from the pain associated with her trauma by "repressing...the emotional components of [the] experience, but not the informational components" (p. 146). In identification (answer A), the individual adopts "the values and feelings of a person who causes anxiety in an attempt to increase self-worth" (p. 146). In projection (answer B), one attributes "personally unacceptable impulses or desires to the external world" (p. 146). Denial (answer C) is a "defense mechanism by which a person disavows or refuses to acknowledge the external source of anxiety" (p. 146). See Reference: Cara & MacRae. (2013). Andonian, L, Cara, E and MacRae, A: Psychological theories and their treatment methods in mental health practice.

70. (C) The time, date, next meal, and the weather. "Reality orientation is a cognitive intervention that is used primarily for adults with dementia." Reality orientation boards typically list "information such as the time, the, next meal, etc." (p. 256). Illustrated step-by-step instructions (answer A), pictures of family members (answer B), and a list of medications (answer D) are all also interventions that can be used to modify the task or environment for people with dementia. See Reference: Brown & Stoffel. (2011). Brown, C.: Cognitive skills.

71. (A) Involve the individual in a three-member task group. "Grading refers to systematically increasing the demands of an occupation to stimulate improved function or reducing the demands to respond to client difficulties in performance." In this case, the activity should be upgraded by slightly increasing the size of the group, challenging the client to use and develop greater personal interaction skills (p. 323). Progressing from rubber stamping to stenciling (answer B) adds a level of complexity to the task, which can help to develop problem-solving skills. Answers A, B, and C can all be effective adaptations of the task for other goals, but are not geared toward developing interpersonal skills. See Reference:

Schell, Gillen, & Scaffa. (2014). Gillen, G.: Occupational therapy interventions for individuals.

72. (A) In the individual's home. Occupational therapists use "task specific training or rote repetition of a specific task or routine within the natural context to develop habits or functional behavior routines. Repetitive practice reduces demands on cognitive resources needed for task performance and increases automaticity of performance" (p. 781). Because individuals who require task-specific training are unable to generalize learning to other situations (including other garments and other environments), it is important to train the individual in the environment where the task will be performed. This type of training should take place at least five times a week. Training in the OT department (answer B), twice a week (answer C), or only when the client is feeling cooperative (answer D) would all be ineffective. See Reference: Schell, Gillen, & Scaffa. (2014). Toglia, J.P. et al: Cognition, perception, and occupational performance.

73. (A) A harm reduction program. The harm reduction model (answer A) "acknowledges the difficulty of abruptly stopping usage and lifelong abstinence. If...terminating usage is unlikely, small steps are introduced to reduce usage and harm to physical, mental and social functioning. Harm reduction views any changes that lead to reduced usage as positive and healthy" (pp. 847–848). Alcoholics Anonymous (answer B) and Narcotics Anonymous (answer C) are both 12-Step programs that maintain that "abstinence is a prerequisite for successful treatment and once addicted, an individual can never successfully return to even limited usage" (p. 847), and would therefore not be the best match for this individual. Outcomes of both types of programs have been shown to be comparable. Health promotion programs (answer D) focus on developing a healthy lifestyle and typically address nutrition, exercise, participation in meaningful activity, and social participation. While a health promotion program may be useful in the long run, a program directly addressing his addiction will be more important immediately following discharge. See Reference: Cara & MacRae. (2013). Hoppes, S., Bryce, H.R., & Peloquin, S.M.: Substance abuse and occupational therapy.

74. (C) Set down the utensil until the mouth is cleared. Having the individual learn to set down the utensil until the mouth is cleared (answer C) is a method of imposing a restriction on the behavior that can then develop into an established routine to pace himself during feeding. "Many survivors of brain injury are impaired when performing controlled cognitive processes but are not when performing automatic processes. As controlled processing is heavily

involved in the early stages of learning a skill and is less involved as a skill comes to be performed more routinely with practice, those rehabilitation programs that reduce the requirement for controlled processing during learning may be the most effective" (p. 200). Cutting the food into smaller pieces (answer A) and placing food in separate containers (answer D) are examples of environmental adaptations, not habit development. An impulsive person who eats too fast also will have difficulty counting slowly enough to have his mouth cleared by the time the count of 10 is reached (answer B). See Reference: Gillen. (2009. Managing attention deficits to optimize function.

75. (A) Depression and substance abuse. Co-occurring disorders (CODs) "is a term used to describe persons who have one or more substance abuse-related disorders and one or more mental disorders (answer A)... for example, an individual with bipolar disorder who also has an alcohol use disorder or a young adult with schizoaffective disorder who also has cocaine dependence" (p. 211). Answers B, C, and D do not include any substance abuse conditions and therefore do not meet the criteria. See Reference: Brown & Stoffel. (2011). Moyers, P.: Co-occurring disorders.

76. (B) Line-dancing involving movement in three planes. Ross's Five-Stage Group Approach begins with introduction and orientation. When using a sensorimotor approach, the opening is followed by "maximum exertion in movement...incorporating all three planes.... Stage III emphasizes perceptual motor skills.... Stage IV is the time for cognitive stimulation.... Stage V provides resolution and termination" (pp. 261–262). Line-dancing (answer B) is an example of Stage II—maximum exertion and movement. The fruit salad activity (answer A) would fit best under Stage III, the sensory motor activity. Planning for the next session (answer C) is a closing activity that represents Stage V. Introductions (answer D) is an example of Stage I—an opening activity. See Reference: Cole. (2012). Sensorimotor approaches.

77. (B) Decreased arousal and drowsiness. Medication side effects are typically observed and reported by OT practitioners. Anti-anxiety medications reduce anxiety, but also "may have side effects of drowsiness, loss of coordination, or mental slowing, at least initially" (p. 247). Akathisia, extrapyramidal syndrome, and tardive dyskinesia (answers A, C, and D, respectively) are adverse effects commonly linked to antipsychotic medications. See Reference: Falvo. (2009). Falvo, R.: Psychiatric disabilities.

78. (D) Share space while working on a task without disrupting others for 15 minutes. Parallel groups are most appropriate for people who can tolerate being with more than one person at a time, but do not have the ability to interact successfully with other group members. "A parallel group is made up of an aggregate of patients who are involved in individual tasks with minimal necessity for interaction" (p. 396). Therefore, appropriate expectations for parallel groups focus on remaining in the group and working alongside others (answer D). Experimenting with a new group role (answer A) is a goal consistent with egocentric-cooperative groups. Sharing materials with another group member (answer B) is a project group goal. Expressing feelings within a group (answer C) is consistent with a cooperative group. See Reference: Cole. (2012). Mosey, A.C.: The concept and use of developmental groups.

79. (C) Working with the caregivers to help them utilize routines that will facilitate caregiving. This individual clearly has late stage Alzheimer's disease, which is characterized by "profound disturbances in orientation and memory, unable to recognize caregivers/family, severe intellectual deterioration, severely limited verbal communication, [and] unaware of the environment" (p. 1099). In the later stages of Alzheimer's disease, intervention should focus on "adaptation of the environment, safety, and caregiver training" (p. 1099). Caregiver training is designed to "enable caregivers to use routines (answer C), some modifications, and adaptive equipment" (p. 1100). Home modification to ensure safety (answer A) should be done during the early and mid-stages of the disease process, before the individual became so dependent and incontinent. The use of memory strategies (answer B) is another intervention that would be used earlier in the disease process, and is no longer appropriate. Promoting independence (answer D) is also no longer an appropriate goal. See Reference: Schell, Gillen, & Scaffa. (2014). Appendix 1: Common conditions, resources, and evidence.

80. (D) Set personal boundaries appropriate to the therapist-patient relationship. It is important to acknowledge the individual's need for sexual expression while supporting the sense of self and identifying acceptable relationships and behaviors. "The client's sense of masculinity or femininity may be threatened by the disability.... The therapist should not be surprised by flirtations or sexual advances from clients. In response, the OT practitioner should deal with these behaviors and set therapeutic boundaries [answer D] in a positive and professional manner" (p. 298). Outright rejection (answer A) may cause an individual to believe he or she is sexually undesirable or unlovable. Flirting back (answer B) may imply that a sexual relationship between the therapist and the patient is possible or acceptable. Although the individual may need to know how SCI

affects sexual functioning (answer C), the behavior that requires a response is not about a lack of knowledge, but rather about how to appropriately express sexual interest and the need for reinforcement of a sexual identity. See Reference: Pedretti. (2013). Tipton-Burton, M. & Burton, G.U.: Sexuality and physical dysfunction.

81. (B) Performing a simple task. Individuals with severe depression benefit from activities that are "concrete and tangible,... short-term, simple, and success enhancing. The surrounding environment should be carefully arranged so as not to be too distracting. The therapist also should make decisions, provide clearer expectations and parameters for activities, and provide...validation for depressed behavior" (pp. 238–240). Sorting laundry (answer B) is the best example of a concrete, tangible, short-term, and simple activity. Engagement in leisure exploration (answer A), meditation (answer C), and stress management activities (answer D) would eventually be relevant intervention activities for a person with depression. However, in the early stages of depression, attention span, concentration, and energy level may to be too impaired to benefit from these types of activities. See Reference: Cara & MacRae. (2013). Cara, E.: Mood disorders.

82. (D) A workroom with upbeat music and a variety of jobs from which to choose. This individual's behavior is typical of someone who is sensation seeking. "Sensation seekers are easily bored or frustrated in environments that do not meet their elevated needs for sensation.... The sensation seeker desires variety, intensity, and unpredictability in his or her environment, and he or she will benefit from opportunities to explore and take control of the environment to create sensation. Sensations that may be distracting to others might be helpful for the sensation seeker to maintain arousal and focus. If the sensation seeker is required to be in a low stimulus environment, he or she may need breaks to get up and move around, talk, or spend time engaged in higher level of activity" (p. 292). Therefore, a workroom with upbeat music and a variety of jobs from which to choose (answer D) would be the preferred environment for this individual. Individuals with sensory sensitivity would prefer less stimuli, and may be "highly distractible and more likely to experience discomfort in high intensity environments" (p. 292). They may therefore may benefit from a quiet workroom with minimal noise and lowered blinds to reduce lighting (answer A). Individuals who are sensory avoiding prefer "reducing the amount and intensity of sensation and increasing predictability and familiarity...[and] providing a quiet space" (p. 292) and may do better with a job that offers structure and repetition (answer B). Individuals with low registration "tend to miss input that others take in. They may be slow to respond or require repetition and cues.... They are not bothered by sensory stimuli and can typically manage distracting environments quite well" (p. 292). These individuals may benefit from rotation between several job stations, with an alarm to alert them to when it is time to rotate (answer C). See Reference: Brown & Stoffel. (2011). Brown, C. & Nicholson, R.: Sensory Skills.

83. (D) Show a video about nutrition and keep a meal diary for a week. The psychoeducational model utilizes a teacher-student format as opposed to a learning-by-doing approach. It is used "to teach specific information or techniques to clients and their families" (p. 696). Showing an educational video (answer D) is an example of this approach. Answers A, B, and C can all be used to promote healthier eating; however, they all involve learning through occupation-based activities rather than psychoeducational activities. See Reference: Cara & MacRae. (2013). Cara, E.: Groups.

84. (C) Allow the person to perform tasks in a quiet, separate area. An important aspect of intervention for the occupational therapist is the ability to change aspects of the environment to maximize the performance of a client. All of the answer choices are environmental strategies which can have an impact on the ability to become engaged in an activity and can affect performance, but allowing the person to perform tasks in a quiet area (answer C) is most likely allow concentration when a person is easily distracted. Gillen identifies several environmental strategies that can be used to promote attention, including reducing distractions and avoiding crowds (p. 204), both of which can be accomplished by moving the individual to a quiet area. The use of music (answer A) can be very effective to shift a person's attention and decrease agitation, but may provide too much sensory stimulation. Decreasing the lighting (answer B) may help decrease the level of stimulation in the room, but also could encourage relaxation, rather than focused concentration. Adjusting the temperature and ventilation in the clinic (answer D) could enhance the working environment if it were previously too hot and stuffy, but from the question, the human environment seems to be the most distracting feature in the clinic. See Reference: Gillen. (2009). Managing attention deficits to optimize function.

85. (D) Design a program focusing on developing parenting skills, beginning with a module on age-appropriate expectations. The results of the needs assessment suggest that these parents are having difficulty engaging with their children successfully in meaningful activities. Understanding child development (answer D) would enable them to have

more realistic expectations of their children. Future modules could address additional parenting skills, including identifying appropriate play activities, setting limits, encouraging successful communication, and developing coping skills. "The common goals of these programs are to enhance quality of life for parents and their children by enhancing parenting self-efficacy, enhancing child development, strengthening parent-child relationships, decreasing family isolation, and stabilizing parents' mental health" (p. 418). Given that the OT is functioning in the role of a consultant, individualized intervention (answer A) would not be realistic. However, as a consultant, it is likely that the OT would provide educational materials/resources to both clients (answer B) and staff (answer C). See Reference: Brown & Stoffel. (2011). Urish, C. & Jacobs, B.: Families living with mental illness.

86. (D) Acknowledge his feeling of isolation. Communication is enhanced when the individual believes he is being heard. Acknowledgment of a person's feelings (answer D) is an example of empathic listening, which involves "the process of recounting, accepting, and affirming any perception or experience a client offers" (p. 162). Encouraging a personal friendship (answer A) and telling someone you know how he feels (answer B) can be counterproductive to developing a therapeutic relationship. Encouraging more socialization (answer C) is not helpful, because the individual probably would do so if he were able. See Reference: Taylor. (2008). Therapeutic communication.

87. (B) Occupational profile. The occupational therapy profile is designed to be used in a client-centered fashion to gather information about the client, from his/her perspective. The occupational profile includes information on the individual's "occupational history and experiences, such as patterns of daily living, interest, values, and needs. The patient's problems and concerns about performing occupations and daily life activities are stated and priorities are determined" (p. 30). A physical assessment (answer A) would be performed to determine the individual's baseline regarding strength, endurance, and balance. An activity configuration (answer C) could be used to contribute information to the occupational profile. A psychoeducational session (answer D) would be used to provide information about the disease and/or strategies for managing it. See Reference: Hemphill-Pearson. (2008). Page, M.S.: Interviewing in occupational therapy.

88. (A) Get Joe's attention, then return the tool to Sam and ask him whether you may use the tool when he has finished with it. Modeling is a behavioral intervention that recognizes that "learning occurs through observation and imitation of the behaviors of others.... Persons can learn by observing the consequences that people receive for their behaviors" (p. 151). Demonstrating an appropriate way of asking to use the tool (answer A) is an example of modeling. Praising Joe (answer B) is an example of positive reinforcement. Asking Joe to identify another method he might have used (answer C) is an example of a problem-solving approach. Recognizing Joe's frustration (answer D) is an example of an empathizing approach. See Reference: Cara & MacRae. (2013). Andonian, L., Cara, E., & MacRae, A.: Psychological theories and their treatment methods in mental health practice.

89. (B) Identify leisure skill strengths and weaknesses. All of the answers include strategies that are important for individuals in recovery from substance abuse. However, "recognition of the problem [answer B] and willingness to do something about it are important first steps" (p. 109). Following recognition of the problem, additional sessions could address healthy leisure activities (answer A), encouraging problem-solving (answer C), and providing strategies for healthy social interaction (answer D). See Reference: Bonder. (2010). Substance-related disorders.

90. (B) Slow movements Individuals experiencing extrapyramidal disorders "are characterized by hypokinesia or hyperkinesia. Parkinson's disease is characterized by hypokinesia (bradykinesia), cogwheel and lead pipe rigidity, a decrease in or loss of postural mechanisms, and a resting, pill-rolling tremor" (answer, B, p. 479). Answer A, hyperextension or hyperflexion of the wrist and fingers, is associated with dystonia. Answer C, athetoid movements, are "wormlike, arrhythmic movements" that tend to impact distal extremities, and answer D, chorea, (jerky, irregular moments) is more typically associated with individuals with Huntington's disease. See Reference: Pedretti. (2013). Preston, L.A.: Evaluation of motor control.

91. (D) Suggest trying a small birdhouse first. This client "will benefit from direction providing parameters of acceptable behavior, and an honest appraisal of behavior presented in a gentle yet firm, matter-of-fact way" (p. 242), and so suggesting the birdhouse is the most appropriate course of action. Manic individuals are often unaware of their problem areas, and therefore tend to make grandiose or inappropriate choices. This lack of awareness may make it difficult for the individual to recognize or accept that his attention span is too limited (answer B). Whereas a depressed individual may need support for his choices (answer A), a manic individual may need to be redirected. Although sharp tools (answer C) may be contraindicated for individuals with suicidal ideation, in this situation it is not the type of tools, but the qualities of building a clubhouse related to cost,

space, time, complexity, and possibly skill that are inappropriate. See Reference: Cara & MacRae. (2013). Cara, E.: Mood disorders.

92. (B) Yoga, initially in her own room. Yoga, progressive relaxation, and aerobic exercise have all been shown to be effective in managing stress. However, "clients with histories of sexual abuse and issues with body image may initially feel unsafe practicing relaxation in a group atmosphere. Therapeutic intervention should consider the client's need to practice the techniques alone [answer B] and with the therapist prior to joining a group" (p. 323). It may be too challenging initially for the client to relax in an aerobics class (answer D) or progressive relaxation group (answer C). Although sewing and handcrafts (answer A) can be very relaxing, these would not address the client's goal of using physical activity. See Reference: Brown & Stoffel. (2011). Haertl, K. & Christiansen, C.: Coping skills.

93. (C) Interview a reliable informant instead of the individual. Individuals who are unable to think clearly, or who are experiencing memory loss, are often disturbed or frightened by this change, and may confabulate, or "fill in the missing gaps with erroneous information" (p. 558). When an individual is unable or unwilling to provide accurate information, it may be necessary to use a reliable informant (answer C). This is often someone who lives with the individual and is able and willing to provide the necessary information. Using closed-ended questions (answer A) with this individual would not necessarily yield more accurate information, but can be useful when specific information is being sought, or to more effectively structure or control an interview situation. This individual is unlikely to do any better with a written questionnaire than in an oral interview. However, written questionnaires (answer D) may be used effectively with individuals with the requisite cognitive skills. There is no reason to think the individual would be any more reliable the next day (answer B). See Reference: Cara & MacRae. (2013). Phipps, S.: The cognitive, behavioral, and psychosocial sequela of brain injury.

94. (B) Have the group create a list of their favorite holiday songs and set a date for a performance. "Egocentric-cooperative groups are characterized by group members selecting, implementing, and executing relatively long-term tasks through joint interaction. The task remains essential, but satisfaction of some social-emotional needs of fellow group members is encouraged" (p. 396). Cooperatively developing a song list establishes a long-term goal of performing, and practicing over the next few weeks (answer B) incorporates the elements of an egocentric-cooperative group. The one-time sing-along (answer A) and the reminiscence group (answer D) are both one-time occurrences and lack the long-term cooperative element. The emphasis of the cookie swap (answer C). is on making the cookies ahead of time, not as a group, and then having a one-time get-together to swap the cookies. See Reference: Cole. (2012). Appendix B.

95. (C) Rotate frequently from one station to another. This individual's behavior suggests that he has low registration. "People with low registration tend to miss input that others take in. They may be slow to respond or require repetition and cues. Yet, these individuals are highly flexible because they are not bothered by sensory stimuli and can typically manage distracting environments quite well.... For individuals with low registration, it is important to enhance relevant sensory stimuli so that the individual notices what he or she needs to notice. This might include increasing the intensity or amount of sensory input or reducing the speed at which information is presented so the person has time to take in the information. Cues such as signs or a beeping alarm can be helpful for a person with low registration. It is also helpful to reduce the predictability or familiarity of the input,...and the individual may benefit from a change in setting" (p. 292). Therefore, job rotation (answer C) would be an appropriate intervention, as it would enhance the level of stimulation. Noise-canceling headphones (answer A) or a quieter work area (answer B) could be appropriate interventions for individuals with sensory sensitivity, but would make things even more challenging for this individual. Although a job coach could be an appropriate intervention, it does not address his sensory issues. See Reference: Brown & Stoffel. (2011). Brown, C. & Nicholson, R.: Sensory skills.

96. (D) Position the individual with their back to the window. This behavior is indicative of an attention deficit. "Strategies aimed at modification of task and environment have proved to be beneficial for this population" (p. 663). Removing visual distractions (answer D) is an example of an environmental modification that would have an immediate effect. Self-instruction statements (answer A), such as "I must concentrate on what I am doing," are also an effective strategy, but teaching the individual to use them would take some time, as would instructing the individual in the use of orienting procedures (answer B). Time pressure management strategies (answer C) are used with individuals who have deficits in speed of processing information. See Reference: Pedretti. (2013). Gillen, G.: Evaluation and treatment of limited occupational performance secondary to cognitive dysfunction.

97. (D) Provide them with information about the National Alliance on Mental Illness (NAMI). The literature identifies professional competencies that should be possessed by professionals working with families of individuals with mental illness. Providing family members with information about NAMI (answer D) incorporates several of these competencies, including "developing a collaborative relationship with the family, providing information on psychiatric disorders, enhancing coping and stress management skills of family members, [and] assisting family members in navigating the mental health system" (pp. 423–424). These competencies do not say anything about putting the needs of the mentally ill individual first (answer C). Excluding family members (answer B) is not best practice, and, in fact, evidence suggests that "family psychoeducational approaches result in reduced rates of relapse" (p. 424). The situation described does not involve confidentiality, and therefore HIPAA (answer A) is not a concern. See Reference: Brown & Stoffel. (2011). Urish, C. & Jacobs, B.: Families living with mental illness.

98. (B) Journal and diary writing. The psychodynamic frame of reference "provides a framework by which therapists can use expressive techniques in collaboration with the client to develop insights and understanding, and facilitate adaptive behaviors to meet goals.... Studies demonstrate the effectiveness of therapeutic writing techniques, suggesting that personal expression in response to stress and trauma improve overall health and well-being" (pp. 320–321). Although answers A, C, and D would benefit the self-confidence and stress management needs of women struggling with the anxiety and other issues associated with emotional and physical abuse, they are not expressive activities. See Reference: Brown & Stoffel. (2011). Haertl, K. & Christiansen, C.: Coping skills.

99. (A) Time management, ability to accept feedback, following instructions. Evidence suggests that "the best clinical predictors of future work performance are ratings of a person's work adjustment skills" (p. 818), such as appearance, punctuality, ability to accept feedback, following instructions, and productivity (answer A). In addition, individuals who have a work history, are motivated to work, and work in a job they like are more likely to be successful (pp. 817–818). Various occupational performance skills and client factors (answers B and C) should also be assessed to guide intervention, but these are broad areas and they are all not necessarily predictive of success. Likewise, the work environment (answer D) may impact performance, and should be assessed to see whether modifications or additional supports may be warranted. See Reference: Cara & MacRae. (2013). Auerbach, E.S.: Vocational programming.

100. (D) Help him to identify the feelings she is having but is unable to express verbally. Listening for the feelings behind the words will best help to identify and address the needs of the person who has lost the ability to use words effectively (answer D). The resident's searching for her mother may reflect a sense of loneliness. "Rather than reacting to the behavior as a negative attribute of the individual with dementia or a willful attempt to be difficult, health professionals can play an important role in enabling caregivers to view these 'problem behaviors' as the consequence of individuals' inability to express their feelings verbally and directly. If caregivers can identify triggers...for behaviors, they will be more likely to identify effective strategies either for preventing or dealing with such problems when they appear" (p. 239). Explaining the factual truth (answer A) can have the effect of unnecessarily confronting the person with his or her deficits, and she may respond to the news as if hearing it for the first time. Telling the person to stop the behavior (answer B) will not address the need that is being expressed verbally. Answer C, telling a therapeutic fib, might work for a brief period of time, but may backfire if the person continues to question the story given, or if it causes sadness or anger. See Reference: Bonder & Bello-Haas. (2009). Doble, S.: Dementia.

101. (A) Write articles about occupational therapy for local newspapers. In this situation, the target market is potential consumers of occupational therapy, i.e., patients, clients. The best answer for targeting this population would be through local newspapers that reach the general public (answer A). The open house (answer B) and the in-service workshop for nurses (answer C) are good examples of how referral sources may be targeted. Presenting at an occupational therapy conference (answer D) is a good example of a professional development activity, but the impact would be limited to other occupational therapists (p. 135). See Reference: Jacobs & McCormack. (2011). Richmond, T.: Marketing occupational therapy.

102. (A) Rote repetition of packaging task substeps with gradually fading cues. The use of "task specific training or rote repetition of specific task or routines within natural contexts to develop habits or functional behavioral routines" is recommended for individuals with chronic or severe cognitive deficits. "Repetitive practice reduces demands on cognitive resources needed for task performance and increases automaticity or performance" (p. 781). Answers B, C, and D all involved the use of remedial activities designed to address impaired cognitive skills, and require a level of self-awareness. For an individual who is 10 years post-injury, the task-specific training approach is more appropriate. See Reference: Schell, Gillen, & Scaffa. (2014). Toglia, J.P. et al: Cognition, perception, and occupational performance.

103. (B) Show acceptance and understanding regarding the individual's situation. Active listening is a technique that helps to establish the therapeutic relationship. "It involves paraphrasing the speaker's words rather than reacting to them in order to clarify you have caught the intended meaning" (p. 96). The OT paraphrases by repeating in her or his own words what the client has said. Redirection (answer A) is used to promote healthier thoughts and behaviors. Forcing the individual to make a choice (answer C) may be accomplished by providing a question that includes two possible choices. An individual is encouraged to provide additional information (answer D) when the OT asks open-ended questions. See Reference: Davis. (2011). Davis, C.M.: Effective communication.

104. (C) Choose one goal to address in the next session. Individuals in the action stage are ready to implement a plan, such as choosing a specific goal to address in the next session (answer C). Other examples of action activities could include "list the steps to take this week to begin implementation, locate a specific local group to visit: make phone call, get directions, discuss with members what support you need to carry out plans" (p. 274). Identifying concerns about retiring (answer B) would be an activity appropriate for the precontemplation stage. Listing the pros and cons of retiring (answer A) would be an activity appropriate for the preparation stage. Identifying social supports, such as possible groups to join, is also an activity appropriate for the "building social supports" part of the preparation stage. See Reference: Cole & Donohue. (2011). Cole, M.B.: Older adult interventions to facilitate social participation.

105. (A) Appeal to the group to give the individual feedback about how his behavior affects them. Assigning a specific and concrete task allows the individual to focus on the task at hand, while sending the message that the individual is a valued member of the group. "The therapist not only needs to recognize these roles, he or she also should help members take on a variety of roles and to change those roles that are detrimental to the group. It is often through taking on different roles that much of the therapeutic learning takes place in the group setting" (p. 44). Giving the individual control over other group members (answer B) feeds into the individual's issues. Pairing the individual with another group member (answer D) will give that other group member little opportunity for involvement. Limiting participation to observation (answer C) will only increase the individual's frustration and lead to feelings of isolation. See Reference: Cole. (2012). Understanding group dynamics.

106. (C) Use a diary to record each dosage after it is taken. The use of memory notebooks and diaries "has been documented to improve orientation, as well as support everyday living tasks such as morning ADLs and simple IADLs" (p. 667). Using a diary to record each dosage (answer C) would be most effective because it would provide the patient with a written record of when the medication was taken. Answer A, establishing a routine, and answer B, keeping the medications in a special location, could be helpful in reminding the patient to take the medication, but would not be as effective as a diary for remembering whether the medications were taken. Answer D, arranging to have a caregiver remind the patient, would not facilitate independence with medication management. See Reference: Pedretti. (2013). Gillen, G.: Evaluation and treatment of limited occupational performance secondary to cognitive dysfunction.

107. (D) Limit the time available to answer each question, interrupting when possible. Individuals with OCD frequently experience time-consuming compulsions having to do with thoughts and/or actions. Limiting the time available to answer questions and "interrupting when possible" (p. 322) (answer D), using highly structured interviews, and closed-ended questions will help these individuals structure their time and be able to more effectively complete the evaluation process. Open-ended questions (answer B) are useful for eliciting more information, but are more difficult to time limit than are closed-ended questions. Instructing the individual to take as much time as necessary (answer C) may be beneficial for a highly anxious individual. Individuals with attention deficits would most likely benefit from limiting environmental distractions (answer A). See Reference: Cara & MacRae. (2013). Cara, E.: Personality disorders.

108. (B) Identify peer leaders who can model and train their peers to identify adults they can trust. A program that identifies peer leaders (answer B) is most appropriate for this age group, because they "often do not know where to turn, and increasing their comfort in asking for help, or identifying those adults they feel they can trust could potentially save lives" (p. 436). A volunteer program (answer A) would be appropriate for older adults who may be looking to replace the worker role by participating in altruistic activities. Although a filmmaking course (answer C) and after-school tutoring program (answer D) are both age-appropriate, may target interests, and may be meaningful to many adolescents, they do not target suicide prevention. See Reference: Cara & MacRae. (2013). Lambert, W. & Carley, E.: Mental health of adolescents.

109. (D) Point out where on the schedule to find times for buses leaving the center in the morning. "Social skills training (SST) is founded on social learning theory and the principles of operant conditioning.... The key elements of SST include warm-up activities, behaviorally based instructions, demonstration, corrective feedback, and homework assignments" (p. 63). The goal for this session (determining a departure time) has already been introduced, so the next step is demonstration, in this case showing the group how to use the bus schedule (answer D). This is the correct answer, because it follows the behaviorally based instructions. This would then be followed by corrective feedback such as helping participants recognize when they are not respecting the ideas of others (answer A). Finally, a homework assignment such as working with a partner to schedule a return trip (answer B) reinforces the learning. An appropriate warm-up activity for this group, asking who had been to an aquarium and what they remember about the experience (answer C), would precede the demonstration. See Reference: Brown & Stoffel. (2011). Tsang, H.W.H., Siu, A.M.H., & Lloyd, C.: Evidence-based practice in mental health.

110. (A) Involve the group in generating possible solutions for the problem. Responsive social skills training programs follow a specific sequence. First, participants are asked to report on their progress since the previous session and describe problems they have recently experienced or are anticipating. The problem-solving sequence begins with defining the problem, which in this case is concerned about the upcoming interview and how much to reveal. The next step, then, is to "generate possible solutions for the problem" (answer A), which is followed by "identify the pros and cons of each possible solution [answer D], select the best solution or combination of solutions [answer B] and...discuss how to carry out the solution in a social interaction" (p. 309). Once the problem-solving sequence is completed, the group would move on to the social skills training sequence, during which role-playing (answer C) would occur. See Reference: Brown & Stoffel. (2011). Stoffel, V.C. & Tomlinson, J.: Communication and Social Skills.

111. (A) A game of Social Bingo. In a project group, the focus is on "common, short-term tasks that require some interaction, cooperation, and competition.... Mutual interaction outside the task is not expected" (p. 396). These qualities can be found in a game of Social Bingo (answer A). An exercise group (answer B) does not require interaction, and is more appropriate for a parallel group activity, which is also true of attending a church service (answer D). Planning a birthday party (answer C) requires a higher level of interaction than the individuals in this group are ready for. See Reference: Cole. (2012). Appendix B.

112. (D) Creating a budget. The errorless learning approach may be used with individuals with memory impairments. "It is typical for people with memory impairments to remember their own mistakes as results of their own action more successfully than they remember the corrections to their mistakes.... With errorless learning a person learns something by saying or doing it, rather than being told or shown by someone. In addition, the person is not given the opportunity to make a mistake" (pp. 228–229). The tasks of identifying coins (answer A), making change (answer B), and writing a check (answer C) all have correct methods for accomplishing the tasks, and so lend themselves to an errorless learning approach. Creating a budget (answer D), however, can be accomplished many different ways and would not be an appropriate activity for errorless learning. See Reference: Gillen. (2009). Managing memory deficits to optimize function.

113. (B) Incorporate advocacy skill training into the group format. It is important for OTs to "prepare our clients to advocate for their own full participation.... Preparing individuals with disabilities to be self-advocates and to be self-empowered is central to productive living" (pp. 53–54). The sense of empowerment that comes with self-advocacy internalizes the locus of control. These same advantages would not be recognized through a stress management group (answer D). Assessing the site for ADA compliance (answer A) is a possible option, and because the OT leading the group can perform the assessment, it would not be necessary to hire an OT. Suing the facility for noncompliance (answer C) would be a last resort after many other attempts to resolve the situation have been made. See Reference: Brown & Stoffel. (2011). Crist, P.: Psychosocial concerns with disability.

114. (A) Assertive communication skills. Clarifying expectations, honestly defining needs, and providing tactful and constructive feedback are communication skills that promote understanding. Successful communication with the client's children will most likely help them deal with their fears and concerns, increase their understanding of their mother's condition, and elicit greater cooperation, which should help to decrease some stress for the mother. Using assertive communication skills "increases the likelihood that everyone's needs will be met" (p. 117). The mother will be able to get her point across and have her needs met while maintaining a sense of power, thereby reducing the stress she is experiencing with her children. Although time management tech-

niques, deep breathing, progressive muscle relation, and laughter (answers B, C, and D) are all useful and valid stress reduction techniques, they do not address the issue at hand, which is communication between the mother and her children. See Reference: Davis. (2011). Davis, C.M.: Assertiveness skills and conflict resolution.

115. (A) Occupational self-analysis. Lifestyle redesign programs emphasize "the power of occupations by educating participants about the health relevant consequences of their occupation.... Each module begins by guiding small groups of community living older adults through an occupational self-analysis [answer A]" (p. 275). There are eight content areas, including transportation (answer B), safety (answer C), and social relationships (answer D). See Reference: Cole & Donohue. (2011). Cole, M.B.: Older adult interventions to facilitate social practice the patient.

116. (C) Have the individual predict his performance before an activity, then have him self-evaluate the performance. Having the individual predict his performance before an activity (self-estimation) and comparing his predicted performance with a self-evaluation of the actual performance can provide meaningful self-initiated feedback and would be the best way to increase awareness. Simply discussing the individual's perceptions (answer A) would not provide concrete immediate feedback about performance. Reviewing a checklist of necessary skills, answer B, would probably not be effective in increasing awareness because the patient feels he already possesses these skills. Answer D, ignoring the patient's perceptions, would not address the patient's therapeutic need to increase awareness and could lead to increased resistance. See Reference: Pedretti. (2013). Gillen, G.: Evaluation and treatment of limited occupational performance secondary to cognitive dysfunction.

117. (D) Using consumer input, create a list of potential problems. Designing a skills training intervention begins with problem identification (answer D), followed by solution identification (answer A), and finally module development (answer B). In this situation, it would be particularly important to involve the consumers (answer D) in problem and solution identification, because the likelihood of finding literature (answer C) about skills training for dairy farming is slim (p. 669). See Reference: Brown & Stoffel. (2011). Brown, C.: Activities of daily living and instrumental activities of daily living.

118. (C) Institute a participant-led discussion of how the activity made them feel and identification of reasons they deserve to feel so good. At the cooperative group level, "members are encouraged to identify and gratify each other's social-emotional needs in conjunction with task accomplishment.... The therapist acts primarily in the role of an advisor and may not be present at all group meetings" (p. 396). Discussion about how the activity felt and reinforcement of each individual's value (answer C) is the only answer that contains the element of providing social support characteristic of a cooperative group. Getting feedback from the group and planning a future group (answer D) involve the therapist at more than an advisory level. While planning a fashion show (answer A) and taking "glamour shots" (answer B) could both be good follow-up activities, they do not incorporate the social support element integral to a cooperative group, and involve the therapist as a leader more than an advisor. See Reference: Cole. (2012). Appendix B.

119. (A) Encourage other group members to express their frustration with the individual using "I statements." The individual dominated the group with disruptive behaviors. "If the group is able to express its frustration...then she might be helped by learning to control the behaviors that elicit negative feelings from others" (p. 49). Ignoring her inappropriate behavior during group (answer C) disregards the needs of other group members. This individual may not have the skills or insight to treat others with respect at this time, and explaining that the behavior is unacceptable (answer D) may not be enough. Denying her access to groups (answer B) may be a last resort only after all other options have been exhausted. See Reference: Cole. (2012). Understanding group dynamics.

120. (C) Provide meaningful activities that will divert attention from the symptoms. Answer C, providing activities, is the best approach because "people who display positive symptoms, especially hallucinations, benefit from activities that divert attention from their symptoms. In the process, the individuals can learn self-help coping strategies to minimize the intrusiveness of positive symptoms. However, it is only when people can clearly identify activities with personal meaning or purpose that they are able to see them as a viable method of symptom management. While random applications of activities sometimes provide a temporary distraction from hallucinations, it is the use of activities that bolsters the sense of personal achievement and mastery that are consistently deemed as most successful in coping with hallucinations and other positive symptoms" (p. 213). Leaving people experiencing hallucinations alone (answer A) would have no benefit in reducing attention to the hallucination. Completely isolating the person from others (answer B) is not recommended because interpersonal contact can be beneficial for reinforcing reality and reducing hallucinations. Moving the person to a more stimulating environment (answer D) can have the effect of increasing hallucinations if they find the environmental stimuli too stressful. See Reference: Cara & MacRae. (2013). MacRae, A. & Andonian, L.: Schizophrenia.

121. (A) Social interaction skills. Appropriate social interaction skills (answer A) require individuals to conform to implicit and explicit social norms, to assume a manner of acting that tries to establish a rapport with others, and to accommodate other people's reactions and requests. Examples include "displaying no inappropriate aggressive behaviors during peer interactions," "politely asserts one's self," and "obtains and responds to relevant situational cues in the social environment" (p. 457). While poor eye contact may indicate a difficulty with physical, nonverbal communication (answer B) and grabbing may indicate poor self-control (answer C), the combination of behaviors described is most indicative of poor social interaction skills. By developing her interpersonal and coping skills (answer D), the individual may be able to demonstrate improved social conduct. See Reference: Hemphill-Pearson. (2008). Appendix U.

122. (A) Work environment, structure of work tasks, rules, and supervision. Assessment of the work environment, tasks, and supervision (answer A) would be key to making recommendations concerning accommodations for those with mental health issues, including ways to eliminate distraction, and providing frequent supervision, flexible work hours, and breaks. "Adaptations made at the workplace are...considered reasonable accommodations for a qualified individual who can perform the essential functions of the job with certain modifications in either the job, environment, or supervisory process" (p. 831). Assessment of the architectural barriers (answer B) would be irrelevant unless the population had physical disabilities as well. Assessment of work aptitudes, interests, and capacities of the individuals (answers C and D) would be relevant for placement recommendations of individuals, but not accommodation recommendations for the worksite regarding the population. See Reference: Cara & MacRae. (2013). MacRae, A., & Smith, J.: Mental health of the older adult.

123. (B) Making leather lacing change purses from kits. All of the choices are good leisure group activities. However, activities that can be completed in one session, are structured for success, and yield a tangible end product (such as a kit) are very likely to turn out well regardless of the individual's skill level. They are best for promoting a sense of competence and mastery over the environment. "In structured crafts, the limits of a repetitive and predictive project can offer reassurance to the fearful person and help to contain anxiety.... Completing these tasks successfully also provides a sense of mastery and accomplishment and increases clients' perceived sense of effectiveness" (p. 289). Collages (answer A) are useful for expressing thoughts or feelings about a particular theme, such as nutritional foods or leisure activities one enjoys participating in; however, the end product is not always predictable. Going to the movies (answer C) can incorporate goals related to community mobility and money management; however, there is no tangible end product. Putting on a resident talent show (answer D) can promote self-esteem and self-expression; however, it usually requires more than one session to prepare. Given the nature of a drop-in shelter, it would be important to use activities that could be completed in one session. See Reference: Cara & MacRae. (2013). Cara, E: Anxiety disorders.

124. (B) An activity exploring leisure opportunities and problems. The OT practitioner can assist individuals in developing self-knowledge of leisure and play preferences, which is the first step in making choices about leisure and play participation. Once the therapist has collected "data about the past and present interests of the client and the uniqueness of those interests, as well as what makes particular activities important to the client...[then] [t]his information can be applied to interventions designed to help the client explore and create new or alternative activities" (p. 728). Answer B, an activity exploring leisure opportunities and problems, is the best answer because this type of activity could assist this individual in developing knowledge about other leisure opportunities and explore his feelings about engaging in these opportunities. This individual's previous leisure interests are already known, so a leisure inventory assessment (answer A) would be a duplication of information. An activity that encourages the individual to sign up for social activities (answer C) may not be effective because the individual has indicated no interest in these activities so far. Looking at leisure activities available in the community (answer D) is premature at this point because the individual has not identified any goals around which to plan future leisure activities. See Reference: Brown & Stoffel. (2011). Howells, V.: Leisure and play.

125. (A) Use room-darkening curtains and lower the temperature. Environmental adaptations that can facilitate sleep include darkening the room, cooler temperatures (answer A), earplugs or a fan to drown out noise, and comfortable furnishings. "For sleep, a room should be completely dark.... Light triggers the brain to believe it is daytime, and this in-

terferes with sleep" (p. 751). Therefore, raising the temperature (answer B) would probably not be beneficial. Participating in a quiet activity is recommended, but although a glass of wine before bed (answer C) may produce drowsiness initially, once the "alcohol is metabolized, sugar levels drop causing awakening" (p. 750). A CPAP (continuous positive airway pressure) machine (answer D), which is used to control breathing for individuals with sleep apnea, is a medical intervention, not an environmental adaptation. See Reference: Brown & Stoffel. (2011). Pierce, D. & Summers, K.: Rest and sleep.

126. (D) built-up handles. Built-up handles (answer D), without adding extra weight, allow a comfortable grasp that regular utensils (answer A) do not provide. A weighted handle (answer B) would cause more rapid fatigue and strain to the joints. A person with arthritis most likely has adequate grasp and release with a built-up handle, making it easier to use than a universal cuff (answer C). See Reference: Pedretti. 2013. Deshaies, L.: Arthritis.

127. (A) Cold modalities, elevation, and active assist and/or passive range of motion. Cold thermal modalities, elevation, and active assist and/or passive range of motion are all "remedial edema techniques of the biomechanical theory according to phase of healing" (p. 39). In the acute phase, postinjury, with presenting edema, "cold thermal modalities, nonthermal ultrasound, compression garments, compression pumps, compression wrapping, elevation, PROM, AAROM, AROM" (p. 39) are all options to consider to remediate the presenting edema and stiffness. Answers B and D, electrical stimulation, dynamic use of orthosis, and joint mobilization, are all considered treatment techniques for more established joint stiffness. Resistive exercises, weight-bearing, and lifting (answer C) could all potentially contribute to increasing joint stiffness and pain. See Reference: Meriano & Latella. (2008). Proulx-Sepelak, D.: Foundational skills for functional activities.

128. (D) Resting hand. A resting hand orthotic device is indicated for the wrist, fingers, and thumb joints during acute synovitis, answer D. "One of the orthotic devices most frequently fabricated by OTs is the resting pan (also known as the resting hand or functional position orthotic device), which is used to maintain the hand in a functional position. The purpose of this positioning orthotic device is to keep the soft tissues of the hand in midrange to maintain optimal mobility and to prevent shortening of the soft tissue structures around the joints" (p. 780). A wrist stabilization orthosis (answer B) would be indicated for wrist pain and to protect the extensor tendons from rupture. An ulnar drift positioning orthosis (answer C) would be used to prevent ulnar drift, while maintaining joint alignment for grasp and pinch activities. A protective MP joint orthosis (answer A) would assist in keeping the MP joints in normal alignment, while preventing volar subluxation. See Reference: Pedretti. (2013). Kasch, M.C. & Walsh, J.M.: Hand and upper extremity injuries.

129. (C) C6 An individual with C6 quadriplegia has some use of the abductor pollicis longus, extensor pollicis longus, extensor digitorum communis, and extensor carpi ulnaris. The extensor tone of the muscles in conjunction with the orthosis will operate the power for prehension force. "The wrist-driven wrist-hand orthosis, or the flexor hinge orthosis and tenodesis orthosis, is a metal device that transfers power from the extended wrist to the radial fingers, allowing a stronger pinch" (p. 1189). Individuals with Cl or C3 injuries (answers A and B) have higher-level lesions and lack the wrist extension strength needed to operate the wrist-driven flexor hinge orthosis. An individual with a T1 injury (answer D) is able to grasp and manipulate utensils without difficulty or need for assistance. See Reference: Trombly. (2008). Atkins, M.S.: Spinal cord injury.

130. (C) Extension to promote finger flexion, and flexion to facilitate finger extension. "Tenodesis is the reciprocal motion of the wrist and fingers that occurs during active and passive wrist flexion and extension. Tenodesis is the action of wrist extension producing finger flexion, and wrist flexion producing finger extension. It is caused by the lack of change in length of the long finger muscles during wrist extension" (pp. 758–759). The method used to maintain tenodesis in the hand of a person with tetraplegia is to keep the wrist extended to facilitate finger flexion, and flexed to promote finger extension. The other methods would stretch the tendons too much, which would not allow a tenodesis grasp. See Reference: Pedretti. (2013). Lashgari, D. & Yasuda, L.: Orthotics.

131. (A) Stop the activity. Activity should be stopped immediately when symptoms occur during treatment of an acute cardiac patient (answer A). Symptoms, including confusion, shortness of breath, profuse sweating, cold skin, clammy skin, chest pain, nausea, and light-headedness, should be reported to the physician. After the session is over, symptoms should be documented (answer B). Continuing the activity, whether seated or with the patient's permission (answers C and D), is dangerous and may result in further cardiac damage. See Reference: Pedretti. (2013). Huntley, N.: Cardiac and pulmonary diseases.

132. (D) pressure marks or redness from the orthotic device disappear within 20 minutes. A universal and primary concern is that all orthotic devices provided to a patient be checked for correct fit, answer D. This is achieved by making adjustments to areas that present with redness or pressure marks after the orthosis has been removed for 20 minutes. Many types of orthoses may be made without the fingers flexed or the thumb opposed (answers A and B) as in an antispasticity ball orthosis or a dynamic extension orthosis. Most orthoses are not worn at all times, answer C, but are removed for activities such as self-care or exercise. The OT practitioner should issue an orthosis wear schedule at the time that the orthosis is fitted for the patient. See Reference: Pedretti. (2013). Lashgari, D. & Yasuda, L.: Orthotics.

133. (B) Median nerve. The median nerve (answer B) passes through the carpal tunnel at the wrist. Impingement in this region causes sensory changes in the thumb, index finger, long finger, and half of the ring finger. Prolonged impingement in the carpal tunnel results in atrophy of the thenar eminence and weakness of the opponens pollicis. Injury to the radial nerve (answer C) in the wrist area causes sensory damage only. Damage to the ulnar nerve (answer A) at the wrist causes decreased grip strength and complete or partial loss of sensation over half of the fourth digit (ring finger) and all of the fifth digit (little finger), plus the proximal hypothenar region. A brachial plexus injury (answer D) may result in damage to any or all of the UE peripheral nerves. This may cause motor and/or sensory impairments. See Reference: Pedretti. (2013). Kasch, M.C. & Martin Walsh, J.: Hand and upper extremity injuries.

134. (A) Repetition, high force, and awkward joint postures. The term "cumulative trauma disorder should be viewed as a description of the mechanism of injury and not a diagnosis.... Diagnoses associated with cumulative trauma usually fall into one of three categories: tendinitis (such as lateral epicondylitis, tennis elbow or de Quervain's tenosynovitis), nerve compression syndromes (such as carpal tunnel syndrome or cubital tunnel syndrome), or myofascial pain" (p. 1064). Repetition, high force, and awkward joint postures are work-related risk factors that are frequently associated with cumulative trauma disorders. Progressive resistive exercises, joint mobilization, and weight-bearing (answer B) are interventions that OT practitioners may use with a variety of conditions. Answers C and D, inflammation, swelling, pain, fatigue, cramps, and paresthesias, are considered to be potential symptoms of cumulative trauma disorders, not factors that contribute to the condition. See Reference: Pedretti. (2013). Kasch, M.C. & Walsh, J.M.: Hand and upper extremity injuries.

135. (A) Individual will purchase 10 items at the supermarket with supervision. Short-term goals must relate to the long-term goal being addressed. Because the long-term goal being addressed is independence in grocery shopping, the short-term goal must relate to grocery shopping. Answers B and C do not relate to grocery shopping. Answer D is an appropriate treatment intervention, but is written in a way that describes what the OT, not the individual, will do. Answers B and C describe activities related to the task of shopping, but not the shopping itself. See Reference: Schell, Gillen, & Scaffa. (2014). Birge James, A.: Activities of daily living and instrumental activities of daily living.

136. (B) Scoot forward to the edge of the wheelchair seat. After locking the brakes, the OT encourages the client to "scoot to the edge of the surface, and put his or her feet flat on the floor" (p. 255). Having the individual scoot forward to the edge of the wheelchair (answer B) helps the individual position the body over the feet and causes the weight to shift forward during a transfer. The individual is much easier to transfer when the weight is shifted forward. If the person attempts to stand up (answer A) from a regular seated position, and the weight is shifted back during a transfer, it may require more than one person to assist with the transfer. Answer C, unlocking the wheelchair brakes, is incorrect because the wheelchair needs to be stabilized in a locked position before standing. Positioning the wheelchair facing the mat table (answer D) allows no room for the OT to stand and assist with the pivot. See Reference: Pedretti. (2013). Bolding, D., Adler, C., Tipton-Burton, M., Verran, A., & Lillie, S.M.: Mobility.

137. (C) assume the bottom, supine position. Taking the bottom, supine position (answer C) requires the least amount of energy expenditure and should be the primary recommendation. In addition, the OT may encourage experimentation with a variety of positions (answer D). Having sex at times when there is most energy also would be beneficial, but the individual will most likely be more fatigued at the end of the day (answer A). See Reference: Pedretti. (2013). Birge James, A.: Restoring the role of independent person.

138. (B) seating the individual upright on a firm surface with the chin slightly tucked. The best position for feeding an individual with a swallowing disorder is upright and symmetrical with the chin slightly tucked (answer B). Supine, semireclined, and side-lying positions (answers A, C, and D) all place the individual at greater risk for choking and aspiration. See Reference: Pedretti. (2013). Smith, J. Jenks, K.N.: Eating and swallowing.

139. (C) Steps, width of doorways, and threshold heights. The first area of evaluation should be

the steps, width of doorways, and presence and height of door thresholds (answer C) to determine whether the wheelchair user will be able to enter and exit interior spaces in the wheelchair or whether structural modifications are required. Answers A, B, and D reflect areas that also will need to be evaluated; however, they are not as critical to initial interior access. See Reference: Schell, Gillen, & Scaffa. (2014). Rigby, P., Trentham, B., & Letts, L.: Modifying performance contexts.

140. (B) Rolling clay into a 1/4-inch slab using a rolling pin. "Treatment using motor behavior models attempts to make an impact on the neurological system through positioning, normal movement patterns, and tactile and proprioceptive cues. Occupations may involve gross motor body movements, weight-bearing, diagonal movement patterns, and controlled external sensory stimulation. Crafts that involve weight-bearing...are often considered most likely to achieve normal neural reactions. Sautéing, sanding, rolling, rubbing, or mixing can be used to achieve goals in this model" (pp. 20–21). Rolling clay with a rolling pin (answer B) is the best choice because of the high level of deep proprioceptive input that can be achieved through the shoulders and upper extremities. Papier-mâché (answer A) can provide some resistance, as well as experience with variations in texture, which can be valuable for sensory integration/sensory processing. Gluing mosaic tiles (answer C) and stringing beads (answer D) do not provide significant proprioceptive input, but include activity components that can promote grasp, coordination, and a variety of cognitive skills. See Reference: Tubbs & Drake. (2012). The case for crafts.

141. (A) extend the operated leg forward, reach back for the armrests, then slowly sit. By extending the operated leg forward, reaching back for the armrests, and slowly sitting, an effective and safe transfer can be accomplished (answer A). Answers B, C, and D are all contraindicated transfer training techniques for individuals who must adhere to total hip precautions. These precautions restrict flexing of the hip greater than 80 degrees, hip adduction, and internal rotation. See Reference: Pedretti. (2013). Coleman Lawson, S. & Murphy, L.F.: Hip fractures and lower extremity joint replacement.

142. (B) Lateral trunk stability. Criteria for use of a MAS include "adequate power from neck, trunk, shoulder girdle, or elbow muscles," adequate motor control; 0 to 90 degrees PROM in shoulder flexion and abduction, as well as adequate PROM in internal and external rotation, elbow flexion, and pronation; trunk stability; motivation; and a supportive environment. An individual with fair plus (3+) elbow flexion (answer C) would be able to stabilize the elbow on the table to bring the hand to the mouth and would have enough strength to move the arm without the mobile arm support. Although individuals with quadriplegia often meet these criteria (answer A), so do individuals with muscular dystrophy, Guillain-Barré syndrome, ALS, and polio (p. 445). See Reference: Trombly. (2008). Deshaies, L.D.: Upper extremity orthoses.

143. (C) demonstrate adherence to prescribed hip precautions. The ability to stand for 10 minutes (answer A) or to increase hip flexion to 90 degrees (answer B) is not necessary for independence in dressing. However, the adherence to appropriate hip precautions (answer C) is mandated by many physicians for the individual to perform activities safely. "The patient must be reminded that the operated hip is not to be flexed actively or passively or the leg adducted beyond midline" (p. 1118). Energy-conservation techniques (answer D) are appropriate for individuals who demonstrate very low endurance levels, and may be appropriate for some individuals following hip arthroplasty, but hip precautions would need to be observed during energy conservation activities to prevent dislocation of the prosthesis. See Reference: Trombly. (2008). Maher, C. & Bear-Lehman, J.: Orthopaedic conditions.

144. (A) Holding the hammer. Holding the hammer (answer A) is the only activity listed that requires gripping with the entire hand, along with resistance. "Household items...have been used to increase strength of grasp and pinch" (p. 1067); therefore, holding a hammer would require hand grip. Also, "occupational therapists are skilled in collaborating with people with physical disabilities to assist them in resuming a full life" (p. 413). "Crafts that have been found to work well with hand injuries include macramé, Turkish knot weaving, clay molding, leather tooling, and woodworking" (p. 1067). Holding the stamping tools and needle (answers B and D) requires pinch patterns. Squeezing the sponge (answer C) offers less resistance than holding the hammer, and therefore, would be less effective for strengthening and hand grip. See Reference: Pedretti. (2013). Krishnagiri, S. & Southam, M.: Leisure occupations and Kasch, M.C., & Walsh, M.J.: Hand and upper extremity injuries.

145. (B) Showering on a tub bench while incorporating rest breaks. "When patients are taught methods to conserve their energy resources, they will be able to perform at a higher functional level without expending energy.... Rest breaks are scheduled throughout the day.... Standing activity requires more energy than seated activity" (p. 1210), making the tub transfer bench the best option for bathing. Answers A and C would most likely be used by individuals with limited reach and limited grip strength, respectively, whereas use of proper body mechanics (answer D) is important for individuals with back injuries. See Reference: Pedretti. (2013). Huntley, N.: Cardiac and pulmonary diseases.

146. (D) The individual attempts to find coins in a pocket while occluding vision. According to Bentzel, "stereognosis—the ability to identify objects through proprioception, cognition and the sense of touch," such as identifying coins in a pocket (answer D), would be the best choice. Answers A and B do not encourage the use of proprioception and touch, whereas answer C, the use of putty, may be something used to increase proprioception; however, the goal of increasing strength was not identified in this question. See Reference: Trombly. (2008). Bentzel, K.: Assessing abilities and capacities: Sensation.

147. (B) weight-bearing through the upper extremity in sitting or standing. Weight-bearing is the most effective way of normalizing tone, according to the NDT approach for adult hemiplegia. Placing a weighted cuff on the extremity (answer A) would have the effect of increasing muscle tone, making reaching more difficult. Answer C, using only the unaffected upper extremity, would accomplish the reaching task, but would not normalize muscle tone in the affected upper extremity. Answer D, "forced use," is a treatment concept used to encourage functional motor return in hemiplegic upper extremities, but is not a method designed to normalize muscle tone, nor is it a specific technique of the NDT approach. See Reference: Pedretti. (2013). Schultz-Krohn, W., Pope-Davis, S.A., Jourdan, J.M., & McLaughlin-Gray, J.: Traditional sensorimotor approaches to intervention.

148. (B) Implement a pureed diet and allow adequate time for eating. As ALS progresses, speaking and swallowing become more difficult and a pureed diet becomes necessary (answer B). The individual runs the risk of aspiration or choking if meals are rushed. Adaptive equipment (answers A and D) are provided much earlier in the disease process. The independence achieved with adaptive equipment has a positive psychological effect on the individual who most likely sees his or her independence slipping away. Answer C, upper extremity strengthening, would be contraindicated in the late stages of the disease. See Reference: Pedretti. (2013). Smith, J. & Jenks, K.N.: Eating and swallowing.

149. (D) Dynamometer. This individual exhibits difficulty in the area of strength. A "standard adjustable-handle dynamometer is recommended for assessing grip strength" (p. 1047). A volumeter (answer C) is a container used to measure edema in the hand by measuring the amount of water displaced when the hand is placed into the container. A goniometer (answer A) is a tool with two arms used to measure movement at a joint. One arm is held stationary while the other arm moves around an axis of 360 degrees. An aesthesiometer (answer B) measures two-point discrimination with a moveable point attached to a ruler that has a stationary point at one end. See Reference: Pedretti. (2013). Kasch, M.C. & Walsh, J.M.: Hand and upper extremity injuries.

150. (C) Increase swimming time to 25 minutes or to tolerance. This individual's goal is to maximize strength and endurance. Although ALS is a progressive degenerative disease, improvements in strength and endurance are possible if the individual was not previously functioning at maximum capacity. The correct answer (answer C) increases the duration of the activity while recognizing the importance of avoiding fatigue. This individual's performance indicates potential for further improvement. Therefore, the program should be upgraded, not downgraded (answer B). Methods for improving endurance include increasing the frequency, intensity, or duration of the activity. Answer A continues the program at a maintenance level. Using adaptive equipment (answer D), such as a flotation belt, is an energy-saving strategy that would be appropriate if the individual were experiencing fatigue during swimming. See Reference: Pedretti. (2013). Schultz-Krohn, W., Foti, D., & Glogoski, C.: Degenerative diseases of the central nervous system.

151. (B) Temperature and pain. The sensations of pain and temperature are carried along small, unmyelinated nerve fibers, which recover more rapidly than senses carried by larger, myelinated fibers. The sensations of pain and temperature also are part of the protective or primary sensory systems, which are the receivers of simple information. More complex information is carried through the discriminative or epicritic system. The senses carried on this system are vibration, light touch, proprioception, and tactile localization. See Reference: Trombly. (2008). Bentzel, K.: Assessing abilities and capacities: Sensation.

152. (C) Altering the task. When the task method is altered, the same task objects are used in the same environment, but the method of performing the task is modified to make the task feasible given the client's impairments (p. 501). One example is substituting one-handed techniques for someone who previously used both hands (i.e., one-handed shoelace tying for an individual who recently had an above-elbow amputation). Problem-solving (answer A) is the ability to organize information from several levels to generate a solution to a problem. Retraining (answer B) teaches the same activity skills to the individual who previously had mastery of those skills (e.g., having an individual with hand weakness practice tying knots). Compensation (answer D) would be avoiding performance of the activity entirely by using an alternative piece of equipment or method. See Reference: Schell, Gillen, & Scaffa. (2014). James, A.B.: Activities of daily living and instrumental activities of daily living.

153. (B) environmental hazard analysis and falls risk during performance of ADL. Answer B, occupational therapy, may include "treatment that helps to prevent falls [that] includes detecting and removing environmental hazards, optimizing motor control, recommending appropriate adaptive devices, and teaching safety measures to patient and family" (p. 1023). Statistical analysis of data (answer A) might be performed by risk management or human resources personnel. Answer C, evaluation of gait and mobility device use, is an area of specialized expertise for the physical therapist. Medical and/or pharmacology personnel (such as the nurse, physician, or pharmacist) would most likely assess the impact of medication on fall incidence (answer D). See Reference: Trombly. (2008). Woodson, A.M.: Stroke.

154. (B) Pinch gauge. "Pinch strength should also be tested, using a pinch gauge. The pinch gauge has been found to be the most accurate.... As with the grip dynamometer, three successive trials should be obtained and compared bilaterally" (p. 1048). A pinch gauge is used to measure the strength of a three-jaw chuck grasp pattern (also known as palmar pinch, as well as key (lateral) pinch and tip pinch. All of these pinch patterns require thumb opposition. For each of these tests, the individual performs three trials, which the evaluator averages together; the result is compared with a standardized norm. An aesthesiometer (answer A) measures two-point discrimination. A dynamometer (answer C) measures grip strength, but is not particularly sensitive to thumb opposition. A volumeter (answer D) measures edema in the hand. See Reference: Pedretti. (2013). Kasch, M.C. & Walsh, J.M.: Hand and upper extremity injuries.

155. (D) Early morning and again at another time of day. "As with assessment of function, the time of day and anti-inflammatory or analgesic medications taken should be noted because these factors may influence results.... The clinical evaluation may take considerable time.... The OT may need to perform the assessments over several sessions.... Morning stiffness should be considered" (answer D, pp. 1013–1014). Evaluating the individual only in the morning (answers A and C) or only in the afternoon (answer B) accurately reveals the individual's functional level at only one time of day. Individuals with arthritis have many changes in functional status after morning stiffness has disappeared. See Reference: Pedretti. (2013). Deshaies, L.: Arthritis.

156. (C) ask another person for assistance. It is often necessary to procure assistance when transferring individuals who are mobidly obese (answer C). Trying to attempt this transfer alone could result in injury to the patient and/or the therapist, even if proper body mechanics are used (answer A). Asking someone else to do a difficult task (answer B) is not professional. If the patient needs to be transferred, not transferring him (answer D) is not an option. See Reference: Pedretti. (2013). Bolding, D., Adler, C., Tipton-Burton, M., Verran, A., & Lillie, S.M.: Mobility.

157. (D) volar wrist. "Tapping at the volar wrist elicits Tinel's sign, which is a sensation of tingling or electric shock if the median nerve is compromised" (p. 1148). Answers A, B, and C are inappropriate choices for eliciting Tinel's sign. See Reference: Trombly. (2008). Cooper, C.: Hand impairments.

158. (D) Obtain a narrower wheelchair because this one is now too wide. "Measure the individual across the widest part of the thighs or hips while the client is sitting in a chair comparable with the anticipated wheelchair.... Wheelchair clearance: Add 1/2 to 1 inch on each side of the hip or thigh measurement taken. Consider how an increase in the overall width of the chair will affect accessibility" (p. 248). If the seat is 2.5 inches wider than the individual, it is too wide (answer D), not too narrow (answer A). In addition, the width of the wheelchair should be kept as narrow as possible. The narrower the wheelchair, the easier it is to maneuver. Because a narrower wheelchair would be better, padding the sides (answer C) is a less desirable option. The need to lose or gain weight (answer B) should be discussed first with an individual's physician. See Reference: Pedretti. (2013). Bolding, D., Adler, C., Tipton-Burton, M., Verran, A., & Lillie, S.M.: Mobility.

159. (A) Moderate exercise in uninvolved muscles and active range-of-motion exercise. "Early interventions should target the individual's symptoms as these affect their occupations.... Stage I, activities to maintain motor function,...moderate exercise in unaffected muscles, active range of motion (ROM) exercise" (p. 1094). Progressive resistive exercises (answer B) may cause cramping and fatigue, and therefore are not recommended for individuals with ALS. Use of orthosis and adaptive equipment (answer C) will be required in later stages to prevent contractures, support weak muscles, and assist with function. Passive range-of-motion activities and use of orthosis (answer D) also will be required later as

the disease progresses to prevent contractures and maintain strength. See Reference: Trombly. (2008). Forwell, S.J., Copperman, L.F., & Hugos, L.: Neurogenerative diseases.

160. (B) Outpatient. Outpatient therapy (answer B) is appropriate for individuals who are "medically stable and able to tolerate a few hours of therapy and a trip to an outpatient clinic" (p. 35). A patient with such high levels of function is not an appropriate candidate for a home health referral (answer A). Work-hardening programs (answer C) are for individuals who are severely deconditioned as a result of disease or injury, or for those who have significant discrepancies between their symptoms and objective findings. If the individual has potential for further functional improvement, continuation rather than discontinuation (answer D) of services is indicated. See Reference: Pedretti. (2013). Schultz-Krohn, W. & McHugh Pendleton, H.: Application of the occupational therapy practice framework to physical dysfunction: treatment contexts.

161. (C) fluctuating weakness and/or further decline. "Generally, equipment, environmental, and behavioral modifications help patients compensate for weakness. Powered wheelchair mobility devices, such as scooters or electric wheelchairs, are frequently effective in limiting fatigue and aiding functional limitations related to weakness and spasticity. Powered mobility devices that are capable of adaptation [for issues such as fluctuating decline, correct answer C] later, such as adding a tilt feature to an electric wheelchair, accommodate the changing status" (pp. 1088–1089). Improved wheelchair mobility and gains in strength (answers A and D) are not characteristic of progressive degenerative diseases. When ordering a wheelchair for a pediatric or adolescent client, it is important to anticipate growth of the individual (answer B). See Reference: Trombly. (2008). Forwell, S.J., Copperman, L.F., & Hugos, L.: Neurogenerative diseases.

162. (D) perform only gentle active range of motion. Gentle active range of motion allows the individual to control the movement and avoid overstretching inflamed joint tissues. Brisk active range of motion (answer A) and the addition of resistance (answer B) are likely to cause further damage to the joints by increasing stress, which results in increased inflammation. The individual must understand the importance of joint protection during exercise. Eliminating all range-of-motion exercise (answer C) would result in further joint stiffness and loss of range of motion. See Reference: Trombly. (2008). Yasuda, Y.L.: Rheumatoid arthritis, osteoarthritis and fibromyalgia.

163. (B) Demonstrate the procedure on the un-affected extremity, then occlude the individual's vision and test the affected side. The presentation of stimuli in sensory evaluation is extremely important. Because of the compensation that may occur with vision, it is necessary to occlude the individual's vision. Also, the unaffected extremity should be assessed before the affected extremity, the opposite of answer A, to reduce anxiety in the individual. Stimuli should be presented in a random proximal-to-distal pattern. A rapport (answer C) should be established before beginning any evaluation procedure, which would also reduce anxiety. An individual may not be aware of any deficit areas (answer D); therefore, the whole extremity should be assessed to ensure accuracy. Picture cards are helpful in assessing individuals with expressive aphasia. See Reference: Trombly. (2008). Bentzel, K.: Assessing abilities and capacities: Sensation.

164. (C) Toothbrush with built-up handle. An individual with C7 to C8 quadriplegia has the hand strength to hold a toothbrush with a built-up handle, answer C. An alternate method can be to position the toothbrush between the fingers. An individual with a C5 injury may require a mobile arm support for brushing teeth (answer A). Other individuals with injuries at the C5 to C6 level may be able to use a universal cuff (answer B), or a wrist support with a utensil holder (answer D) to hold the toothbrush. See Reference: Pedretti. (2013). Adler, C.: Spinal cord injury.

165. (B) practicing the whole task of putting on a shirt in a setting similar to the real environment. Retention of a skill will be enhanced if the task is practiced in its entirety during each performance trial (answer B), because whole task performance is easier to recall than separate steps. "Breaking a task into its component parts for teaching purposes is useful only if the task can naturally be divided into discrete, recognizable units. This is so because continuous skills (or whole task performance) are easier to remember than discrete responses. For example, once a person has learned to ride a bicycle, this motor skill will be retained even without practicing for many years. Continuous skills should be taught in their entirety rather than segments" (p. 113). Answer A, practice of each segment of the process, may be useful for improving performance of the activity segments practiced, but will not enhance retention and generalization of the skill. Providing simulation activities (answer C) may improve some performance components involved in the dressing process, but will not enhance learning of the whole task of putting on a shirt. Answer D, showing a videotape and providing written directions, is a useful instructional technique for client education from a cognitive perspective, but they do not provide the motor component necessary for learning a motor skill. See Reference: Pedretti. (2013). Richardson, P.: Teaching activities in occupational therapy.

166. (A) A craft activity using increasingly heavy hand tools. Progressive resistive exercise is the most effective method for increasing strength in a muscle with fair plus strength. Mild resistance would be used initially, increasing resistance as appropriate. Mildly resistive activities that are stopped as soon as the individual begins to experience fatigue (answer B) are appropriate for maintaining or improving strength in individuals with conditions in which fatigue should be avoided (e.g., MS, ALS, and Guillain-Barré syndrome). Electric stimulation (answer C) is appropriate for increasing strength in very weak muscles. A craft activity that can be performed against increasing resistance for prolonged periods of time would be more effective than resisted active range of motion (answer D), which is usually performed only once or twice a day. See Reference: Trombly. (2008). Trombly Latham, C.A: Occupation as therapy: Selection, gradation, analysis, and adaptation.

167. (B) Playing hook and loop checkers to tolerance. Gentle, repetitive, and resistive exercises such as playing Velcro checkers (answer B) help maintain strength and endurance in weakened muscles. A wrist support (answer A) compensates for loss of muscle strength, but does not help to maintain strength. Exercising without resistance once a day (answer C) also will not help maintain strength. Exercising against maximal resistance (answer D) is contraindicated for individuals with ALS. See Reference: Trombly. (2008). Forwell, S.J., Copperman, L.F., & Hugos, L.: Neurogenerative diseases.

168. (A) coughing or choking. Coughing and choking are motor problems that are commonly noted in patients with dysphagia. Disorientation and confusion (answer B) are related to cognitive problems, and pain and decreased smell and taste (answers C and D, respectively) are related to sensory problems in patients with dysphagia. See Reference: Trombly. (2008). Avery, W.: Dysphagia.

169. (B) examine the results of a job-demand analysis. "Assessing the physical demands of a job by JDA (job demand analysis) is often beneficial in the rehabilitation process inasmuch as recommendations for initiation of return to work require objective information about both the client's abilities and the job itself" (p. 344). The job demand analysis is a detailed description of the physical, sensory, and psychological demands of a job. The job analysis may be performed by an occupational therapist or other professional involved in the case. Examples of performance requirements include tasks such as lifting, walking, sitting, standing, and reaching as well as seeing, hearing, and interpersonal skills. Interviewing the individual (answer A) is useful to obtain information about his or her perception of the injury, motivation for returning to work, and sense of responsibility for rehabilitation. However, the worker may not be able to give an objective, detailed, and concise analysis of the job. *The Dictionary of Occupational Titles* (answer C) provides generic job descriptions, but does not contain as much specific information as a job analysis. A physician (answer D) is unlikely to have the depth of information necessary or the time available to provide the necessary information. See Reference: Pedretti. (2013). Haruko Ha, D., Page, J.J., & Wietlisbach, C.M.: Work evaluation and work programs.

170. (D) Low-impact aerobics three times a week for 1 hour. "Treatment of clients with arthritis must take into account the progressive nature of the disease. The overarching goal of therapy is to decrease pain, protect joints, and increase function.... The intervention plan should be designed for the individual client and based on the stage of the disease, the severity of symptoms, general health status, lifestyle, and mutually agree upon goals" (p. 1019). Based on the information provided, the low-impact aerobics activity is the most client-centered of the choices. Answer A, lifting weights, is considered to be an activity that promotes hyperextension and resistance, possibly leading to increased pain, immobility, and further damage to the joints, in addition to joint pain and fatigue. Answer B, the use of relaxation tapes, would be an appropriate selection for assisting an individual to cope with the potential psychosocial aspects of arthritis. Answer C, vocational retraining, is not indicated based on the information provided. See Reference: Pedretti. (2013). Deshaies, L.: Arthritis.

171. (B) determine whether there are any motivational or cultural issues interfering with orthosis-wear compliance. Prior to fabricating another orthosis, the OT practitioner must determine whether the individual is likely to comply with a new use of orthosis program (answer B). Some individuals refuse to wear orthoses owing to cultural norms, whereas others are simply embarrassed to wear an orthosis in public. Some people demonstrate a low motivational level in regard to regaining function, whereas others may overdo their use of orthosis program in the hopes that it will facilitate healing. "OTs deal with humans as a whole, not just as a hand, a toe, or a shoulder. With the human hand, even the smallest impairment may affect function.... An orthosis is one of the most important tools thera-

pists can use to minimize or correct impairment and to restore or augment function. Little else so readily calls attention to the hand as a splint [orthotic device].... The decision to provide or fabricate a splint [orthotic device] requires an in-depth understanding of the pathologic condition to be affected and of the many splint [orthotic device] choices available" (p. 757). In the given case, it would not be indicated to fabricate a new orthosis, answer A, unless the individual agrees to adhere to the wearing schedule. Answer C, requesting that the individual find the orthosis or you will threaten to call his physician, would not be the first step to take in the process. Contacting the physician regarding the individual's noncompliance, as well as providing documentation of performance, is indicated, but is not something to be used to threaten the individual. Answer D, discharging the individual, would not be appropriate until the therapist discusses the case with the physician and individual. See Reference: Pedretti. (2013). Lashgari, D. & Yasuda, L.: Orthotics.

172. (D) Use a dust mitt to keep fingers fully extended. "An effective means of maintaining functional motion and strength with arthritis is to have clients perform daily occupations.... As the client's condition improves, usual life activities should be resumed because this will help promote physical status and psychological well-being.... Analysis of activity demands and activity contexts is a critical component in helping clients maintain, restore, or enhance their engagement in desired activities and occupations" (p. 1027). Using dust mitts prevents prolonged finger flexion and allows the fingers to remain straight while dusting. Pushing the vacuum (answer A) forward by straightening the elbow completely, then pulling it back close to the body requires long strokes and promotes good elbow and shoulder range of motion. When ironing (answer B), trying to get the elbow into full extension helps to maintain elbow range of motion. Keeping lightweight objects (answer C) on high shelves encourages reaching, which helps maintain shoulder range of motion. See Reference: Pedretti. (2013). Deshaies, L.: Arthritis.

173. (B) Avoid internal rotation and adduction of the involved hip. Following hip arthroplasty, positions such as flexion of the hip past a prescribed range (usually 60 to 90 degrees), internal rotation, and adduction can result in dislocation of the hip. Therefore, answer B, avoid internal rotation and adduction of the involved hip, is the priority set of instructions to convey. OT practitioners instruct individuals in hip precautions and provide them with adaptive equipment so they can safely perform self-care, work, and leisure activities. Answers C and D may help an individual comply more easily with hip precautions. Sitting during LE dressing (answer A) also is recommended. See Reference: Pedretti. (2013). Coleman Lawson, S. & Murphy, L.F.: Hip fractures and lower extremity joint replacement.

174. (A) Independent with a transfer board. An individual injured at the C7 to C8 level should be able to perform transfers independently either with or without sliding board. "Level C7—C8 bed/wheelchair transfers...Level...independent, with or without transfer board" (p. 972). They do not typically require minimal to moderate assistance (answer B). Stand-pivot transfers (answer D) are appropriate for individuals who can come to a standing position and bear some weight on the lower extremities. Individuals with injuries C4 or higher are unable to provide physical assistance during transfers but may provide verbal direction (answer C). See Reference: Pedretti. (2013). Adler, C.: Spinal cord injury.

175. (B) Sterilize it before using it again. "The Occupational Safety and Health Administration (OSHA) issues regulations to protect the employees of health care facilities.... In the clinic, general cleanliness and proper control of heat, light, and air are important for infection control. Spills should be cleaned up promptly. Work areas and equipment should be kept free from contamination. To decontaminate is to remove, inactivate, or destroy blood-borne pathogens in a surface or item to the point where they are no longer capable of transmitting infectious particles and the surface or item is rendered safe for handling, use, or disposal" (p. 147). Other examples are using sharps containers, eyewash stations, and biohazard waste containers. Answers A, C, and D would not meet guidelines set forth by OSHA regarding equipment that has come into contact with open wounds. See Reference: Pedretti. (2013). George, A.H.: Infection control and safety issues in the clinic.

176. (A) When the OTA consistently obtains the same results as the OT. The term service competency relates to "the specific knowledge, skills, and attitudes to perform at an expected level that matches the requirements of the area of practice or service" (answer A, p. 1241). "Service competency is the process of teaching, training, and evaluating in which the OT determines that the OTA performs tasks in the same way that the OT would and achieves the same outcomes" (p. 1084, AOTA, 2009, in Schell, Gillen, & Scaffa). Service competency is determined by skill level, not by years of experience (answer D). Passing the NBCOT examination (answer B) establishes entry-level competence, not service competence in a particular area. OT practitioners have a professional responsibility to maintain competence, and continuing education (answer C) is one

method for maintaining competence and promoting lifelong learning. See Reference: Schell, Gillen, & Scaffa. (2014). Youngstrom, M.J.: Supervision.

177. (A) Pureed foods such as pudding or applesauce. "To minimize the risk of aspiration, pureed foods are chosen for clients with decreased oral motor control and chewing difficulties or apraxia" (answer A). Soft foods and mechanical soft-textured foods (answers B and C) may increase risk of aspiration and would be introduced if pureed foods do not present an issue. Thin liquids (answer D), such as juice and water, would be contraindicated at this point of intervention, as they "are the most difficult to control because they require intact oral motor strength and coordination, and an intact swallow to prevent aspiration" (p. 691). See Reference: Pedretti. (2013). Smith, J. & Jenks, K.N.: Eating and swallowing.

178. (C) restoration of function. Individuals admitted to a rehabilitation unit need to be able to participate in 3 hours of therapy a day. Therefore, goals for these individuals "involve restoration [answer C] and support of function within a rehabilitation model of care (i.e., learning to live with and adapt to changes in functional abilities)" (p. 1220). Palliative care (answer A) is provided to individuals in the advanced stages of cancer and focuses on comfort, symptom management (answer D), and ease of participation in activity. Prevention programs (answer B) focus on educating people about risky behaviors that can result in illness or injury and focus on developing healthy habits. See Reference: Pedretti. (2013). Burkhardt, A. & Schultz-Krohn, W.: Oncology.

179. (D) indicate whether the body part is being moved up or down. The response of the client would be to "indicate whether the body part is being moved 'up' or 'down'" (p. 583, answer D). Answers A, B, and C are not indicative of the assessment of proprioception. "Conscious proprioception derives from receptors found in muscles, tendons, and joints and is defined as awareness of joint position in space. It is through cerebral integration of information about touch and proprioception that objects can be identified by tactile cues and pressure. If proprioception is impaired, it may be difficult to gauge how much pressure to use when holding a paper cup" (p. 583). See Reference: Pedretti. (2013). Cooper, C. & Canyock, J.D.: Evaluation of sensation and intervention for sensory dysfunction.

180. (C) Remove the threshold altogether. Removing the threshold altogether would be the simplest and safest solution. Door thresholds may have a maximum height greater than 0.5", and these must be beveled; keeping it as it is (answer A) would provide a barrier to wheelchair accessibility and a safety hazard for people with visual deficits. Placing a throw rug to cover the threshold (answer B) would not improve accessibility and would present a slipping hazard. Because the threshold height is more than half an inch, placing a ramp over the threshold (answer D) would be required if the threshold could not be removed. The best solution would still be to remove the threshold altogether to provide the most accessible surface. See Reference: Trombly. (2008). Sabata, D.B., Shamberg, S., & Williams, M.: Optimizing access to home, community, and work environments.

181. (D) Strength. Exerting enough pressure to twist off a jar lid requires strength, which it appears the client is lacking, making answer D correct. The client demonstrates adequate range of motion (answer A) when he grasps the knife. He demonstrates adequate coordination (answer B) by spreading peanut butter on the bread and accurately positioning the lid on to the jar opening, and he demonstrates adequate endurance (answer C) by standing during the entire activity of making a peanut butter sandwich. See Reference: Pedretti. (2013). Preston, L.A.: Evaluation of motor control.

182. (D) Ethnography. The choice that would best capture the information related to understanding the people in this research project is answer D, ethnography. "Ethnography is a primary research approach in anthropology concerned with description and interpretation of cultural patterns of groups, as well as the understanding of the cultural meanings people use to organize and interpret their experiences" (p. 350). Answer A, participatory action research, is an "approach that directly involves study participants in each of the 10 research essentials; that is, it involves study participants that contribute to formulating the research questions, or query, study design, and approach to analysis" (p. 353). Answer B, grounded theory, is a method of naturalistic inquiry that is used to "generate theory, primarily employing the deductive process of constant comparison" (p. 350), whereas answer C, phenomenology, aims to "uncover the meaning of how humans experience phenomena through the description of those experiences as they are lived by the individual" (p. 353). See Reference: DePoy & Gitlin. (2011). Glossary.

183. (B) Discuss precautions necessary for sex. "Questions may be raised regarding how or if a person with an indwelling catheter can have sex. Sex is possible for both men and women, but some precautions should be taken. If the catheter becomes kinked or closed off (which will definitely happen in the case of a catheterized man having vaginal intercourse), pressure should not be placed on the bladder. The bladder should be fully voided before sexual activity.

Urine flow should be restricted for as short a time as possible and no more than 30 minutes. Damage to the bladder and kidneys could result if these precautions are not followed" (p. 305). Sexuality is a part of human performance that OT practitioners should be knowledgeable about and comfortable in discussing (answer B, also making answer D incorrect). When uncomfortable discussing the topic, the therapist may refer the patient to another team member, which may include the physician (answer A). It is not necessary to remove an indwelling catheter for participation in sexual activity and it is not within the scope of OT practice to teach an individual how to remove one (answer C). See Reference: Pedretti. (2013). Tipton-Burton, M. & Umphred Burton, G.: Sexuality and physical dysfunction.

184. (A) Elevate the affected extremity. Positioning, the use of a compression glove, edema massage, and PROM exercises are all effective methods for reducing edema and preventing further edema. "Even in the absence of motor recovery, normal movement is an important model for movement reeducation. Passive and assisted active movement can be incorporated into activities, with the patient experiencing and concentrating on movement in a functional context.... Hand edema is a frequent complication of hemiplegia. Edema control techniques include elevation of the hand...and use of pressure gloves.... Prolonged hand edema can lead to limited passive range of movement, pain, and soft tissue contractures" (p. 1027). The goal is to promote the movement of fluid back into normal circulation, rather than allowing it to collect in one area or body part. Gentle PROM is necessary to help maintain joint structure and provide nutrients to the joint. The actual movement of the extremity may serve as a "pump" to assist in moving excess fluid back into the body. These techniques are contraindicated for individuals who have deep vein thrombosis. Edema is caused in part by the loss of movement in an extremity because there is no contraction of muscles, which helps to pump the fluid to the heart. Use of orthosis (answer B) is effective for proper positioning and preventing deformity, but elevation and compression gloves are more effective in reducing edema. Taking no action (answer C) could result in permanent damage to the tissue of the involved extremity. Having the individual attempt to squeeze a ball (answer D) would be inappropriate because the left arm is flaccid. See Reference: Trombly. (2008). Woodson, A.M.: Stroke.

185. (A) Textured material, rubbing, tapping, and prolonged contact. "A program of desensitization generally includes repetitive stimulation of the hypersensitive skin with items that provide a variety of sensory experiences, such as textures ranging from course to soft " (p. 717), much like the graded tactile stimuli listed in answer A. Treatment is most successful when carried out and controlled by the individual. With a severe injury such as a burn, it also is necessary to train the individual in protective precautions. Answers B and C, techniques that provide an ungraded or nonspecific level of touch, would not be well tolerated by a person with hypersensitivity because much of the input would facilitate sensory stimuli and would be interpreted as painful. Visual compensation and functional use of the extremity (answer D) are techniques used with individuals who have impaired sensation. See Reference: Trombly. (2008). Bentzel, K.: Optimizing sensory abilities and capacities.

186. (A) Isometric muscle contractions. Isometric muscle contraction involves contracting the muscle without joint movement or a change in muscle length. Isometric strengthening is "exercise in which a weak muscle is isometrically contracted to its maximal force 10 times with rest periods between each contraction" (p. 585). Isotonic contractions (answer B) shorten the muscle length with accompanying joint movement. Progressive resistance (answer C) is a type of isotonic exercise that uses an increase in weight during consecutive exercise repetitions. A person who has a cast that is obstructing movement would be unable to perform either type of isotonic exercise. Passive movements (answer D) are performed by an outside force to the arm and involve joint motion, but no muscle contraction. Passive movement could not be performed with a casted joint. See Reference: Trombly. (2008). Flinn, N.A., Jackson, J., McLaughlin Gray, J., & Zemke, R.: Optimizing abilities and capacities: Range of motion, strength, and endurance.

187. (C) produce a flyer identifying risk factors for cumulative trauma disorders. Cumulative trauma disorders are viewed as a mechanism of injury for tendonitis, nerve compression syndromes, and myofascial pain. Associated risk factors include repetition, high force, awkward joint posture, direct pressure, vibration, and prolonged static positioning. The term "cumulative trauma disorder should be viewed as a description of the mechanism of injury and not a diagnosis.... Diagnoses associated with cumulative trauma usually fall into one of three categories: tendinitis (such as lateral epicondylitis, tennis elbow or de Quervain's tenosynovitis), nerve compression syndromes (such as carpal tunnel syndrome or cubital tunnel syndrome), or myofascial pain" (p. 1064). Repetition, high force, and awkward joint postures are work-related risk factors that are frequently associated with cumulative trauma disorders. Answer A, osteoarthritis disorders, frequently

present with stiffness, redness, and edema, and are not caused by cumulative trauma. Answer B, peripheral vascular disease, is unrelated to the diagnoses mentioned in the question and is more commonly associated with the vascularity of the client. A neuroma (answer D) is specifically related to an amputation, nerve injury, or suture. See Reference: Pedretti. (2013). Kasch, M.C.& Walsh, J.M.: Hand and upper extremity injuries.

188. (B) A key guard. A key guard is a device that covers computer keys and provides a guide for a finger or stick without punching extra keys. A moisture guard (answer A) is a flexible plastic cover that protects the keys from drool, moisture, or dirt. An auto-repeat defeat mechanism (answer C) stops repetition of letters or numbers caused by overlong or involuntary depression of keys. One-finger-access software (answer D) allows the user to lock out keys such as Shift or Enter. This enables an individual who uses only one finger or a stick to type capital letters or perform other keyboard functions that require simultaneous depression of more than one key. See Reference: http://www.myhandicap.com/handicap-computer-keyguards.html http://www.myhandicap.com/handicap-computer-keyguards.html.

189. (C) have the individual repeatedly squeeze with the hand against increasing amounts of resistance. The biomechanical approach is a treatment approach used when a person has a deficit in strength, endurance, or range of motion, but has voluntary muscle control during performance of activities. The biomechanical approach focuses on decreasing the deficit area to improve the person's performance of daily activities. Eliciting functional grasp using reflex-inhibiting postures (answer A) is a neurophysiological approach, which emphasizes an understanding of the nervous system in a person with brain damage and how to elicit a desired response from that person. Muscles can be stimulated through a variety of neurodevelopmental techniques (answer B) using an understanding of the nervous system to elicit a response in a developmental sequence. Building up utensils (answer D) is an example of the rehabilitative approach, which teaches a person how to compensate for a deficit on either a temporary or permanent basis. See Reference: Pedretti. (2013). Breines, E.B.: Therapeutic occupations and modalities.

190. (B) Statins. Beta blockers (correct answer C) such as atenolol and propranolol are "common cardiac medications...with the purpose and use to decrease heart rate and cardiac output, lower blood pressure, and make the heart beat more slowly and with less force" (p. 1201). These medications are frequently used to control hypertension and heart failure. Diuretics, answer A, are used to "lower blood pressure...[and] reduce edema in lungs and extremities." In answer B, "statins, lower LDL and raise HDL, and lower triglyceride levels." In answer D, "antiplatelet agents prevent clots after MI; with unstable angina, ischemic stroke, plaque" (p. 1201). See Reference: Pedretti. (2013). Matthews, M.M.: Cardiac and pulmonary diseases.

191. (C) Strength, range of motion, coordination. "The understanding of kinematics and kinesiology serves as the foundation for the biomechanical frame of reference. The clinician views the limitations in occupational performance from a biomechanical perspective, analyzing the movement required to engage in occupation" (answer C, p. 40). The biomechanical approach is based on enhancing strength, range of motion, and endurance. The rehabilitative approach (answer A) emphasizes making an individual as independent as possible, compensates for limitations, and incorporates the use of adaptive equipment (answer A). The neurodevelopmental approach (answer B) is used for individuals who are born with a central nervous system dysfunction, have experienced an illness, or have had an injury to the neural system. The neurodevelopmental approach is based on using sensory input and developmental sequences to promote function. Evaluation focuses on tone, reflex development, and automatic reactions. The Model of Human Occupation recognizes that human performance is organized and directed by volition, habituation, and mind-brain-body subsystems. This model emphasizes the importance of habits, values, roles (answer D), interests, and personal causation. See Reference: Pedretti. (2013). Schultz-Krohn, W. & McHugh Pendleton, H.: Application of the occupational therapy practice framework to physical dysfunction.

192. (B) cognitive status. The individual's ability to learn how to safely perform ADLs and IADLs is directly related to cognitive status (answer B). "The primary cognitive capacities of orientation, attention, and memory largely reflect the neuroanatomical and physiological integrity of the brain. They are thought to be prerequisite to higher level thinking abilities and to influence metaprocessing" (p. 262). Although it also is important to know what type of support the individual will have upon returning home, which can include marital status (answer A), this information could be obtained from the medical chart or other sources. Leisure interests and work responsibilities (answers C and D) are important areas to identify, but are secondary to cognitive status because of its relationship to safety. See Reference: Trombly. (2008). Radomski, M.V.: Assessing abilities and capacities: Cognition.

193. (D) a cotton swab to apply light touch to a small area of the skin. The senses included in the somatosensory system are touch, movement, pain, and temperature. The auditory, olfactory, visual gustatory, and vestibular systems are special systems that directly give input into the brain. Answer D, the use of "a cotton ball or swab, fingertip, pencil eraser" (p. 223), is a test commonly used to determine a client's ability to feel light touch, whereas answer A is a component for the assessment of deep pressure. Answer B is typically used to determine pain perception and answer C is a technique commonly used to distinguish the client's ability to perceive temperature. See Reference: Trombly. (2008). Bentzel, K.: Assessing abilities and capacities: Sensation.

194. (C) Make a report to appropriate authorities. Answer C, making a report, is correct. OTs are "mandated by federal law to report suspected cases of abuse and neglect to state child protective agencies" (p. 409). All agencies serving children have policies and procedures for reporting injury in these situations. Answers A, B, and D delay or prevent proper assistance to the child and family. See Reference: Case-Smith & O'Brien. (2010). Davidson, D.A.: Psychosocial issues affecting social participation.

195. (B) State licensure board. State regulatory boards (SRBs) "safeguard and promote the public welfare by ensuring that qualifications and standards for professional practice are properly evaluated, applied, and enforced" (p. 422). Only SRDs (answer B) have the power to prevent an individual from practicing through disciplinary action such as revoking the license. Because NBCOT (answer A) certification is voluntary after initial certification, sanctions imposed by NBCOT can only prevent an individual from practicing in cases in which certification is mandatory. The role of the AOTA Ethics Commission is to recommend ethical standards for the profession and "educate members and consumers regarding ethics standards" (p. 422). Disciplinary actions may be imposed only on members of the AOTA, and because membership is voluntary, the sanctions will not prevent an individual from practicing. Reporting the individual to a facility administrator (answer D) could result in them losing their job, but would not necessarily prevent them from practicing in another environment. See Reference: Schell, Gillen, & Scaffa. (2014). Doherty, R.F.: Ethical practice.

196. (B) is medically necessary. "Generally, Medicare payments are based on the type of service provided.... Part B also covers some durable medical equipment" (p. 1059). Medicare Part B does not typically cover assistive device items such as elevated toilet seats, grab bars, or adaptive equipment because they are not considered to be medically necessary. Answers A, C, and D may all be a part of the broader statement of medical necessity not pertaining to Medicare Part B. See Reference: Schell, Gillen, & Scaffa.

(2014). Braveman, B.: Management of occupational therapy services.

197. (C) Ease the child to a lying position, remove or pad nearby objects, and loosen clothing. The most important action to take is to protect the child during the seizure by preventing injuries that can occur from falling or hitting objects during movements. Other protective measures include loosening clothing that is restrictive, and placing a blanket or cushion underneath the child if possible (p. 162). Answer A is incorrect because checking breathing would not be done until the seizure has stopped. Answer B is incorrect because any attempt to restrain the child could result in injury. Although it is important to let the seizure end without any interference, answer D, taking no action except observation, would not help to protect the child from environmental hazards. See Reference: Case-Smith & O'Brien. (2010). Rogers, S.L.: Common conditions that influence children's participation.

198. (C) Creating effective communication via weekly staff meetings, voice mail, and faxes. "When the OT and OTA work as a team, they are able to use and build on each other's skills and expand the number and kinds of services that can be provided to clients.... Indirect methods include communicating...via phone, e-mail, or written correspondence" (answer C, pp. 1082–1083, p. 35). Countersignature alone for documentation (answer B) does not necessarily constitute adequate supervision. Individual states may have additional specific guidelines. A handout (answer D) may provide useful information to the client and caregivers about OT services but is not a critical component in establishing a collaborative relationship. Determining reimbursement criteria (answer A) would be something that should transpire as a result of effective communication/collaboration between the OT and OTA. See Reference: Schell, Gillen, & Scaffa. (2014). Youngstrom, M.J.: Supervision.

199. (C) Obtain a physician's plan of care identifying services to be provided. Within the home care setting, the therapist must have a physician's order (answer C), which identifies the services that are to be provided. After the OT's evaluation, identification of deficits as well as short- and long-term goals (answers A and B) can be established. The individual's history of the current illness (answer D) is contained within the initial assessment. See Reference: Schell, Gillen, & Scaffa. (2014). No chapter/Pamphlet.

200. (A) Assisting with routine dressing, after training and competency have been demonstrated. Aides must be very closely supervised, are expected to receive site-specific training in selected activities determined by the supervising OT practitioner, and must be utilized in accordance with state regulations. "When performing delegated client-related tasks, the supervisor must ensure that the aide (a) Is trained and able to demonstrate competency in carrying out the selected task and using equipment;...(b) Has been instructed on how to specifically carry out the delegated task with the specific client; and (c) Knows the precautions, signs, and symptoms for the particular client that would indicate the need to seek assistance from the occupational therapist or occupational therapy assistant" (p. 178). Activities and levels of supervision in answers B, C, and D are all beyond the scope of the OT aide. "Aides do not provide skilled [i.e., billable] [answer C] occupational therapy services" (p. 177). An aide could order but does not have the knowledge or judgment to determine which tub bench is appropriate (answer D). When introducing a new piece of equipment (answer B), the predictable outcome required for an aide to engage in the activity cannot be ensured. See Reference: AOTA Reference Manual of Official Documents. AOTA Guidelines for Supervision 2009.

Bibliography

American Occupational Therapy Association. (2013). *The reference manual of the official documents of the American Occupational Therapy Association, Inc.* (18th ed.). Bethesda, MD: Author.

Bonder, B. (2010). *Psychopathology and function* (4th ed.). Thorofare, NJ: SLACK.

Bonder, B., & Dal Bello-Haas, V. (2009). *Functional performance in older adults* (3rd ed.).Philadelphia, PA: F.A. Davis Company.

Bracciano, A. G. (2008). *Physical agent modalities: Theory and application for the occupational therapist* (2nd ed.). Thorofare, NJ: SLACK.

Brown, C., Stoffel, V., & Muñoz, J. P. (2011). *Occupational therapy in mental health: A vision for participation.* Philadelphia, PA: F.A. Davis Co.

Cara, E., & MacRae, A. (2013). *Psychosocial occupational therapy: An evolving practice* (3rd ed.). Clifton Park, NY: Delmar Cengage Learning. Retrieved from http://catdir.loc.gov/catdir/toc/ecip0418/2004013041.html

Case-Smith, J., & O'Brien, J. C. (2010). *Occupational therapy for children* (6th ed.). St. Louis, MO: Elsevier Mosby.

Champagne, T. (2011). *Sensory modulation and environment: Essential elements of occupation* (3rd ed.). Sydney, Australia: Pearson Australia Group.

Cole, M. B. (2012). *Group dynamics in occupational therapy: The theoretical basis and practice application of group intervention* (4th ed.). Thorofare, NJ: SLACK.

Cole, M., & Donohue, M. (2011). *Social participation in occupational contexts: In schools, clinics, and communities.* Thorofare, NJ: SLACK.

Cottrell, R. P. F. (2000). *Proactive approaches in psychosocial occupational therapy.* Thorofare, NJ: SLACK.

Depoy, E., & Gitlin, L. (2011). *Introduction to research: Understanding and applying multiple strategies* (4th ed.). St. Louis, MO: Mosby.

Dunn, W., & Dunn, W. (2011). *Best practice occupational therapy for children and families in community settings* (2nd ed.). Thorofare, NJ: SLACK.

Falvo, D. R. (2009). *Medical and psychosocial aspects of chronic illness and disability* (4th ed.). Sudbury, MA: Jones & Bartlett.

Gateley, C., & Borcherding, S. (2012). *Documentation manual for occupational therapy: Writing SOAP notes* (3rd ed.). Thorofare, NJ: SLACK.

Gillen, G. (2009). *Cognitive and perceptual rehabilitation: Optimizing function.* St. Louis, MO: Mosby Elsevier.

Hemphill-Pearson, B. J. (2008). *Assessments in occupational therapy mental health: An integrative approach* (2nd ed.). Thorofare, NJ: SLACK.

Jacobs, K., & McCormack,G. (2011). *The occupational therapy manager* (5th ed.). Bethesda, MD: AOTA Press.

Kramer, P., & Hinojosa, J. (2010). *Frames of reference for pediatric occupational therapy* (3rd ed.). Philadelphia, PA: Wolters Kluwer Health/Lippincott Williams & Wilkins. Retrieved from http://www.loc.gov/catdir/enhancements/fy0902/2008046747–d.html

Meriano, C., & Latella, D. (2008). *Occupational therapy interventions: Function and occupations.* Thorofare, NJ: SLACK.

Parham, L. D., & Fazio, L. S. (2008). *Play in occupational therapy for children* (2nd ed.). St. Louis, MO: Mosby Elsevier.

Pendleton, H. M., & Schultz-Krohn, W. (Eds.). (2012). *Pedretti's occupational therapy: Practice skills for physical dysfunction* (7th ed.). St. Louis, MO: Elsevier/Mosby.

Pollard, D. (2010). *How to begin using Allen's Cognitive Levels.* Monona, WI: Cantankerous Cow Books

Radomski, M. V., & Latham, C. A. T. (2008). *Occupational therapy for physical dysfunction* (6th ed.). Philadelphia, PA: Lippincott Williams & Wilkins. Retrieved from http://www.loc.gov/catdir/toc/ecip076/2006101666.html

Sames, K. M. (2010). *Documenting occupational therapy practice* (2nd ed.). Upper Saddle River, NJ: Pearson Education.

Schell, B. A. B., Gilen, G., & Scaffa, M. E.. (2014). *Willard & Spackman's occupational therapy* (12th ed.). Philadelphia, PA: Wolters Kluwer Health/Lippincott Williams & Wilkins. Taylor, R. R. (2008). *The intentional relationship: Occupational therapy and use of self.* Philadelphia, PA: F.A. Davis Co.

Thomas, H. (2012). *Occupation-based activity analysis.* Thorofare, NJ: SLACK.

Tubbs, C., & Drake, M. (2012). *Crafts and creative media in therapy* (4th ed.). Thoroface, NJ: SLACK.

▪ Website References

1. Pub 100–02 Medicare benefit policy: http://www.cms.gov/Regulations-and-Guidance/Guidance/Transmittals/Downloads/R165BP.pdf

2. Sex after stroke: Our guide to intimacy after stroke http://www.heart.org/HEARTORG/Conditions/More/ToolsForYourHeartHealth/Sex-After-Stroke-Our-Guide-to-Intimacy-After-Stroke_UCM_310558_Article.jsp

3. *Medicare benefit policy manual.* Covered medical and other health services (Chap. 15): http://www.cms.gov/manuals/Downloads/bp102c15.pdf

4. *Medicare and home health care*: http://www.medicare.gov/Publications/Pubs/pdf/10969.pdf

5. *Occupational therapy private practice advocacy resources*: http://www.aota.org/~/media/Corporate/Files/Advocacy/Reimb/Pay/Private/OTPPP%20%201-08%20finaloptimized.ashx

6. Accreditation: Why does accreditation matter? http://www.carf.org/Accreditation/

7. Keyboard keyguards: http://www.myhandicap.com/handicap-computer-keyguards.html

8. *Guidelines for supervision, roles, and responsibilities during the delivery of occupational therapy services*: http://www.aota.org/~/media/Corporate/Files/Practice/OTAs/Supervision/Guidelines%20for%20Supervision%20Roles%20and%20Responsibilities.ashx

9. American Occupational Therapy Association. (2009). Guidelines for supervision, roles, and responsibilities during the delivery of occupational therapy services. *American Journal of Occupational Therapy, 63,* 173–179.

10. AOTA code of ethics 2010: https://www.aota.org/-/media/Corporate/Files/AboutAOTA/OfficialDocs/Ethics/Code%20and%20Ethics%20Standards%202010.ashx

11. AOTA ACOTE standards 2011: http://www.aota.org/education-careers/accreditation/standardsreview.aspx

12. AOTA standards of practice 2010: http://www.aota.org/~/media/Corporate/Files/Practice/OTAs/ScopeandStandards/Standards%20of%20Practice%20for%20Occupational%20Therapy%20FINAL.ashx

13. AOTA Physical Agent Modalities 2010: http://www.aota.org/-/media/Corporate/Files/Secure/Practice/OfficialDocs/Position/Physical-Agent-Modalities-2012.PDFent%20Modalities.ashx